ANATOMY & PHYSIOLOGY

for Allied and Healthcare Students

ANATOMY & PHYSIOLOGY

for Allied and Healthcare Students

SECOND EDITION

GD Mogli

PhD MBA FHRIM (UK) FAHIMA (USA)

(Father of Medical Records of India and the Middle East)

IFHIMA (World) recognized him as the "Champion of Developing Countries"

CEO & MD Mogli's Management Education & Research

Centre for Health Excellence (Dr Mogli's MERCHE)

Visiting Professor, Medical Informatics,

MGIM Sciences, Sevagram, Maharashtra, India

Ex. WHO Consultant, Sr. eHealth Management, HEARTCOM (USA)

Sr. Consultant/Adviser to Ministries of Health,

India, Afghanistan, Iran, Kuwait, Saudi Arabia, Oman, Bahrain, Qatar & UAE

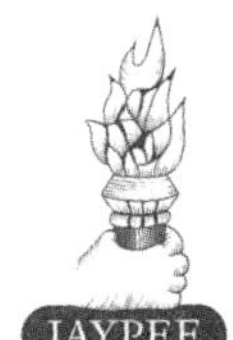

JAYPEE BROTHERS MEDICAL PUBLISHERS

The Health Sciences Publisher

New Delhi | London

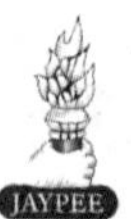

Jaypee Brothers Medical Publishers (P) Ltd

Headquarters
EMCA House
23/23-B, Ansari Road, Daryaganj
New Delhi 110 002, India
Landline: +91-11-23272143, +91-11-23272703
+91-11-23282021, +91-11-23245672
Email: jaypee@jaypeebrothers.com

Corporate Office
4838/24, Ansari Road, Daryaganj
New Delhi 110 002, India
Phone: +91-11-43574357
Fax: +91-11-43574314
Email: jaypee@jaypeebrothers.com

Overseas Office
J.P. Medical Ltd
83 Victoria Street, London
SW1H 0HW (UK)
Phone: +44 20 3170 8910
Email: info@jpmedpub.com

EU GPSR Authorised Representative
Logos Europe, 9 rue Nicolas Poussin
17000, La Rochelle, France
Phone: +33 (0) 6 67 93 73 78
E-mail. Contact@logoseurope.eu

Website: www.jaypeebrothers.com
Website: www.jaypeedigital.com

Inquiries for bulk sales may be solicited at: jaypee@jaypeebrothers.com

Anatomy and Physiology for Allied and Healthcare Students

First Edition: 2019

Second Edition: **2026**

ISBN: 978-93-6616-077-1

Printed in India at: Purewell Ventures Pvt Ltd

Dedicated to

The Medical, Nursing and Paramedics including allied healthcare professionals, such as students of paramedics, nurses, to serve as textbook in their academic programs, professional career building, besides reference guide throughout. This work is also dedicated to the medical laboratory technologists, radiology technologists, medical assistants, cardiovascular technicians, respiratory therapists, dental assistants, physiotherapists, occupational therapists, optometrists, audiometer technicians, medical social workers, medical records personnel, medical secretaries, patient relationship coordinators, legal professionals, medical representatives, insurance professionals, and healthcare software developers.

Preface to the Second Edition

The preface for the 2nd edition *Anatomy and Physiology for Allied and Healthcare Students* is a continuation of the first edition of *Anatomy and Physiology for Paramedical Students*. The Ministry of Health and Family Welfare, through the National Commission for Allied and Healthcare Professions (NCAHP), has recommended that the term "Allied and Healthcare" be used in place of the traditional term "Paramedical," to ensure uniformity and to appropriately recognize the essential roles and contributions of these professionals.

The first edition of the book was a bestseller and was greatly appreciated by readers due to its comprehensive content, simple explanations that made each chapter easy to understand, and excellent diagrams illustrating even minute anatomical parts. These features made the book user-friendly and greatly aided both learning and teaching, making knowledge acquisition more practical and accessible.

The publisher and author felt that there was scope for further improvement and thus added more quality content, especially by focusing on the readers' interests. The book, which originally had 329 pages, has been expanded to 396 pages, and the number of chapters has been reduced from 20 to 16. One might wonder if reducing the number of chapters could result in the loss of vital information. However, instead of omitting any content, the author has added more valuable information and restructured the material to form 14 main chapters. Each of these chapters includes a summary and answers, followed by review questions and one-word answer exercises.

The 15th chapter deals with human body identification exercises and their answers, while the 16th chapter is dedicated to recapitulation, containing chapter-wise brainstorming questions and answers. Through this approach, the reader becomes engaged from beginning to end, repeatedly practicing the subject to gain mastery.

What is new in the 2nd edition is that each chapter contains a summary with questions and answers, followed by review exercises with one-word answers, helping the reader to grasp the content thoroughly and gain confidence in each chapter.

Constructive suggestions and positive criticism to further enhance future editions are welcome and can be shared at: *gdmogli@yahoo.com*.

GD Mogli

Preface to the First Edition

In the study and practice of paramedics, there is constant need for guiding principles, brief summaries of subjects related to the allied medical sciences, and explanations of techniques and procedures. It is evident that any medical, nursing or paramedics students cannot become proficient in his/her respective fields without having solid foundation of anatomy and physiology. Yet, there is a variation among these professions; some need much depth knowledge of all the systems and some require to master only related systems, while some should have basic level. This book has been written to serve the professionals to grasp the medical field in a comprehensive manner, absorb the concept of the human body, structure and functions. Precisely, this book is a combination of anatomy and physiology with description of pictures and tables.

In the course of my four-decade career as medical record administrator, educator, consultant and adviser, dealing with health professionals in diverse organizations, in nine different countries, I felt the need for such a concise book. Without losing the main information part to develop a simple, tractable, handbook for the present users who with too many subjects to learn, hardly find time to scan a variety of books on a single subject available in the market. With this objective, a considerable amount of time and effort have gone in preparing this book. This classical book deals with human anatomy and physiology fully illustrated and apt to the need of allied science professionals, it is the ultimate book for understanding how we work.

I have realized the need for the basic knowledge of anatomy and physiology which is foundation of any medical or paramedical professionals to practice, has synthesized the subject, developed this book, to meet the facets of the requirement of the allied healthcare professionals, such as students of paramedics including nurses, medical laboratory technologists, radiology technologists, medical assistants, cardiovascular technicians, respiratory therapists, dental assistants, physiotherapists, occupational therapists, optometrists, audiometer technicians, medical social workers, medical records managers, medical secretaries, law professionals, medical representatives, insurance companies, and healthcare software developers to serve as textbook in their academic programs and professional career building, besides reference guide throughout.

The special feature of this book is descriptive illustrations, selective structure parts' names that will be grasped by the learners' mind much faster to enable him/her to coordinate with the structure and functions of the human body that will lead to the diagnosis or to the treatment and its related issues. Classification of systems of human body with related concise information will add to the memory power of the learners. Precisely, this is a concise handbook for medical, nursing and especially all allied health professionals besides other professionals who deal with medical and healthcare issues. The book has 20 chapters. Unto 14 chapters, at the beginning of each chapter contains the learning skills, e.g., after completion of the chapter, what the learners are able to know/do. (Similarly, for each chapter, brainstorming exercise questions and answers are given at the end of the textbook). The 3 chapters (15, 16 and 17), dedicated to brainstorm exercises; Chapter 15 deals with brainstorm exercise on anatomical structures to make the users grasp thoroughly the parts of cell, tissues, organs and systems and its relationship with physiology, and Chapter 17 encompasses the brief revision of physiology with 58 questions to make the readers recapitulate knowledge of all the systems easily. And also anatomical pictures with the parts for identification of names; this will give readers, good grasp of the subject and thorough knowledge with the names and parts of the body. Answers to the exercises are provided in 18, 19 and 20 chapters, respectively.

It is hoped that this will serve the purpose for which it was prepared; nevertheless, there is always scope for improvement. I would be extremely indebted to receive any suggestions to improve further.

GD Mogli

Acknowledgments

My sincere gratitude to State Health Ministers and Deputy Ministers of Gulf Cooperation Council (GCC) countries and other administrators, and professional colleagues of India, Afghanistan, Iran, Kuwait, Kingdom of Saudi Arabia, Oman, Bahrain, Qatar and United Arab Emirates (UAE), for their support, encouragement and cooperation. My special thanks to all the medical, nursing professionals including juniors and seniors, with whom I was associated as Senior Consultant Adviser to the Ministries of Health, India, Afghanistan, Iran, Kuwait, Saudi Arabia, Oman, Bahrain, Qatar, and UAE in developing healthcare management system including patient care at outpatient, emergency and inpatients. Their encouragement and support helped greatly in preparation of related paramedical handbooks for teaching and learning purposes for healthcare professionals.

While preparing this *Anatomy and Physiology for Allied and Healthcare Students*, I had the opportunity of taking the help of many senior clinicians of varied specialties, their expertise and using many reference books. For example, 'Medical Terminology (1983)' by Barbara A Gyles and Mary Ellen Wedding of University of Toledo Community and Technical College, Toledo, Ohio, and also many pertinent books and references were scanned to get appropriate information for the benefit of health-care providers. I am indebted to all those authors, for their wonderful work that has equipped me with preparation of this comprehensive *Anatomy and Physiology for Allied and Healthcare Students.*

My special thanks to Narendar Sampath, Medical Record Manager, Welcare Hospital, Dubai, UAE; Ramalingam Selva Kumar, Clinical Coder, Aberdeen Royal Infirmary Hospital, Aberdeen Scotland, United Kingdom, and Mary Stella Alexander, Medical Record Manager, Hamad General Hospital, Doha, Qatar.

I am very grateful to the whole team of M/s Jaypee Brothers Medical Publishers (P) Ltd, New Delhi, India, who helped and guided me, Shri Jitendar P Vij (Group Chairman), Mr Ankit Vij (Managing Director), Mr MS Mani (Group President), Dr Madhu Choudhary (Director–Educational Publishing), Ms Pooja Bhandari [Director-

Production (Books and Journals)], Mr Ajay Kumar Sharma [Deputy General Manager (Books and Journals)], Ms Sunita Katla (Executive Assistant to Group Chairman and Publishing Manager), Ms Samina Khan (Executive Assistant to Director -Educational Publishing), Mr Vijay Kumar Bhatia (Manager-Production), Ms Seema Dogra (Cover Visualizer), Ms Neha Verma (Graphic Designer-Cover), Mr Bishan Singh (Production Manager), Mr Vakil Khan (Proofreader), Mr Akshay Thakur (DTP Operator), Mr Satender Singh (Graphic Designer) and their team members, for all their support to work in this project and make it a success. Without their cooperation, I could not have completed this project.

The author expresses his gratitude for the valuable input from Dr Jasmeet Kaur (Senior Development Editor) of M/s Jaypee Brothers Medical Publishers (P) (Ltd), which has made the book even more appealing to readers.

And lastly, I owe my sincere gratitude to my family, for their encouragement and support.

Contents

1. Cell **1**

- Structure of Cell *1*
- Functions of the Cell *3*
- Cell Division *4*
- Tissue Fluid *5*
- Tissues *5*
- Organs *8*
- Systems *9*
- Body Cavities *12*
- Anatomical Divisions of the Body *12*
- Clinical Divisions of the Abdomen *14*
- Anatomical Divisions of the Back (Spinal Column) *14*
- Planes of the Body *16*
- Positional and Directional Terms of the Body *17*

2. Musculoskeletal System **21**

- Properties of Muscle *21*
- Muscular Tissue *23*
- Functions of Muscles *24*
- Skeletal System *28*
- Joints *40*

3. Cardiovascular System **53**

- Arteries *54*
- Veins *54*
- Capillaries *54*
- Heart *55*
- Pulmonary and Systemic Circulation *61*
- Blood Pressure *63*
- Pulse *63*
- Electrical Conduction of the Heart Pulses *64*

4. Blood and Lymphatic System **74**

- Blood *74*
- Plasma *76*
- Erythrocytes (Red Blood Cells) *77*
- Leukocytes (White Blood Cells) *78*
- Blood Clotting Mechanism *80*
- Blood Group *80*

- Lymphatic System *81*
- Immunity *84*

5. Nervous System **95**
- Structure of Nervous System *96*
- Central Nervous System *97*
- Peripheral Nervous System *102*

6. Digestive System **117**
- Organs of Digestive System *118*
- Accessory Organs of Digestion *128*
- Metabolism *131*

7. Endocrine System **142**
- Hormones *142*
- Different Endocrine Glands Present in Human Body *142*

8. Respiratory System **160**
- External and Internal Respiration *160*
- Parts of the Respiratory system *160*
- Mechanism of External Respiration *164*
- Vital Capacity *166*
- Factors Influencing the Respiratory System *166*

9. Sense Organs **174**
- Eye *174*
- Ear *178*
- Skin *181*
- Tongue *185*
- Nose *186*

10. Excretory System **198**
- Parts of Urinary System *199*
- Excretion Process of Urine *202*

11. Reproductive System **208**
- Male Reproductive System *208*
- Female Reproductive System *212*
- Pregnancy *216*

12. Oncology **226**
- Differences between Malignant and Benign Neoplasms *226*
- Different Types of Tumors *226*
- Staging *227*
- Grading *228*
- Cancer Treatment *229*

13. Psychiatry **232**
- Psychiatry Disorders *232*

14. Medical Psychology **237**
- Abnormal Psychology *238*
- Biological Psychology *239*
- Clinical Psychology *239*
- Cognitive Psychology *240*
- Community Psychology *240*
- Comparative Psychology *241*
- Counseling Psychology *241*
- Critical Psychology *242*
- Developmental Psychology *242*
- Educational Psychology *243*
- Evolutionary Psychology *243*
- Forensic Psychology *244*
- Global Psychology *244*
- Health Psychology *245*
- Industrial/Organizational Psychology *245*
- Legal Psychology *245*
- Occupational Health Psychology *246*
- Personality Psychology *246*
- Quantitative Psychology *247*
- Mathematical Psychology *247*
- Social Psychology *247*
- School Psychology *248*
- Research Methods *249*
- Qualitative and Quantitative Research *250*
- Practice *250*

15. Human Body Part Identification Exercises and Answers **254**
- Exercises *254*

16. Recapitulation **297**

Chapter 1: Cell 297
- Levels of Organization *297*
- Anatomical Position *298*
- Planes of the Body *298*
- Body Cavities *298*
- Directional Terms *299*

Chapter 2: Musculoskeletal System 300
- Anatomy and Physiology of Musculoskeletal System *300*
- Skeletal System *301*

- Structure and Types of Bones *301*
- Divisions of Skeletal System:
  Axial and Appendicular Skeleton *302*
- Muscles *305*
- Connective Tissue Covering *306*
- Attachments *307*

Chapter 3: Cardiovascular System 307
- Anatomy and Physiology of Cardiovascular System *307*
- Vascular System *308*
- Heart *309*

Chapter 4: Blood and Lymphatic System 313
- Anatomy and Physiology of Hematic and Lymphatic Systems *313*
- Blood *313*
- Blood Groups *318*
- Lymphatic System *319*

Chapter 5: Nervous System 320
- Anatomy and Physiology of Nervous System *320*
- Divisions of Nervous System *320*
- Nervous Tissue *322*

Chapter 6: Digestive System 325
- Anatomy and Physiology of Digestive System *325*
- Mouth (Oral Cavity, Buccal Cavity) *326*
- Stomach *327*
- Small Intestine *327*
- Accessory Organs and Digestion *329*

Chapter 7: Endocrine System 330
- Anatomy and Physiology of Endocrine System *330*
- Pituitary Gland *330*
- Thyroid Gland *331*
- Parathyroid Glands *332*
- Adrenal Glands *332*
- Pancreas (Islets of Langerhans) *334*
- Pineal Gland *334*

Chapter 8: Respiratory System 334
- Anatomy and Physiology of Respiratory System *334*
- External Respiration *334*
- Internal Respiration *335*
- Structures Associated with Breathing *335*

Chapter 9: Sense Organs 336
- Anatomy and Physiology of Special Senses *336*
- Eye *337*
- Ear *339*

Chapter 10: Excretory System 340
- Anatomy and Physiology of Urogenital System *340*
- Urinary System *340*

Chapter 11: Reproductive System 342
- Anatomy and Physiology of Urogenital System *342*
- Male Reproductive System *342*
- Female Reproductive System *343*
- Menopause *346*
- Pregnancy *346*

Chapter 12: Oncology 347
- Characteristics of Neoplasms *347*

Brainstorming Questions 349

Annexure 1 *355*
Annexure 2 *358*
Annexure 3 *382*

Index *397*

Introduction to Anatomy and Physiology

Upon completion of this topic, you will be able to:

- Define anatomy and physiology
- Distinguish main differences between anatomy and physiology
- Classify two main subdivisions of anatomy
- Explain histology and cytology
- Elucidate the process of cell to system

Anatomy and physiology are closely related concepts that are often studied together. In few words, anatomy is a study of the physical structure of an organism, while physiology involves the study of the functions of individual structures and systems within an organism, as well as the function of an organism as a whole. An understanding of anatomy is vital to the study of physiology and learning about physiology is important to people who want to understand how anatomical structure work.

The study of anatomy focuses on learning about the size, shape and location of structure in the body. It is usually centers around dissection, in which examples are carefully cut up to reveal the structure within. Physical structures can be identified with the naked eye or observe under magnification with a microscope for more detail.

Anatomy could be considered a fixed study, while physiology is more dynamic, involving the chemical, physical and electrical processes that regulate heart rate to the complex system involved in visual perception.

In order to study physiology, it is necessary to work with living organisms or tissue to fully understand physical processes, such as the release of neutron transmitters in the brain and storage of energy in cells. Both anatomy and physiology can be studied with the use of dissection, medical imaging techniques and laboratory analysis of samples from specimens.

Medical undergraduates study these fields extensively over the course of their educations, so that they understand how the body works as a whole, and the different systems within the body relate to each other. The allied healthcare professionals such as students of paramedical including nurses, medical laboratory technologists, radiology technologists, medical assistants, cardio-vascular technicians, respiratory therapists, dental assistants, physiotherapists, occupational therapists, optometrists, audiometer technicians, medical social workers, medical records managers/ administrators, medical secretaries, patient relationship coordinators, law professionals, medical representatives, insurance companies and healthcare software developers need knowledge of anatomy and physiology to perform their work effectively. Also to serve as textbook in their academic programs, professional career building, besides reference guide throughout. Human anatomy is the scientific study of human body structures, while physiology, which is the study of why and how certain structures functions, anatomy deals with human parts, including molecules, cells, tissues, organs, systems and the way they interact. It also deals with outward characteristics, such as shape, structure, pattern, color and composition. Together with physiology and biochemistry, human anatomy is considered as a basic medical science.

The anatomy can be classified into two subdivisions; gross and microscopic anatomy. Gross anatomy refers to the study of human organs that can be seen without magnification. Microscopic anatomy refers to the study of anatomic parts that can only be seen with a microscope. Histology, the study of tissue organization and cytology, the study of cellular organization, neurophysiology is the study of how the nervous system functions are microscopic anatomy fields.

Summary: In precise, anatomy is the study of the structure and relationship between body parts and the body as a whole.

Organization of living systems: Living system can be redefined from various perspectives, from the broad (looking at the entire earth) to the minute (individual atoms). Each perspective provides information about how or why a living system functions.

At the chemical levels, atoms, molecules (combination of atoms) and the chemical bonds between atoms provide the framework upon which:

- The cell is the smallest unit of life. Organelles within the cell are specialized bodies performing specific cellular functions. Cells themselves may be specialized. Thus, there are nerve cells, bone cells and muscle cells.

- A tissue is a group of similar cells performing a common function. Muscle tissue, for example, consists of muscle cells.
- An organ is a group of different kinds of tissues working together to perform a particular activity. The heart is an organ composed of muscle, nervous, connective and epithelial tissues.
- Any system is two or more organs working together accomplish a particular task. The digestive system, for example, involves the coordinated activities of many organs, including the mouth, stomach, small and large intestines, pancreas, and liver.
- An organism is a system possessing the characteristics of living things—the ability to obtain and process energy, the ability to respond to environmental changes and the ability to reproduce.

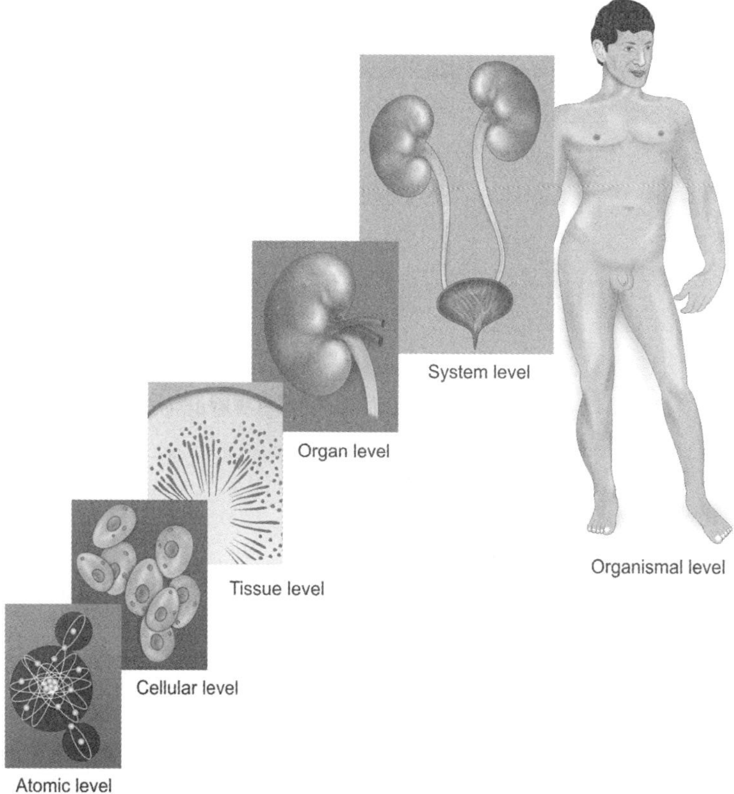

Evolution of the human body

1

CHAPTER

Cell

On completion of this chapter, the student will be able to:

- Explain the structure of the human body cell
- Elucidate briefly the structure and functions of the cell
- Explain cell division and its various types
- Describe tissue and its type
- Record various systems and their organs of the body
- List body cavities and organs present in them
- Specify anatomical and clinical divisions of the abdomen
- List the planes, positional and directional terms of the body

INTRODUCTION

A cell is mass of protoplasm containing a nucleus. It is the unit structure and fundamental part of life, which carries various functions such as reproduction, respiration, excretion and adaptation to the environment. The human body is made up of a trillion number of cells of different types. The size of the cell is about 10–30 mm in diameter.

All cells are similar in that they contain a gelatinous substance composed of water, protein, sugar, acids, fats and various minerals. This substance is called protoplasm. Several parts of a cell are described below and pictured schematically.

STRUCTURE OF CELL (FIGS. 1.1 AND 1.2)

- *Cell membrane:* It is the covering or outer layer of the cell, which protects the internal environment and determines what passes in and out of the cell.
- *Protoplasm:* It is a white fluid like the yolk of an egg, which consists of water, electrolytes, proteins, lipids and carbohydrates. The protoplasm forms cytoplasm and nucleus.
- *Cytoplasm:* It is the protoplasmic material outside the nucleus. It triggers the work of the cell such as contraction in the muscle cell and transmitting impulses in the nerve cell. The cytoplasm

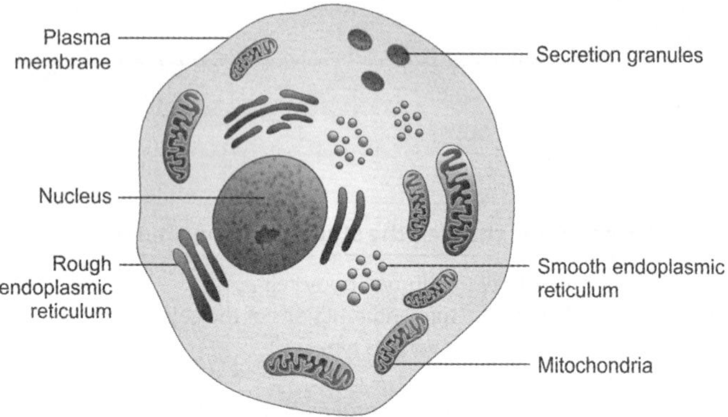

FIG. 1.1 Structure of cell

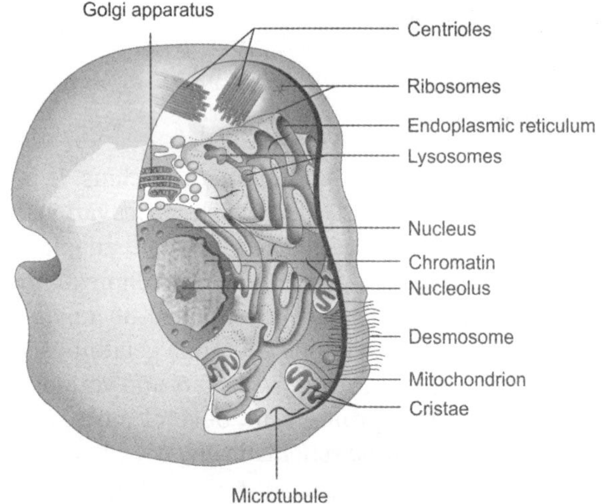

FIG. 1.2 Component parts of the cell

contains mitochondria, endoplasmic reticulum, ribosomes, lysosome, Golgi bodies and the centrosome.

- *Mitochondria:* It is responsible for the production of energy in the cell by breaking up the complex food structure into simpler substances. This process is called catabolism. It is also called kitchen cell (powerhouse).
- *Endoplasmic reticulum:* A tubule-like structure. It contains small bodies called ribosomes, which help make substances (proteins) for the cells, this process is called anabolism.

- *Nucleus:* It is the controlling structure of the cell. It controls the cell reproduction, and contains genetic material which determines the functioning and structure of the cell.
- *Chromosomes:* There are 23 pairs of chromosomes; each chromosome consists of a chain of small units called genes made up of deoxyribonucleic acid (DNA) (hereditary information) and ribonucleic acid (RNA). Out of 23 pairs of chromosomes, 22 pairs are autosomes and one pair is sex chromosome, which decides the sex. A female has 2 X (X, X) chromosomes, whereas the male has 1X, 1Y chromosomes.
- *Lysosomes:* Cell organs or organelles that contain various enzymes capable of breaking down all of the main components of cells; lysosomes destroy bacteria by digesting them.
- *Ribosomes:* Cell organs or organelles that synthesize proteins; often called cell's 'protein factories.'
- *Golgiosome:* Plate-like structure which makes up the Golgi complex of the cell; the plate-like structure consists of stacks of flattened vessels (cisternae) more commonly known as dictyosomes.
- *Chromtin:* More rapidly stainable portion of the cell nucleus, forming a network of a nuclear fibrils within the a chromatin of a cell. It is a DNA attached to a protein (primarily histone) structure base and is the carrier of the genes in inheritance.
- *Desmosome:* A small, discrete, circular, dense body that forms the site of attachment between certain epithelial cells especially those of stratified epithelium of the epidermis.
- *Crista (pl. cristae):* A projection or projecting structure, or ridge, especially one surmounting a bone or its border also called crest and ridge.

FUNCTIONS OF THE CELL

- *Absorption:* The ability of the cell to absorb or take in oxygen and food substances
- *Nutrition:* The intake of food substances by the cell
- *Growth:* It provides the metabolic process to enable the cell to grow to its full size and will be able to function correctly
- *Reproduction:* On reaching maturity, the cell will divide to form two smaller cells

- *Removal of waste products:* The removal of waste products produced during metabolism
- *Movement:* Many cells have the power of movement.

CELL DIVISION

Division of cells is for the growth of the organism and for the replacement of damaged cells. There are two types of cell division.

Mitosis

A process of cell division, which produces two new daughter cells (identical to the parent cells), e.g. plants. This involves a series of changes in which there is a rearrangement of centrioles and chromosomes so that each of the two new cells has a nucleus with 23 pairs of chromosomes. Mitosis is the common type of cell division that occurs in the body cells. It consists of four phases—prophase, metaphase, anaphase and telophase.

Prophase

The centrosome divides and the centrioles move to the opposite poles of the cells with the spindle fibers.

Metaphase

The chromosomes align themselves at the center of the nucleus and become attached to the spindle fibers.

Anaphase

Each chromosome splits into two chromosomes. The separated chromosomes move towards the opposite poles of the cell. The centrioles are divided to form new centrosome.

Telophase

A new nuclear membrane forms around each set of chromosomes, and the spindle fiber disappears. The cytoplasm and cell membrane constrict. Finally, the cell splits into two identical cells.

Meiosis

Cell division occurring in maturation of sex cells, wherein over two successive cell division occur. Each daughter nucleus receives half the number of chromosomes typically to the somatic cells of the species.

The cell division occurring in the human reproductive system is called meiosis. Male or female has 23 pairs of chromosomes comprising of 22 pairs of autosomes and one pair of sex chromosomes or somatic chromosomes. In the meiosis cell division, the daughter cell receives equal number of chromosomes from the parent cells, i.e. 22 pairs of autosomes from father and mother, the male has XY sex chromosomes. Whereas the mother has X and X chromosomes. The sex of a child clearly depends on whether it inherits X or Y chromosome from its father.

TISSUE FLUID

Tissue fluids are of two types—intracellular and extracellular. The fluid inside the cell is called intracellular fluid, while the fluid outside the cell is called extracellular fluid. Tissue fluid acts as a sort of middle man between the blood and tissues, supplying food and oxygen to the cell and removing waste products from the cell.

TISSUES

A tissue is a group of similar cells working together to do a specific job. A histologist is one who specializes in the study of tissues. Tissues can be classified into four major types:

1. Epithelium.
2. Connective tissue.
3. Muscular tissue.
4. Nervous tissue.

Epithelium

The various types of epithelial tissues are as detailed below.

Simple Squamous Epithelium

A single layer of flat cells found in alveoli of lungs, the lining of the interior of the heart and blood vessels and the lymphatic vessels.

Stratified Squamous Epithelium

Stratified squamous epithelium is composed of cells, which are flat and round. It is found in all parts of the body. The skin is composed of stratified squamous epithelium.

Transitional Epithelium

Cells, which provide water tightness. It is found on the lining of urinary tract.

Columnar Epithelium

Cylindrical-shaped cells found in the secretory glands of the body.

Ciliated Epithelium

The free surface of each cell surrounded by fine hair-like structures called cilia. It is found in the lining of (nasal cavity, trachea and bronchi) the respiratory system.

Connective Tissue

Connective tissues are fat (also called adipose tissue), cartilage (elastic, fibrous tissues attached to bones), bone or blood tissues. They are present in different forms in the body. It is a jelly-like substance and hard.

Fibrous Tissue

There are two types of fibrous tissues:

1. White fibrous tissue.
2. Yellow elastic tissue.

White fibrous tissue: It consists of bundles of white fibers, which cannot stretch. It is found in tendons, ligaments, dura mater and outer layer of the pericardium.

Yellow elastic tissue: It consists of fibers, which can stretch. It is found in the walls of arteries, bronchi and alveoli of lungs.

Areolar Tissue

Supporting tissue of the body. Found under the skin, mucous membrane and surrounding blood vessels and nerves.

Adipose Tissue

Found in all parts of the body where fat is deposited or stored, especially under the skin and around the eyes, heart and kidneys.

Cartilage

Cartilage is a flexible tissue found mainly in the skeleton. There are three different types of cartilage:

1. Hyaline cartilage.
2. Fibrocartilage.
3. Yellow elastic cartilage.

Hyaline cartilage: It is bluish white tissue with a smooth glassy surface. It is found covering the ends of the bones, where they form joints (articular cartilage).

Fibrocartilage: It contains white fibrous tissue. It is found in intervertebral disks and semilunar cartilage of the knee joint where great strength combined with certain amount of elasticity is required.

Yellow elastic cartilage: It contains yellow elastic fibers and it is found in the epiglottis and pinna of the ear.

Muscular Tissue

The muscles are structures, which give the power of movements. Muscles are composed of thousands of elongated cells, called muscle fibers. Each contains a small nucleus. Bundles of muscle fibers lie side by side-like threads. There are three different types of muscle tissue; they are voluntary, involuntary and cardiac.

Voluntary Muscles

Voluntary muscles are found in arms, legs and parts of the body where movement is voluntary. All the muscles attached to the skeleton are of this type and their functions are to move the bones at their respective joints and to help in maintaining the posture of the limbs and body as a whole. The microscopic structure of this muscle is striped in structure, i.e. white and black bands, hence it is also called striated muscle.

Involuntary Muscles

Involuntary muscles are found in the internal organs and structures of the body, such as stomach, intestine, bladder, bronchi, blood vessels, and is, therefore, sometimes called visceral muscles. It cannot be consciously controlled and its nervous supply comes from the involuntary or autonomic nervous system. It is also called nonstriated or plain muscle.

Cardiac Muscle

Cardiac muscle is a special type of muscle found only in the heart. Although, it is an involuntary muscle, it has the form of striated muscle. It has the special property, not observed in other varieties of muscles, of automatic rhythmic contraction, which can occur independently of its nervous supply.

Nervous Tissue

Nerve tissues conduct impulses all over the body. The muscles are structures, which give the body the power of movements; almost every movement is governed by some portion of the nervous system, which acts as a medium between brain and muscle.

ORGANS (FIG. 1.3)

Organ structures are composed of several types of tissues. For example, an organ like stomach is composed of muscular tissues, nerve tissues, and glandular epithelial tissues. The medical term for internal organ is viscera (singular form is viscus). The examples are as follows:

- Eye
- Heart
- Hand
- Ear
- Lung
- Leg
- Nose
- Stomach

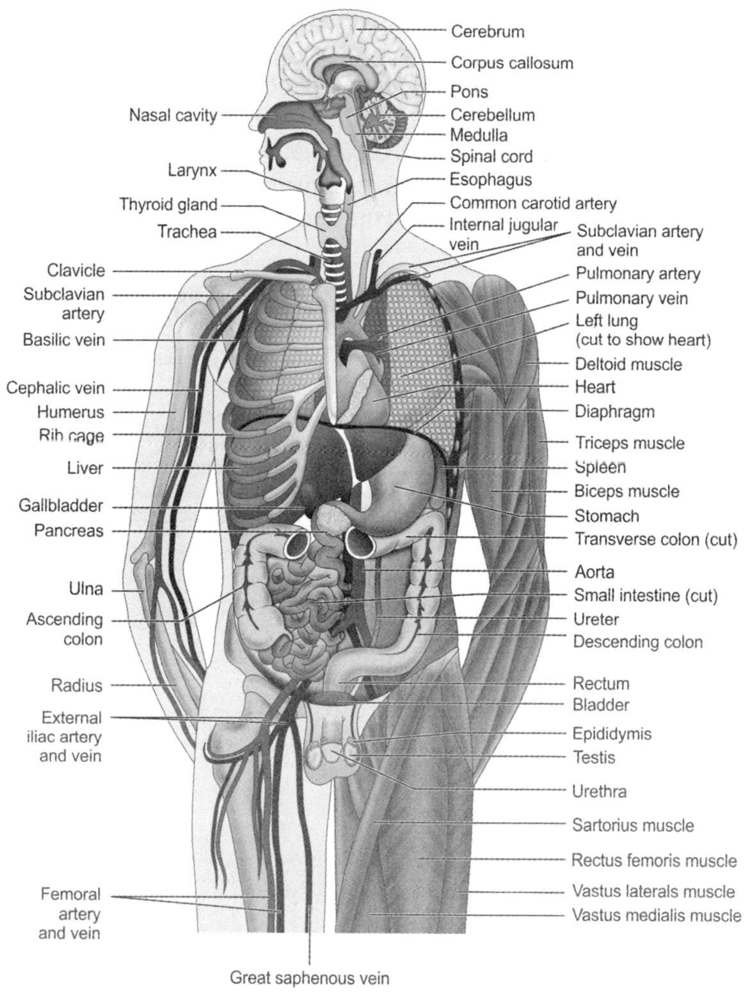

FIG. 1.3 Overview of body structure and organs

- Liver
- Tongue
- Intestine
- Spleen

SYSTEMS

Systems are groups of organs working together to perform essential fundamental functions of the individual (*refer* Fig. 1.3). The different types of systems are skeletal, muscular, nervous, endocrine, circulatory, lymphatic, respiratory, digestive, urinary, and reproductive systems. Although some systems are functioning individually, the functions of various systems are very closely connected and are dependent on each other. For example, mouth, esophagus, stomach and small and large intestines are organs, which compose the digestive system. The main systems and their organs of the body are as given in Table 1.1.

TABLE 1.1 Main systems and their organs

System	Organs/Parts
Muscular system	There are three types of muscle tissues: • Skeletal, voluntary or striated muscle • Visceral, involuntary or smooth muscle • Cardiac muscle
Skeletal system	Bones—there are 206 bones in an adult skeletal system • Joints • Fibrous or fixed joints • Cartilaginous or slightly movable joints • Synovial or freely movable joints
Nervous system	• Brain • Spinal cord • Nerves
Sense organs	• Eye • Ear • Nose • Tongue • Skin or integumentary system
Endocrine system (ductless gland)	• Pituitary gland • Thyroid gland • Parathyroid glands • Thymus gland: Pancreas (islets of langerhans) • Adrenal gland • Sex glands (ovaries and testes)
Cardiovascular system or circulatory system	• Heart • Aorta, artery and arteriole • Vena cava, vein and venule • Capillaries

Contd...

Contd…

System	Organs/Parts
Blood and blood groups	• Blood composition – Plasma – Blood cells ♦ Leukocytes or white blood cells ♦ Erythrocytes or red blood cells ♦ Thrombocytes or platelets • Blood groups – Blood group 'A' – Blood group 'B' – Blood group 'AB' – Blood group 'O' – Rhesus factor (Rh) ♦ Rhesus factor positive (+) ♦ Rhesus factor negative (–)
Lymphatic system	• Lymph vessels • Lymph nodes and other lymphatic tissues • Spleen • Thymus gland
Respiratory system	• Nose • Nasal cavities and paranasal sinuses • Pharynx • Larynx • Trachea • Bronchi (singular form is bronchus) • Bronchioles • Alveoli (singular form is alveolus) • Lung capillaries (bloodstream)
Digestive system	• Oral cavity (mouth) • Pharynx • Esophagus • Stomach • Enteron (small intestine): – Duodenum – Jejunum – Ileum • Colon (large intestine): – Cecum – Ascending colon – Transverse colon – Descending colon – Sigmoid colon – Rectum

Contd…

Contd...

System	Organs/Parts
	• Anus • Accessory organs: – Salivary glands – Liver – Gallbladder – Pancreas
Urinary system	• Kidneys • Ureters • Urinary bladder • Urethra
Reproductive system	*Male:* • Testes • Scrotum • Seminiferous tubules • Epididymis • Vas deferens • Seminal vesicles • Ejaculatory duct • Prostate gland • Penis • Urethra *Female:* • Ovaries • Fallopian tubes • Uterus • Vagina • Vulva • Cervix • Labia majora • Labia minora • Hymen • Mammary glands (accessory organ)

BODY CAVITIES (FIG. 1.4)

A body cavity is a space within the body, which contains internal organs (viscera). Some of the important viscera contained within those cavities are listed in Table 1.2.

ANATOMICAL DIVISIONS OF THE BODY

Anatomical divisions of the abdomen are labeled in Figure 1.5. These divisions are used in anatomy texts to describe the regions in which

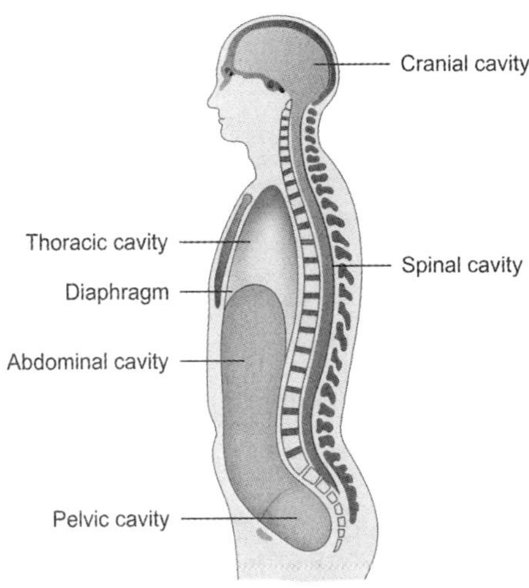

FIG. 1.4 Body cavities

TABLE 1.2 Some of the important viscera contained within body cavities

Name of the cavity	Organs/parts
Cranial cavity	The cranial cavity contains the brain, and the spinal cavity, which contains the spinal cord
Thoracic cavity	Lungs, heart, esophagus, trachea, thymus gland, aorta; the thoracic cavity can be divided into two smaller cavities: 1. The pleural cavity—the areas surrounding the lungs: Each pleural cavity is lined with a double-folded membrane called pleura; visceral pleura is closer to the lungs and parietal pleura is closer to the outer wall of the pleural cavity 2. The mediastinum cavity—the area between the lungs: It contains the heart, aorta, trachea, esophagus and thymus gland
Abdominal cavity	Stomach, small and large intestines, spleen, liver, gallbladder and pancreas
Pelvic cavity	Ureters, urinary bladder, urethra; uterus and vagina in the female
Spinal cavity	Nerves of the spinal cord runs through vertebrae

organs and structures are found, while documenting the patient care. The regions are detailed below:

- Right hypochondriac region (upper lateral regions beneath the ribs)
- Epigastric region (regions of the stomach)

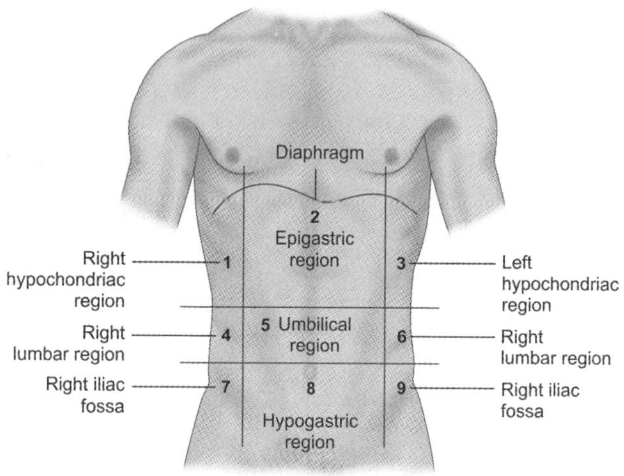

FIG. 1.5 Anatomical divisions of the body (9 divisions)

- Left hypochondriac regions (upper lateral regions beneath the ribs)
- Right lumbar region
- Umbilical region (region of the navel or umbilicus)
- Left lumbar region
- Right iliac fossa
- Hypogastric region (lower middle region below the umbilicus)
- Left iliac fossa.

CLINICAL DIVISIONS OF THE ABDOMEN (FIG. 1.6)

The following terms are used to describe the divisions of the abdomen when a patient is examined in clinic or bedside:

- Right upper quadrant (RUQ)
- Left upper quadrant (LUQ)
- Right lower quadrant (RLQ)
- Left lower quadrant (LLQ).

ANATOMICAL DIVISIONS OF THE BACK (SPINAL COLUMN)

For anatomical divisions of the back, refer to Table 1.3 and Figure 1.7.

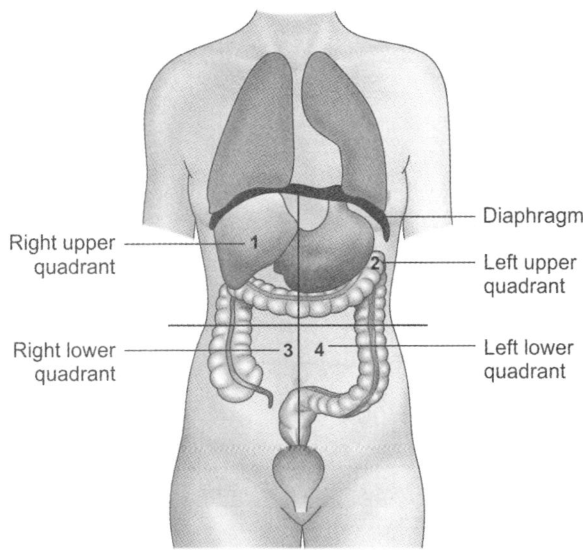

FIG. 1.6 Clinical divisions of the abdomen (4 divisions)

TABLE 1.3 Anatomical division of the back (spinal column with location and abbreviation terms)

Division of the back	Abbreviation	Location
Cervical vertebrae	C	Neck region. There are seven cervical vertebrae (C1-C7)
Thoracic vertebrae	T or D (dorsal)	Chest region. There are 12 thoracic vertebrae (T1-T12). Each bone is joined to a rib
Lumbar vertebrae	L	Loin or flank region (between the ribs and the hip bone). There are five lumbar vertebrae (L1-L5)
Sacral vertebrae	S	Five bones (S1-S5) are fused to form one bone, the sacrum
Coccygeal	Nil	The coccyx (tailbone) is small bone composed of four fused pieces

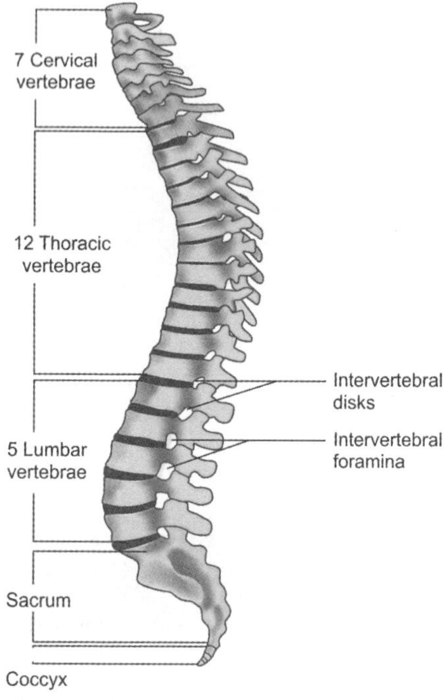

FIG. 1.7 Anatomical divisions of the back (spinal column)

PLANES OF THE BODY (FIG. 1.8)

A plane is an imaginary flat cross-section. The following terms are used to describe the planes of the body (Table 1.4).

TABLE 1.4 Planes of the body

Name of the planes	Explanation
Frontal	Vertical plane, which divides the body or structure into anterior and posterior portions
Sagittal	Lengthwise vertical plane, which divides the body or structure into right and left portions; the midsagittal plane divides the body into right and left halves
Transverse	Plane running across the body parallel to the ground (horizontal); it divides the body or structure into upper and lower portions

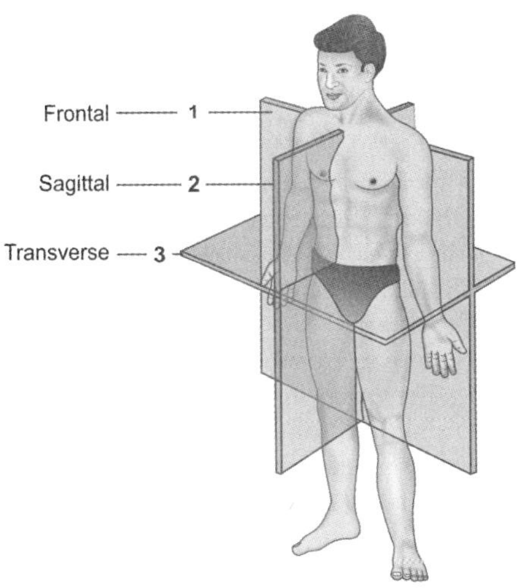

FIG. 1.8 Planes of the body (3 planes)

POSITIONAL AND DIRECTIONAL TERMS OF THE BODY

Positional and directional terms of the body are detailed in Table 1.5.

TABLE 1.5 Positional and directional terms of the body

Position	Description of the position
Anterior	In front of the body
Posterior	At the back of the body
Central	Pertaining to the center
Deep	Away from the surface
Superficial	Near the surface
Distal	Away from the beginning of the structure or away from the center
Proximal	Pertaining to the beginning of a structure
Inferior	Below another structure
Superior	Above another structure
Lateral	Pertaining to the sides
Medial	Near to the median of the body (structure)
Supine	Lying on the back
Prone	Lying on the belly
Afferent	Towards the structure
Efferent	Away from the structure

Chapter Summary

The cell is the essential unit of (1).................... As such, it carries on all the functions associated with life, which include functions such as reproduction, respiration, excretion and adaptation to the environment. In highly complex organisms, cells are modified to carry on a specific activity, in addition to all of the other basic life functions. Muscle cells are designed for contraction; nerve cells transmit electrical impulses; and red blood cells carry oxygen to body tissues.

Cells of same group perform the same basic activity are called (2).........................The types of tissues are epithelial (covering), connective (supporting and protecting), muscular (contracting) and nervous (conducting impulses) tissues. In addition, a variety of cell types compose the specialized tissue of blood. Tissues of the same group work in close association and perform a special function are called (3) ....

In addition to performing a specialized function, organs also have a more or less definite shape. For example, the shape of the stomach somewhat resembles a sac. The stomach is composed mainly of muscle and epithelial tissues. The muscle tissue provides for the mixing of ingested food with gastric juices. These juices are secreted from the epithelial tissue to help in the digestive process.

The next level after cells, tissues and organs is a (4)....................

A system is composed of a group of organs that work together to perform a common function. For example, the mouth, pharynx, esophagus, stomach, small intestine and colon, along with accessory organs, constitute the gastrointestinal system. Each of these organs performs one or more activities associational with digestion. Other body systems are as follows—human body, musculoskeletal, cardiovascular, blood and lymphatic, nervous, endocrine, respiratory, sense organs, excretory and reproductive system.

The human body, which is the highest level of organization is the organism, which is a living entity, composed of all of the body systems. These systems provide for all of the processes associated with life. They are responsible for its autonomous existence.

The levels of organization can be represented as follows:

Cells → Tissues → Organs → Systems → Organism

Answers

1. Life
2. Tissues
3. Organs
4. System

Review Questions

Exercise 1: Answer in One Word

1. The cell is the fundamental unit of ________.
2. Cell functions are reproduction, respiration, excretion, and ________.
3. Muscle cells are designed for ________.
4. Nerve cells transmit electrical ________.
5. Red blood cells carry ________ to body tissues.
6. Groups of cells that perform the basic activity are called ________.
7. Groups of tissues which perform a special function are called ________.
8. A system is made of group of ________.
9. Systems provide for all the processes associated with the ________.
10. Cells → Tissue → Organs → ________ → Organism.
11. The body is divided into ________ major cavities.
12. The dorsal cavities include the ________ cavity.
13. Cranial cavity contains the brain, and the ________.
14. Spinal cavity contains the ________.
15. The ventral cavities include the ________ cavity.
16. Thoracic cavity contains the heart, and ________.
17. The abdominopelvic region may be divided into ________ sections.
18. Movement toward the median plane of the body is called ________.
19. Movement toward the head or upper portion of a structure is called ________.
20. Movement near the front of the body is called ________.
21. Movement near the attachment of an extremity to the trunk or a structure is called ________.
22. Movement near the back of the body is called ________.

Exercise 2: Complete the Following

1. The basic unit of the life is ________.
2. Groups of similar cells working together to do a specific job is ________.
3. Several ________ combine to form a system.
4. There are ________ chromosomes in a mature sex cell.
5. The three types of muscle tissues are ________, ________ and ________.
6. The four planes of the body are ________, ________, ________ and ________ planes.

7. The vertical plane, which divides the body or structure into anterior and posterior portions is _________.
8. The directional term 'efferent' refers to _________ the structure.
9. The directional term 'afferent' refers to _________ the structure.
10. The medical term for one thousand is _________.

Answers

Exercise 1

1. Life
2. Adaptation
3. Contraction
4. Impulses
5. Oxygen
6. Tissues
7. Organs
8. Organs
9. Life
10. Systems
11. Four
12. Cranial
13. Spinal cavity
14. Spinal cord
15. Thoracic
16. Lungs
17. Nine majors
18. Adduction
19. Superior (Cranial)
20. Anterior (Ventral)
21. Proximal movement
22. Posterior (Dorsal) movement

Exercise 2

1. Cell
2. Tissue
3. Organs
4. 23
5. Skeletal, voluntary or striated; visceral, involuntary, nonstriated or smooth; cardiac, involuntary or striated
6. Frontal or coronal; median, midsagittal or midline; sagittal; transverse
7. Frontal
8. Away from
9. Toward the
10. Milli

CHAPTER 2

Musculoskeletal System

On completion of this chapter, the student will be able to:

- Explain the functions of the skeletal system
- Describe different types of bones
- Explain different types of bone structure
- Enlist the bones of different regions of the body
- Elucidate different types of muscular tissues
- Describe characteristics and different functions of muscles

INTRODUCTION

The musculoskeletal system includes the bones, muscles and joints. The skeleton (group of bones) forms a supportive framework and consists of a series of bony levers capable, by virtue of the joints and muscles, to move upon one another. Muscles provide major support for movements of the body. Muscles and bones make up for most of the body's weight. The muscles have the special characteristics of elongation and contraction by which they produce movements of the different parts of the body. The muscle gives the posture of the human body and supports it to withstand against the gravity. The muscles, which are attached to the skeleton, are called skeletal muscles. The skeletal muscle cells have various nerve endings, which produce chemical reaction during contraction and that results in generation of heat. Hence, muscular activity plays an important role in maintaining the body temperature (Fig. 2.1).

PROPERTIES OF MUSCLE

Power of Contraction

Voluntary muscles contract as a result of stimuli reaching them from the nervous system and many nerves have their endings in muscles.

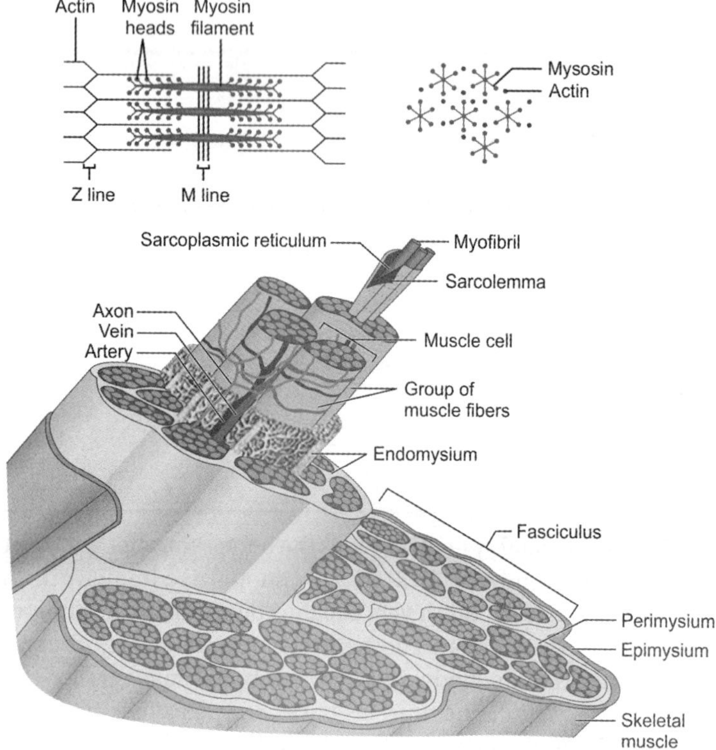

FIG. 2.1 Cross-section of skeletal muscle with names of important parts of the muscle

Elasticity

Muscle tissue is elastic and can be stretched by a weight, when the weight is removed, the muscle returns to its normal position.

Fatigue

When a muscle contracts, it loses energy. This energy is derived from the glucose stored in the muscle as glycogen.

Muscular Tone

Even when a muscle appears to be at rest, it is always partially contracted and ready for immediate action. This state of partial contraction is called muscle tone and it is important in maintaining body posture.

MUSCULAR TISSUE

The muscles are structures, which give the power of movement. Muscles are composed of 1,000 of elongated cells, called muscle fibers, each containing a small nucleus. Bundles of muscle fibers lie side by side like threads in a skin. Three types of muscular tissues are found in the body, which are as follows.

Voluntary/Striated/Skeletal Muscles

Voluntary muscle is attached to the skin. It is under the control of the will and is formed from long multinucleated cells, which show a striped or striated pattern of dark and light bands in their cytoplasm. Voluntary muscles plays an important role for movement, power and strength of the body.

Involuntary/Smooth/Nonstriated/Visceral Muscles

These muscles are found in the internal organs and structures of the body such as the stomach, intestine, bladder, uterus, bronchi and blood vessels. Hence, it is also called internal muscles or visceral muscles. It cannot be controlled by the will. It consists of a series of elongated spindle-shaped cells. It has a single nucleus. Smooth muscle forms sheets of fibers as it wraps around tubes and vessels.

Cardiac Muscle

This is a special type of muscle found only in the heart. It is striated in appearance, but nonstriated in action. Cardiac muscle fibers are cylindrical with centrally placed nuclei and connected strongly with adjacent fibers at intercalated disks. Its movements cannot be consciously controlled.

Characteristics of Muscular Tissue

- *Irritability or excitability:* Property of receiving stimuli and responding to them.

- *Contractility:* Capacity of muscles to become short in response to suitable stimulation.
- *Extensibility:* Muscle can be stretched, i.e. the property of individual cells.
- *Elasticity:* Muscle readily returns to original shape.

Attachment of Muscles

At the extremities of the muscles, the connective tissues are present, which form strong fibrous, nonelastic cards called tendons. Tendon attach a muscle to the bone. Sometimes, they form a broad, flat expansion called aponeurosis.

FUNCTIONS OF MUSCLES

Skeletal (striated) muscles are the muscles, which move the bones of the body. When a muscle contracts, one of the bones to which it is joined, remains virtually stationary as a result of other muscles, which holds it in place:

- Provide the framework
- Support the body and give shape
- Give attachment to bones and tendons
- Permit movements of the body as a whole and of parts of the body, by forming joints that are moved by muscles.

Important muscles of upper and lower limb, head, neck and trunk are detailed in Table 2.1, and their functions detailed in Table 2.2. The anterior and posterior muscles are shown in Figures 2.2 and 2.3.

Functions of Different Muscles

- Flexors : Muscles, which bend a limb at a joint
- Extensor : Muscle, which straighten a limb at a joint
- Abductor : Muscle, which moves the limb away from the midline of the body
- Adductors : Muscle, which moves the limb towards the midline of the body
- Elevators : Muscle, which raises the part of the body
- Depressors : Muscle, which lowers a part of the body.

TABLE 2.1 Important names of muscles of upper and lower limb, head, neck, shoulder and trunk

Head, neck and shoulder	Trunk	Upper limb	Lower limb
• Frontalis • Orbicularis oculi • Orbicularis oris • Masseter • Depressor anguli and depressor labii • Sternohyoid • Sternocleido-mastoid • Trapezius	• Pectoralis major • Serratus anterior • Teres major and minor • Latissimus dorsi • Rectus abdominis • Transversus • External oblique • Internal oblique • External abdominis • Gluteus maximus • Gluteus medius	• Deltoid • Biceps • Triceps • Brachialis major • Carpi radialis • Carpi ulna • Long and short extensors of thumb	• Gluteus maximus • Adductor • Hamstring • Rectus femoris major • Sartorius major • Biceps • Gastrocnemius • Anterior tibial major

TABLE 2.2 Muscles and their functions

Region	Name of the muscle	Function
Scalp	Epicranial or occipitofrontalis	Move the scalp
Head	• Platysma • Sternomastoid Capitis (3)	Flex head on the chest Extends the head
Eyes	• Orbicularis oculi • Levator palpebrae superioris	Closes the eyes tightly Raises the eyelid
Lips	• Orbicularis oris • Buccinator	Closes lips tightly Opens the lips
Mastication	• Masseter • Temporalis	Helps in chewing Chewing and grinding objects
Tongue	• Genioglossus • Styloglossus	Pulls the tongue forward Pulls the tongue backward
Scapula	• Serratus anterior • Trapezius	Abducts the scapula (extends the reach) Adducts the scapula and raises the shoulder

Contd...

Contd...

Region	Name of the muscle	Function
Shoulder joint	• Deltoid • Supraspinatus • Pectoralis major • Coracobrachialis • Teres major • Latissimus dorsi • Teres minor • Infraspinatus	Abducts the humerus (arm) Rotates cuff of the shoulder Adducts the humerus (arm) Pulls arm across chest (flexes arm) Extends arm Rotates humerus inwards Rotates the humerus (outwards) Externally rotate the humerus and stabilize the shoulder joint
Inspiration	• Intercostal – Internal – External – Diaphragm	Helps in inspiration Responsible for forced exhalation Responsible for forced and quiet inhalation Separates the abdominal cavity from the thoracic cavity
Expiration	• Rectus abdominis • External oblique • Internal oblique • Transverse	Helps in expiration Rotate trunk and pulling chest downward to compress the abdominal cavity Provide spinal stability and it flexes and rotates Compresses the ribs and viscera providing thoracic and pelvic stability
Back	• Sacrospinalis • Quadratus lumborum	Holds spine erect Helps spine erect
Floor of pelvis	• Levator ani • Coccygeus	Form floor of pelvis Support all organs located in the pelvis
Hip	• Iliopsoas – Psoas major – Iliacus • Sartorius • Gracilis • Gluteus maximus	Flexes thigh on the trunk Outer rotation of the hip Movement of the lumbar spine, pelvis and hip Flex hip knee joint Abducts the thigh and rotates the leg medially at the knee Extends femur

Contd...

Contd…

Region	Name of the muscle	Function
	• Gluteus medius – Brevis • Adductor – Longus – Magnus • Gluteus minimus • Piriformis	Abduct femur Motor function of the foot Adducts femur Abducts the thigh Contacts and pulls Rotates femur inwards Rotates femur outwards
Knee	• Hamstring – Semitendinosus – Semimembranosus – Biceps femoris • Sartorius • Gracilis • Quadriceps femoris – Rectus femoris – Vastus medialis – Vastus intermedius – Vastus lateralis	Flex the knee and medially (inward) rotate the lower leg when the knee bent Flexes the knee and extend the hip Rotate the knee, tibia medially femur when the knee is fixed Internal and external rotation, and hip extension Flexes the knee joint Hip abduction and knee flexion Flexor of the hip Extend the thigh Extend the knee joint Extend the knee Extension of the lower leg
Forearm	• Brachialis • Biceps brachii anterior • Triceps brachii posterior • Pronator teres (upper end) • Pronator quadratus (lower)	Flexes the forearm Movement of elbow and shoulder Extend the forearm Supinate the hand Pronate the hand Pronate (turn so palm faces downwards) the hand
Fingers	• Flexors • Extensors posterior • Forearm	Flex fingers Extend fingers Extension at the wrist and fingers
Thumb	Thenar group	Controls movement of the thumb
Feet	• Anterior tibialis • Gastrocnemius	Flexes the foot Inverts the foot Flexing the foot and leg at the knee joint

Contd…

Contd...

Region	Name of the muscle	Function
	• Soleus	Extends the foot in walking
	• Posterior tibialis	Extends the foot helps in invert the foot
	• Peroneus (3)	Evert the foot Help to flex the foot
	• Tibialis (anterior)	Dorsiflexion and inversion of the knee
	• Tibialis (posterior)	Contracts to produce inversion and assists in the plantar flexion of the foot at the ankle.

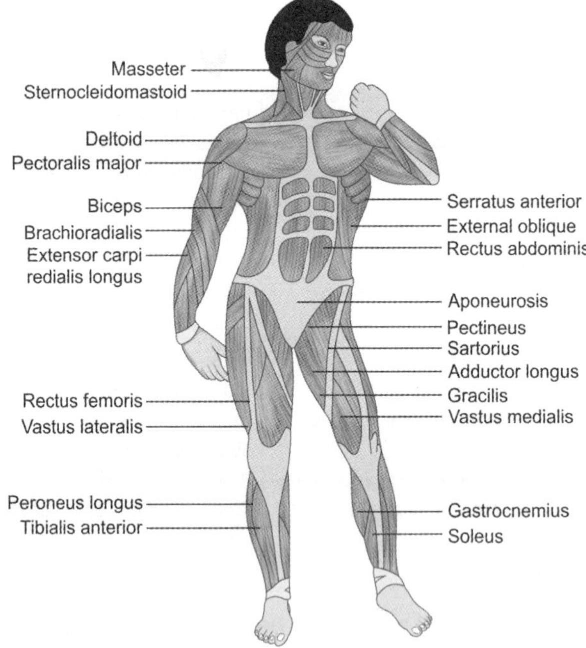

FIG. 2.2 Muscles (anterior view)

SKELETAL SYSTEM

Bones are organs composed of connective tissues called osseous (bony) tissue with a rich supply of blood vessels and nerves. Osseous tissue consists of osteocytes (bone cells), which forms bones by

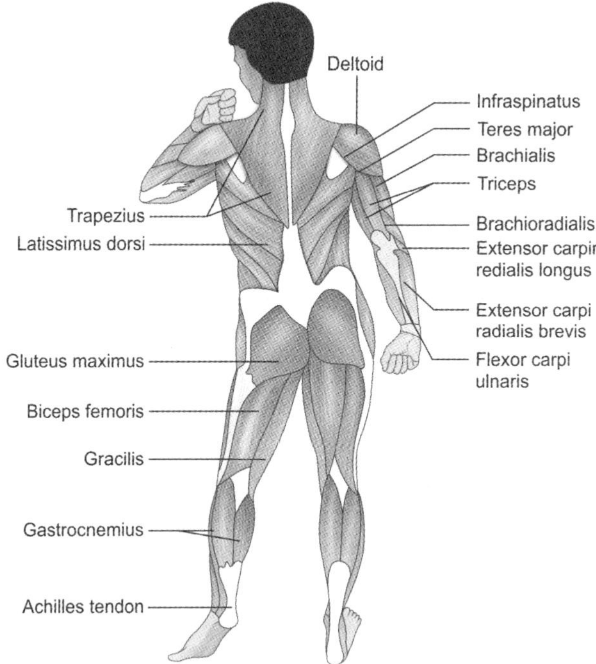

FIG. 2.3 Muscles (posterior view)

ossification. The inner core of bones is composed of hematopoietic tissue (red and yellow bone marrow, manufacturers of blood cells), while other parts are storage areas for minerals necessary for growth, such as calcium and phosphorus. This is the hardest of all the connective tissues. Osteology is the study of the bones.

Formation of Bone

The bones are developed during the fetal stage of the human being, during that time it is made of cartilage tissue, which will be less dense. Gradually, the calcium and immature bone cells are deposited on the cartilage tissues, while the child grows and thus the bone becomes harder and forms the body structure. The development of bones depends on proper supply of calcium, phosphorus and vitamin D to the bone tissue. In long bones, a primary center of ossification forms the shaft (diaphysis) and secondary center forms the ends (epiphysis).

When the adult length of the bone is reached, the epiphyseal cartilage is ossified to form strong bones.

Functions of Bones

- Provide the framework.
- Support the body and give shape.
- Give attachment to muscles and tendons.
- Permit movement of the body as a whole and of parts of the body, by forming joints that are moved by muscles.
- Form the boundaries of the cranial, thoracic and pelvic cavities, protecting the organs they contain red bone marrow in which blood cells develop.
- Provide a reservoir of calcium, potassium, phosphorus and sodium.

Types of Bone (Figs. 2.4 and 2.5)

The bones of the skeleton are classified according to their shape into long, short, flat and irregular bones.

Long Bones

Long bones are found in the limbs or extremities of the body and consist of long shaft with two extremities. The bones of the arm, forearm, thigh and legs are typical examples. The shaft consists of a cylinder of compact bone containing yellow bone marrow. The extremities are formed by a thin outer shell of compact tissue with an interior network of spongy or cancellous bone containing red bone marrow.

Short Bones

Short bones have no shaft, but consist of smaller mass of spongy bones surrounded by a shell of compact bone. They are roughly box-like in shape. They are found in the small bones of the wrist (carpals) and ankle (tarsal).

Flat Bones

Flat bones provide broad surfaces for muscular attachment and extensive protection for internal organs. It is made of cancellous bone

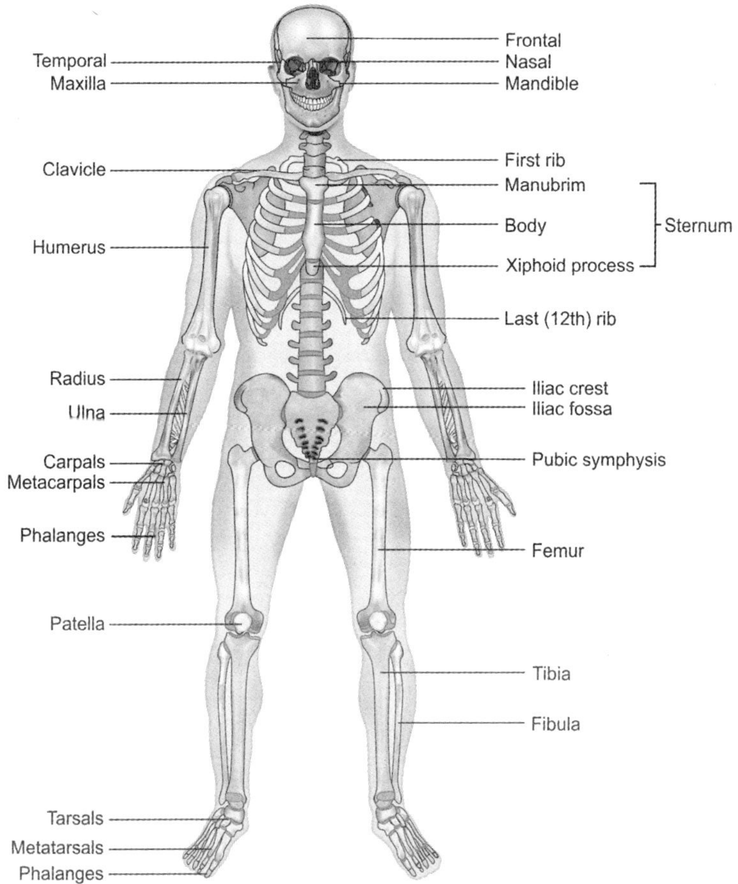

FIG. 2.4 Bones (anterior view)

sandwiched by two compact bones. Examples are bones of skull, shoulder blades (scapula) and sternum.

Irregular Bones

Irregular bones cannot be classified under any of the previous types, because of their peculiar shapes. Examples are bones of the face and the vertebra.

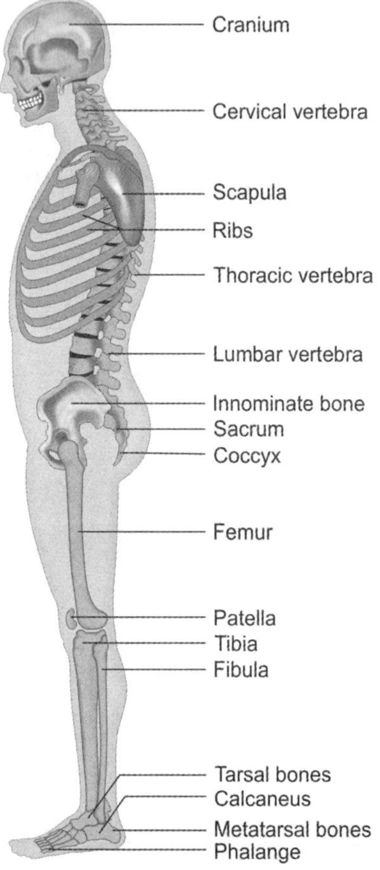

FIG. 2.5 Bones (lateral view)

Sesamoid Bones

Bones that are developed in the tendons of the muscles and are found in the vicinity of a joint. The patella is the largest sesamoid bone to quote as an example.

Structure and Terms Used to Describe the Bones

- *Bone process:* The portion of the bone that projects is called bone process.
- *Bone head:* Rounded end of a bone separated from the body of the bone by a neck.

- *Tubercle:* Small, rounded process, which serves as a site of tendon or muscle attachment.
- *Trochanter:* Large projection on femur, which serves as a site of attachment for muscles.
- *Condyle:* Rounded knuckle-like process at the joint.
- *Epicondyle:* A small projection adjacent to a condyle usually giving attachments to the ligaments.
- *Tuberosity:* Large, round process, which serves as a site of muscle or tendon attachment.
- *Crest:* An elevated ridge of the bone.
- *Facet:* A small articulating surface of the bone.
- *Process:* A projection from a bone.

Bone Depressions

The openings or hollow regions in a bone, which help to join one bone to another, and serve as passageways for blood vessels and nerves. They are:

- *Fossa:* Depression or cavity of a bone.
- *Foramen:* Opening for blood vessels and nerves.
- *Fissure:* Narrow, deep, slit-like opening.
- *Sulcus:* Groove or furrow.
- *Sinus:* Air cavity within a bone.
- *Articulation:* A joint between two bones.
- *Border:* The edge separating two surface of the bone.

Bones of Different Locations (Table 2.3)

The human skeleton contains 206 bones present in the adult. The classification of the bones according to the parts are detailed below.

The skull consists of cranium, face and lower jaw. The trunk consists spinal column, ribs and sternum. The limbs consist of upper and lower limbs together with shoulder and pelvic girdles.

Cranial Bones

The bones of the skull protect the brain and structures related to it, such as eye, ear and nose. The cranial bones of a newborn child are not completely joined. There will be gaps of unossified tissue in the skull, these are called soft spots.

TABLE 2.3 Types of bones

Names of the regions/bones		Total number(s)
Axial skeleton		
Skull		
• Frontal		
• Parietal 1 × 2		
• Temporal × 2		
• Occipital		
• Sphenoid		
• Ethmoid	8	
Face		
• Inferior nasal concha × 2		
• Lacrimal × 2		
• Maxilla × 2		
• Nasal × 2		
• Palatine × 2		
• Zygomatic × 2		
• Vomer		
• Mandible	14	
Ear		
• Malleus × 2		
• Incus × 2		
• Stapes × 2	6	
Neck		
• Hyoid	1	29
Thoracic cavity		
Vertebral columns		
• Cervical 7		
• Thoracic 12		
• Lumbar 5		
• Sacrum 1		
• Coccyx 1	26	

Contd…

Contd...

Names of the regions/bones		Total number(s)
Chest		
• Sternum 1		
• Ribs 12 × 2	25	51
Upper limb		
Shoulder		
• Scapula 2		
• Clavicle 2	4	
Upper arm		
• Humerus 2	2	
Lower arm		
• Radius 2		
• Ulna 2	4	
Hands		
• Carpal 8 × 2 (16)		
• Metacarpal 5 × 2 (10)	26	
Fingers		
• Phalanges 14 × 2 (28)	28	64
Lower limb		
• Pelvis 2		
• Femur 2		
• Patella 2		
• Tibia 2		
• Fibula 2		
• Tarsal 7 × 2 (14)		
• Metatarsal 5 × 2 (10)		
• Phalanges 14 × 2 (28)	62	62
	Total	**206**

Frontal Bone

Forms the forehead and bony sockets, which contain the eyes.

- *Parietal bone:* Two parietal bones, which form the roof and upper part of the sides of the cranium.

- *Temporal bone:* Two temporal bones forms the lower sides and base of the cranium. Each bone encloses an ear and contains a fossa for joining with the mandible. The mastoid process is a round process of the temporal bone behind the ear.
- *Occipital bone:* Forms the back and base of the skull, and joins the parietal and temporal bones, forming a suture. The inferior portion of the occipital bone has an opening called foramen magnum through which the spinal cord passes.
- *Sphenoid bone:* The bat-shaped bone extends behind the eyes and forms part of the base of the skull.
- *Ethmoid bone:* Thin delicate, spongy and cancellous bone supporting the nasal cavity and forms part of the orbits of the eyes.

Facial Bones

Most of the facial bones are immovable bones joined by sutures. The only movable bone is mandible for chewing:

- *Nasal bones:* Two nasal bones supporting to form the bridge of the nose.
- *Lacrimal bones:* Two paired lacrimal bones are located one at the corner of the each eye.
- *Maxillary bones:* Two large bones compose the massive upper jaw bones.
- *Mandibular bone:* This bone forms the lower jaw. Both the maxilla and mandible contain the sockets called alveoli in which the teeth are embedded. The mandible joins the skull at the region of the temporal bone, forming the temporomandibular joint on either side of the skull.
- *Zygomatic bones:* Two bones, one on each side of the face, form the high portion of the cheek.
- *Vomer:* The thin, single, flat bone forms the lower portion of the nasal septum.

Bones of Vertebral Column

The vertebral column is composed of 26 bone segments, called vertebrae, arranged in five divisions:

- *Cervical vertebrae:* The first seven bones of the vertebral column, forming the neck bone.

- *Thoracic vertebrae:* The second set of 12 bones, which joins to the 12 pairs of ribs.
- *Lumbar vertebrae:* The third set of five vertebral bones. They are strongest and largest of the backbones.
- *Sacrum:* The set of four bones slightly curved, triangularly shaped bone. At birth it is composed of five separate segments, these gradually become fused in the young child.
- *Coccyx:* This is the set of five bones and it is the tailbone of the spinal or vertebral column fused together.

Bones of Thorax, Pelvis and Extremities (Figs. 2.6 and 2.7)

- *Clavicle:* This is collar bone, one on each side of the body, connecting the breastbone to each shoulder bone.
- *Scapula:* Shoulder bone, two flat and triangular bones, one on each dorsal side of the thorax.
- *Sternum:* Breast bone, a flat bone extending down the midline of the chest. The uppermost part of the sternum joins on the sides with the clavicle and ribs. The lower portion of the sternum is called xiphoid process.

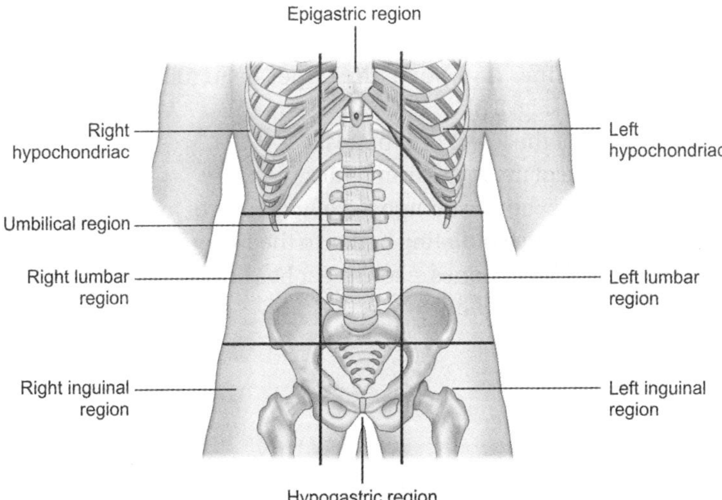

FIG. 2.6 Anatomical divisions of the abdominopelvic region with location of hypochondriac, lumbar and inguinal regions

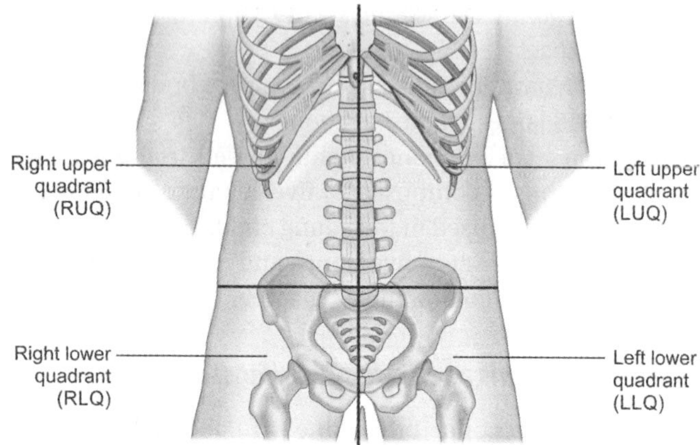

FIG. 2.7 Anatomical division of upper, lower, right and left quadrants

- *Ribs:* There are 12 pairs of ribs. Out of 12 pairs, the first seven pairs (1–7) joins the sternum, which are called true ribs, the ribs (8–10) are called false ribs, these ribs join the 7th rib anteriorly, instead of the sternum. Ribs 11 and 12 are the floating ribs, as they are completely free at their anterior extremity.

Bones of Arm and Hand

- *Humerus:* Upper arm bone, the upper head joins with scapula and clavicle (Fig. 2.8).
- *Ulna:* One of the lower arm bones.
- *Radius:* One of the lower arm bones.
- *Carpals:* Wrist bones, composed of two rows of four bones each.
- *Metacarpals:* Five radiating bones to the finger.
- *Phalanges:* Finger bones, each finger has three phalanges, except the thumb that has only two.

Bones of Pelvis

Pelvic Girdle

Hip bone, large bone supporting the trunk of the body and joins the thigh bone and sacrum. The ilium is the uppermost large portion, ischium is the posterior part of the pelvis. Pubis is the anterior part

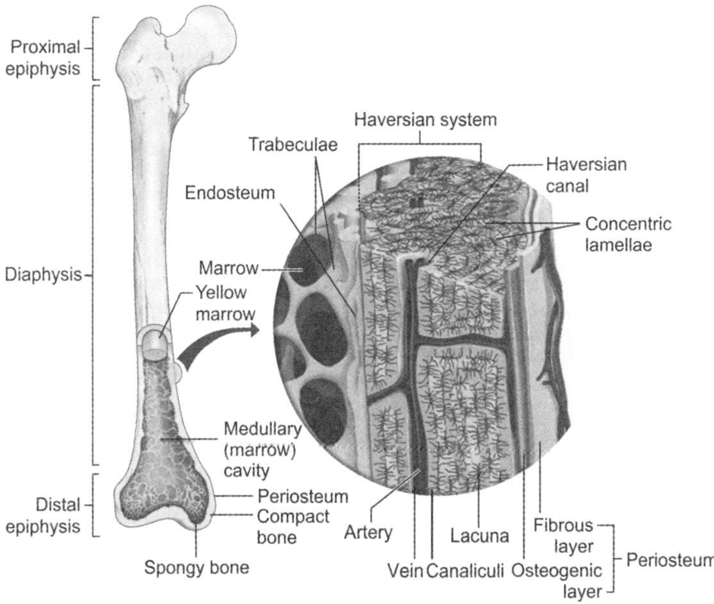

FIG. 2.8 Longitudinal section of a long bone with names of different inner parts of the long bone

TABLE 2.4 Differences between male and female pelvic bones

Name of the bone	Male	Female
Ilium	Narrow and heavy	Broad and light
Inlet	Round	Oval
Pubic	Less than 90°	Greater than 90°
Sacrum	Long and narrow	Short and broad

of the pelvis. Differences between male and female pelvic bone are depicted in Table 2.4.

Bones of Leg and Foot

- *Femur:* Thigh bone, this is the longest bone in the body. The head of the bone joins the socket of the hip bone. This socket is called acetabulum (refer Fig. 2.8).
- *Patella:* Kneecap, this is small, flat bone that lies in front of the joint between the femur and tibia.

- *Tibia:* The largest of the two lower bones of the leg, it joins with femur and patella at the upper end, and with ankle at lower end. The tibia is commonly called shin bone (refer Fig. 2.8).
- *Fibula:* Smaller of two lower leg bones, this is thin bone.
- *Tarsals:* Ankle bones, there are seven short bones that resemble carpal bones of the wrist, but slightly larger. The calcaneus is the largest of these bones and also called heel bone.
- *Metatarsals:* There are five metatarsal bones, each leading to the toes.
- *Phalanges of the toes:* Toe bones—each toe has three phalanges, except the big that has only two.

JOINTS

The joints are the places where two or more bones meet. This is also called articulation. They are concerned with growth, rigidity and movement. There are three types of joints:
1. Fixed joints/Immovable joints/Synarthrosis/Fibrous
2. Slightly movable joints/Amphiarthrosis/Cartilaginous
3. Freely movable joints/Diarthrosis/Synovial.

Fixed or Synarthrosis or Fibrous Joints

Synarthrosis, fibrous or fixed joint is a joint that does not permit movement at all. Bones come together and are bound or united, by a layer of fibrous tissue that does not permit movement. Examples of synarthrosis or fibrous or fixed joints are:
- Suture joints of the skull.
- Peg and socket—the teeth in their socket.

Slightly Movable or Amphiarthrosis or Cartilaginous Joints

Amphiarthrosis or cartilaginous or lightly movable joint is an articulation, which permits slight movement. The bone surfaces of the joint are connected by elastic fibrocartilage and are partially movable.

Examples of amphiarthrosis or cartilaginous or lightly movable joints are found between the vertebrae and between the small bones of the ankle and wrist.

Freely Movable or Diarthrosis or Synovial Joints

A diarthrosis or synovial joint is a freely movable joint. Examples are ball and socket joint (hip joint), and hinge joint (elbow joint).

The bones in a diarthrotic joint are separated by a joint capsule, composed of fibrous cartilage tissue. Ligaments (fibrous bands or sheets of connective tissue). Often they anchor the bones together around capsule to strengthen it. The surface of the bones at the joint is covered with a smooth cartilage surface called articular cartilage. The synovial membrane lies under the joint capsule and lines the synovial cavity, which is filled with a special type of lubricating fluid called synovial fluid produced by synovial membrane.

Varieties of Synovial Joints

- *Gliding or plane:* Two flat surfaces glide over each other, e.g. carpus and tarsus.
- *Ball and socket:* One rounded extremity fits into a cavity in another bone, e.g. hip joint and shoulder.
- *Hinge joint:* One rounded surfaces of the bone fits another, so that movement is only possible in one place, e.g. elbow joint.
- *Condyloid joint:* Similar to hinge joint, but moves into two planes, e.g. the wrist joint.
- *Trochoid or pivot:* Where rotation only is possible, e.g. the head where the atlas rotates around axis.
- *Saddle joint:* Concave-convex surface is received by another convex-concave surface, e.g. the thumb.

Bursae

Bursae are closed sacs of synovial fluid lined within the synovial membrane. They are formed in the space between tendons (connective tissue binding muscle to the bones), ligaments (connective tissue binding bones to bones) and bones. It lubricates these areas where friction would normally develop close to the joint capsule.

Movements of Joints

- *Gliding movements:* Two flat surfaces move on each other.

- *Angular movements:* Described according to the direction in which the movement takes place.
- *Flexion:* Bending or doubling up.
- *Extension:* Stretching or straightening out.
- *Adduction:* Movement towards the medial aspect of the body.
- *Abduction:* Movement away from the medial aspect of the body.
- *Circumduction:* A combination of rotation and angular movement.

Chapter Summary

The musculoskeletal system consists of (1)....................

Bones are the principal organs of support and protection for the body. Joints are the places at which two bones meet (articulate). Because bones are incapable of movement without the help of muscles, contraction must be provided by muscular tissue. In the human skeleton, muscles are usually attached to two articulating bones, and during contraction, one bone is drawn toward another. Muscles, therefore, produce movements by exerting a force on the bones to which they are attached. Stated more simply, skeletal muscles produce movement by pulling on bones. This chapter deals with study of bones, joints and muscles.

Skeletal System

Besides support and protection of the vital organs from injury, the skeletal system provides a number of other important functions. Movement is possible because bones act as points of attachment for muscles, joints, tendons and ligaments. Bone marrow, which is found within the larger bones, is responsible for (2)....................

Bone marrow continuously produces millions of red and white blood cells to replace worn out cells. The bones serve as a storehouse for minerals, particularly phosphorus and calcium. When the body experiences a deficiency in a mineral salt, such as calcium during pregnancy, it is withdrawn from the bones.

Structure and Types of Bones

Bones consist of mineral deposits embedded with living cells that must continually receive food and oxygen. Bone cells also require a system to carry away accumulated waste products. In order to provide these vital functions, there is an extensive vascular system within bones. Fundamentally, all bones are composed of same basic substances, but bones vary in both size and shape. Thus they are distinguished from each other by classifying them in four main categories, (3).................... Long bones are found in the extremities of the body; e.g. arms and legs. Typical long bones consist of the following parts:

1. Diaphysis: Which is the shaft or long main portion of the bone, consists mainly of compact bone.

2. Epiphyses: Which are the two ends, extremities of the bone, have a somewhat bulbous shape to provide space for muscle and ligament attachments near the joints. Proximal and distal epiphyses are two terms used for the ends of a long bone.
3. Articular cartilage: It is a thin layer of resilient hyaline cartilage. The elasticity of the hyaline cartilage provides the joints with a cushion against jars and blows.
4. Periosteum: Which is a dense white fibrous membrane that covers the remaining surface of the bone contains numerous blood and lymph vessels and nerves. In growing bones, the inner layer contains the bone-forming cells or osteoblasts. Since the blood vessels and osteoblasts are located here, the periosteum provides a means for bone repair and general bone nutrition. It also serves as a point of attachment for muscles, ligaments and tendons.

Flat Bones

Provide broad surfaces for muscular attachment and extensive protection for internal organs. Examples are bones of the skull, shoulder blades and sternum.

Short Bones

Short bones are irregular shaped and consist of a core of (4)................. bone enclosed in a thin layer of compact tissue. Examples are bones of the ankles, wrists and toes.

Irregular Bones

Irregular bones are all of the other bones that cannot be grouped under the previous headings because of their peculiar shapes. Examples are the bones of the (5).....................

Axial and Appendicular Skeleton

The skeleton can be divided into two main parts, i.e. the axial skeleton and the appendicular skeleton. The axial skeleton comprises the bones of skull, thorax and vertebral column. These ones contribute to the formation of the body cavities and provide protection for internal organs. The appendicular skeleton consists of bones of shoulder, upper extremities, hips, lower extremities. They attach to the axial skeleton as appendages.

Vertebral Column

The vertebral column of the adult is composed of (6)..................... The vertebral column supports the body and provides a protective bony canal for the passage of the spinal cord. Vertebrae as separated by flat, round structures or intervertebral disks, which are composed of a fibrocartilaginous substance with a gelatinous mass in the center (nucleus pulposus). When the disk material protrudes into the neutral canal, pressure on the adjacent nerve root is manifested by pain. This condition is referred to as herniation of an intervertebral column into five groups of bones and each group derives its name from its location within the spinal column. The seven cervical vertebrae form the skeletal frame work of the neck. The first cervical vertebra is called atlas and supports the skull. The second cervical vertebra, the axis, makes possible rotation of the skull on the neck. Under these are the twelve thoracic or dorsal vertebrae, which support the chest and serve as a point of articulation for the ribs. The next five vertebrae, the lumbar vertebrae, are situated in the lower back area and carry most of the weight of the torso. Below this, five sacral vertebrae are fused into a single bone in the adult and are known as sacrum. The tail of the vertebral column consists of four or five fragmented vertebrae fused together are known as coccyx.

Thorax

Two of the most important internal organs of the chest are (7). .... Together with other soft tissue, they are enclosed and protected by the thorax or rib cage.

The ribs, the sternum or chest plate and the thoracic vertebrae form the skeletal framework of the rib cage. The normal set of ribs in both sexes consists of (8)....................

Twelve ribs are situated on each side of the thoracic cavity. The true ribs are the first seven pairs of ribs. These are attached directly to the sternum by a strip of costal cartilage (hyaline cartilage). The costal cartilage of the next five pairs of ribs is not fastened directly to the sternum. These are known as false ribs. The last two pairs of the false ribs are not joined, even indirectly, to the sternum, but attached posterior to the thoracic vertebrae and are known (9) ....

Pelvic Girdle (Pelvis)

The pelvic is basin-shaped structure that supports the sigmoid colon, the rectum, the urinary bladder and other soft organs of the abdominopelvic cavity. It also provides a point of attachment for the legs.

Male and female pelvises differ considerably in size and shape. Some of the differences are attributable to the function of the female pelvis during the stages of childbearing. The female pelvis is shallower than the male pelvis, but wider in every direction. Not only does the female pelvis support the enlarged abdomen as the fetus matures, but it also must provide a large enough opening to allow the infant to pass through during the process of birth.

Both the male and female pelvises are divided into the (10)............... These are fused together in the adult to form a single bone called innominate bone. However, the individual names are retained in order to identify the respective areas of the bones. The bladder is located behind the symphysis pubis; the rectum is in the curve of the sacrum and coccyx. In the female, the uterus, fallopian tubes, ovaries and vagina are located between the bladder and rectum.

Joints

In order to allow body movements, all bones must have articulating surfaces. These surfaces form joints or articulations, with various degrees of mobility. Some are freely moveable (diarthroses); others are only slightly movable (amphiarthroses) and the remaining are totally immovable (synarthroses). All three types are necessary for smooth, coordinated body movements. Every joint is covered with connective tissue and cartilage. The ligament and connective tissue in this area permit bones to be connected to each other. Muscles attached to freely movable joints permit a great deal of body movement. The synovial membrane that lines in the joint cavity secrets (11)....................., which acts as a lubricant of the joints. The bones in a synovial joint are separated by a joint capsule. It is strengthened by ligaments (fibrous bands or sheets, of connective tissues) that often anchor bones to each other. All of the above factors, working together in a complementary manner, make various body movements possible.

Muscles

Muscular tissue refers to all of the contractile tissue of the body. It includes the cardiac muscle of heart, smooth muscles that compose viscera and skeletal muscles that attach to the bones. The first two categories of muscles are referred to as involuntary, because there is no discretionary control over them. In contrast, the skeletal muscles are voluntary, since their contractions are fully controllable. Some examples of other types of voluntary muscles are those that move the tongue or eyeballs and those that control facial expressions. All muscles through contraction provide body with motion or body posture. The less apparent motions provided by muscles are the passage and elimination of food through the digestive system, propulsion of blood through the arteries and contraction of the bladder to eliminate urine.

Motions such as running and lifting originate with the skeletal muscle, which act upon the system of levers formed by the bones and joints. This engineering relationship needs further explaining. One end of a muscle, usually the proximal end (also called origin), must attach to a rather immovable bone surface, while its remaining part spans across a joint. The other end of the muscle, the distal end (or insertion) is attached to a movable bone. As the muscle contracts, the insertion pulls towards the origin and draws the second bone toward the immovable or first bone. This produces motion. Often, motion is produced when several muscles spanning over the same joint are contracted. Each of these muscles provides for slight variations in a particular movement.

When acting singly or in groups, the muscle or muscles that produce the movement are referred to as prime movers or agonists. Once a motion has occurred, such as bending an arm at the elbow, the arm does not return to its original position even after the contraction has stopped. Instead, an opposing muscle, called antagonist, must contract to bring the arm back to its original position. The need for both agonist and antagonist muscle implies that muscles possess only contracting or pulling, capabilities, not those of pushing. This means that prime mover is not able to reverse its activity and push a bone away from the origin. Opposite motions are accomplished by muscles that act antagonistically to the prime movers. When other muscles contribute indirectly to a specific movement, they are called synergists. They assist the prime movers indirectly in their activity. Fixator is a muscle that stabilizes or fixes one end of a muscle so that all of the force exerted by it occurs only at one end.

Connective Tissue Coverings

Skeletal muscles are enclosed in a sheath of connective tissue. This connective tissue is a part of the deep fascia of the body, which is continuous with adjacent muscles, periosteum and subcutaneous connective tissue. The other sheath of the muscle is the epimysium. Within a given muscle, a perimysium surrounds small bundles of muscles. The endomysium covers each single muscle fiber. These layers of connective tissue contain the nerves and supply blood to muscles.

Attachments

Muscles attach to bones either by fleshy or fibrous attachments. In fleshy attachments, muscle fibers arise directly from bone. These fibers distribute force over wide areas, but a fleshy attachment is weaker than fibrous attachment. In fiber attachments, the connective tissue of the epimysium, perimysium and endomysium converges at the end of the muscle to become continuous and indistinguishable from the periosteum. In some instances, this connective tissue penetrates the very bone itself. When these connective tissue fibers form a cord or strap, it is referred to as tendon. This provides a great deal of force to be localized in a small area of bone. Ligaments are composed of connective tissue and attach one bone to another. When the fibrous attachment spans over a large area of a particular bone, the attachment is called aponeurosis. Such attachments are found in the lumbar region of the back.

Answers

1. Bones, joints and muscles
2. Blood cell formation or hematopoiesis
3. Long bones, short bones, flat bones and irregular bones
4. Cancellous or spongy
5. Ear and the vertebrae
6. 26 bones called vertebrae
7. Heart and lungs
8. 12 pairs or a total of 24 ribs
9. Floating ribs
10. Ilium, ischium and pubis
11. Synovial fluid

Review Questions

Exercise 1: Answer in One Word

1. The musculoskeletal system consists of bones, joints, and __________.
2. Skeletal muscles produce movement by pulling on __________.
3. Blood cell formation is the responsible of __________.
4. Bone marrow produces red and white blood cells to replace __________.
5. Articular cartilage is a thin layer of resilient hyaline __________.
6. The axial skeleton comprises the bones of the skull, thorax, and __________.
7. The vertebral column of the adult is composed of 26 bones called __________.
8. Basically, the vertebral column is divided into __________ groups of bones.
9. Two of the most important organs of the chest are the heart and __________.
10. Twelve ribs are situated on each side of the __________.
11. The first seven parts of the ribs are called __________.
12. The pelvis is __________ structure.
13. __________ supports the sigmoid colon, the rectum, the urinary bladder.
14. __________ provides a point of attachment for the legs.
15. Female and male pelvis is divided into the ilium, ischium and __________.
16. The bladder is located behind the __________.
17. The rectum is in the curve of the __________.
18. The portion of the bone that projects is called a __________.
19. A condyle is a rounded process at the end of a bone that forms an __________.
20. Fissure is also called __________.
21. Freely movable bones are called __________.
22. Slightly movable bones are called __________.
23. Totally immovable bones are called __________.
24. Every joint is covered with connective tissue and __________.
25. The synovial membrane that lines the joint cavity secretes __________.
26. __________ acts as lubrication of the joints.
27. The bones in a synovial joint are separated by a __________.
28. Muscular tissue refers to all of the __________ tissue of the body.

29. The outer sheath of the muscle is the __________.
30. All muscles through contraction provide the body with motion or __________.

Exercise 2: Complete the Following

1. The skeleton is made up of __________ bones.
2. Bones are classified according to shapes, which are __________.
3. The humerus is an example of a __________ bone.
4. A sharp projection in the bone is called __________.
5. The spinal column is made up of vertebrae, __________, and __________.
6. There are __________ pairs of ribs.
7. All skull bones are immobile except for the __________.
8. The three groups of vertebrae in the spinal column are the __________, __________ and __________.
9. The long bones of the arm are __________, __________ and __________.
10. The patella is the __________.
11. The seven ankle bones are called __________.
12. The eight carpal bones are located in the __________.
13. Fibrous joint allow __________ movement, cartilaginous joints allow __________ movement, and synovial joints allow __________ movement.
14. The bending of joint is called __________.
15. The most movable type of joint in the body is the __________ joint.
16. The study of muscles is called __________.
17. Movement is produced by the ability of muscle to __________ and __________.
18. Three types of muscle tissue are __________, __________ and __________.
19. The buccinator muscle is also called __________.
20. The diaphragm is a muscle of respiration located in the __________.
21. Muscles for chewing are the __________.
22. The auricular group of muscles moves the __________.
23. The muscle around the eye is called __________.
24. A broad, flat, superficial muscle of the back of the neck and trunk is the __________.
25. __________ muscles contract when we cough or sneeze.

Exercise 3: Match the Following

1. Sacrum	A. Extreme tip of vertebral column
2. Clavicle	B. Jawbone
3. Femur	C. Smaller bone of lower leg
4. Humerus	D. Large weight-bearing bone of lower leg
5. Sternum	E. Collar bone
6. Zygomatic (or malar)	F. A nasal bone
7. Patella	G. Shoulder blade
8. Coccyx	H. Next to last vertebral bone
9. Scapula	I. Thigh bone
10. Vomer	J. Kneecap
11. Tibia	K. Medial long bone of the forearm
12. Mandible	L. Breastbone
13. Fibula	M. Lateral long bone of forearm
14. Pubis	N. Small, lower, strongest portion of pelvic bone
15. Ischium	O. Broad upper portion of pelvic girdle
16. Carpals	P. Ankle bones
17. Ilium	Q. Most anterior part of pelvic girdle
18. Tarsals	R. Wrist bones
19. Radius	S. Upper arm bone
20. Ulna	T. A cheek bone

Answers

Exercise 1

1. Muscles
2. Bones
3. Bone marrow
4. Worn out cells
5. Cartilage
6. Vertebral column
7. Vertebrae
8. Five
9. Lungs
10. Thoracic cavity
11. Two true ribs
12. Basin-shaped
13. Pelvis
14. Pelvis
15. Pubis
16. Symphysis pubis
17. Sacrum and Coccyx
18. Process
19. Articulation
20. Sulcus
21. Diarthroses
22. Amphiarthroses
23. Synarhroses
24. Cartilage

25. Synovial fluid
26. Synovial fluid
27. Joint capsule
28. Connective
29. Epimysium
30. Body posture

Exercise 2

1. 206
2. Long, flat, short, irregular
3. Long
4. Spine
5. Sacrum, coccyx
6. 12
7. Mandible (lower jaw bone)
8. Cervical, thoracic, lumbar
9. Humerus, ulna, radius
10. Kneecap
11. Tarsals
12. Wrist
13. No, slight, free
14. Flexion
15. Ball-and-socket
16. Mycology
17. Extend, contract
18. Skeletal, visceral and cardiac
19. Trumpeter (muscle)
20. Thorax
21. Masseters
22. Ear
23. Orbicularis oculi
24. Trapezius
25. Abdominal

Exercise 3

1. H
2. E
3. I
4. S
5. L
6. T
7. J
8. A
9. G
10. F
11. D
12. B
13. C
14. Q
15. N
16. R
17. O
18. P
19. M
20. K

3

CHAPTER

Cardiovascular System

On completion of this chapter, the student will be able to:

- Enlist the organs of cardiovascular system
- Describe arteries and veins
- Recognize important arteries and veins
- Explain anatomy of the heart
- Name the four chambers, and valves of the heart
- Explain the heart cycle
- Differentiate systemic and pulmonary circulation

INTRODUCTION

The various organs in the body need energy from the food substances, which reach them after being taken into the body. Food contains stored energy, which can be converted into the energy for movements and work. This conversion of stored energy into active energy of work occurs when food and oxygen combine in cells during the chemical process of catabolism. It is obvious then that each cell of each organ is dependent on a constant supply of food and oxygen in order to receive sufficient energy to work well. The cardiovascular system plays a vital role in transporting food and oxygen to all organ, and cells of the body through the fluid called blood vessels to carry the blood and the muscular pump called the heart. In addition to this, these blood vessels are used to transport cellular waste materials such as carbon dioxide and urea to the lungs and kidneys respectively, where it is removed from the body. Thus, the cardiovascular system is one of the important systems of the human body.

The cardiovascular system is the transport system, carrying oxygen, nutrition, hormones and other substances to the tissues, and conveying carbon dioxide to the lungs and other waste products to the kidney.

Arteries, arterioles, veins, venules and capillaries, together with the heart form cardiovascular system for the flow of blood.

ARTERIES

Arteries are the blood vessels, which carry oxygenated blood from the heart to the various parts of the body. The microscopic structure of arteries has three layers:

1. *Tunica adventitia:* Outer layer
2. *Tunica media:* Middle layer
3. *Tunica intima:* Inner layer.

Tunica adventitia is composed of fibrous tissue, which gives protection and strength to the vessels. Tunica media is composed of smooth muscle with yellow elastic fibers, which are arranged in circular manner. It contracts and relaxes to maintain the blood pressure. Tunica intima consists of a layer of endothelial cells. Arterioles, a minute arterial branch, one just proximal to a capillary.

Important Arteries (Fig. 3.1)

Generally, the names of the arteries mostly coincide with the names of the bone, organs or cavity, etc. it passes through. However, some of the important arteries are listed in Table 3.1.

VEINS

Veins are the blood vessels, which carry deoxygenated blood from various parts of the body to the heart. It also possesses three layers same as that of arteries, but they are much thinner. The smooth muscle inside their walls are under the control of the autonomic nervous system. Small veins are called venules.

Important Veins (Fig. 3.2)

See Table 3.2.

CAPILLARIES

Capillaries are only one cell thick and are just large enough to allow red blood cells to pass through. It is in the capillaries that the nutrient/ gas exchange (diffusion) takes place. They act as a very important link in the circulatory system because it is the capillaries that serve all the tissues in the body by absorbing the energy (glucose) from the

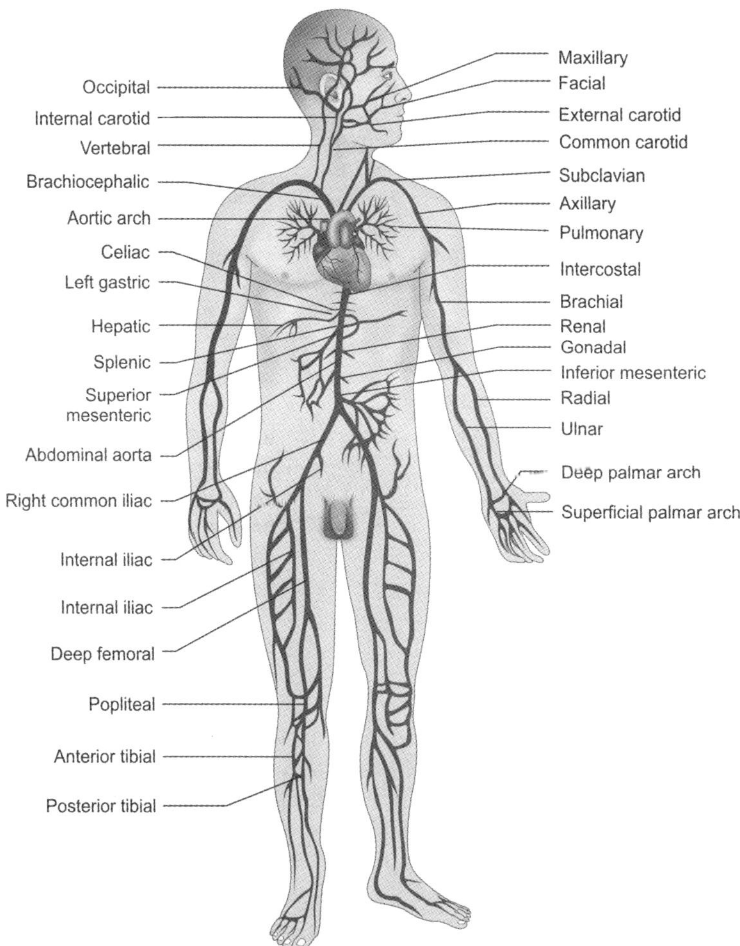

FIG. 3.1 Important arteries

blood of the arteries and transporting the waste materials through the venules to the kidneys.

HEART (FIGS. 3.3 AND 3.4)

Heart is a conical-shaped hollow muscular organ situated in the mediastinum, in between the two lungs in the thoracic cavity. It is slightly tilted towards left side. The heart is made of a special

TABLE 3.1 Important arteries

Head and brain	Upper limb	Lower limb	Chest	Thigh
• Occipital • Cerebellar • Basilar • Temporal • Supraorbital • Supratroch-lear • Maxillary • Carotid • Common carotid • Deep cervical • Vertebral • Thoracic • Subclavian	• Cervical • Vertebral • Common carotid • Suprascapu-lar • Deltoid • Brachial • Radial • Ulnar • Interosseous • Palmar • Digital	• Genicular • Popliteal • Femoral • Tibial • Fibular • Calcaneal	• Subclavian • Brachioce-phalic • Axillary • Pulmonary • Aorta • Ascending aorta • Arch of aorta • Descending aorta • Intercostal • Renal • Inferior mes-enteric • Common iliac • Thoracic • Clavicular • Pectoral	• Abdominal aorta • Common iliac • Middle sacral • Inguinal • Femoral • Perineal • Urethral • Penis • Rectal

type of muscle called the cardiac muscle, composed of striated muscle fibers. The heart has a base above and an apex below and its size will be almost equal to the owner's fist. The heart is divided into two sides, the right and left. The right side of the heart receives the deoxygenated blood and pumps into the lungs for purification and the left side of the heart receives the oxygenated blood from the lung and pumps into the various parts of the body through the aorta and arteries. Each side of the heart is further divided into two chambers, which communicate by means of valves. The upper chambers are the thin-walled atria or atrium, or auricle. The lower chambers are the thick-walled ventricles. Usually, they are represented as right atrium and left atrium, and right ventricle and left ventricle (Fig. 3.3).

The four chambers of the heart are separated by partitions called septa (singular septum). The interatrial septum separates the two upper chambers (atria) and the interventricular septum is a muscular

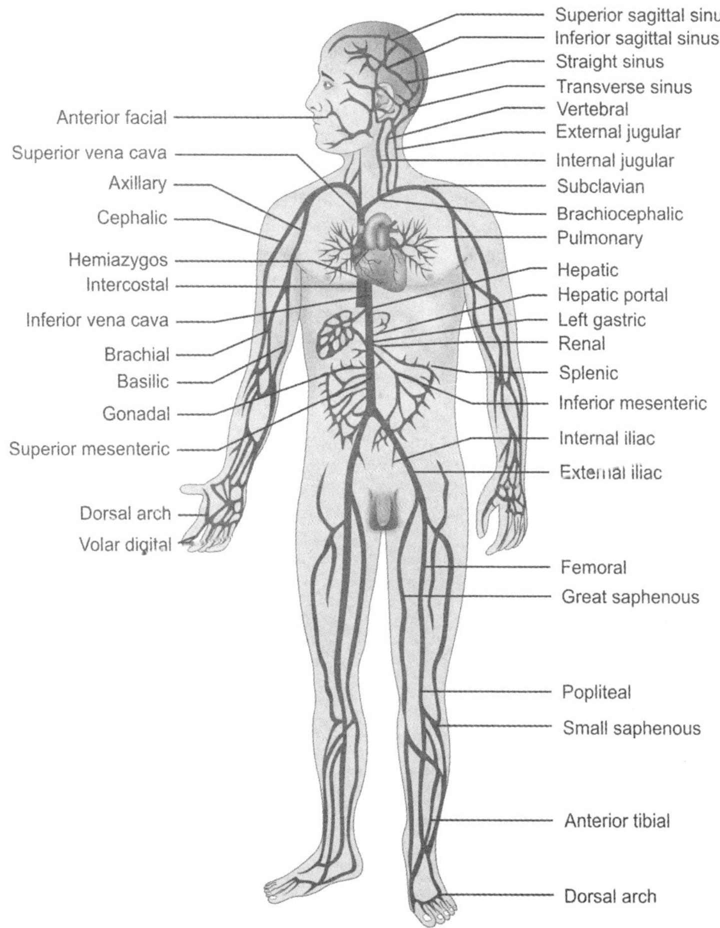

FIG. 3.2 Important veins

wall, which comes between the two lower chambers. The heart wall is composed of three layers. They are:

1. *Endocardium:* Smooth layer of cells, which lines the interior of the heart.
2. *Myocardium*: Middle muscular layer of the heart wall and is the thickest layer.
3. *Pericardium:* Delicate, double-folded membrane, which surrounds the heart like a sac.

TABLE 3.2 Important veins

Head and neck	Upper limb	Lower limb and thigh	Thoracic cavity
• Sagittal sinus • Straight sinus • Transverse sinus • Facial • External jugular • Internal jugular • Subclavia • Brachiocephalic	• Axillary • Brachial • Cephalic • Basilic • Palmar digital	• Superior iliac • Superior epigastric • Femoral • Great saphenous • Popliteal • Small saphenous • Anterior tibial • Dorsal venous arch • Dorsal digital	• Superior vena cava • Left subclavian • Portal • Splenic • Mesenteric • Inferior vena cava • Colic • Superior mesenteric • Ileocolic • Rectal • Deep femoral

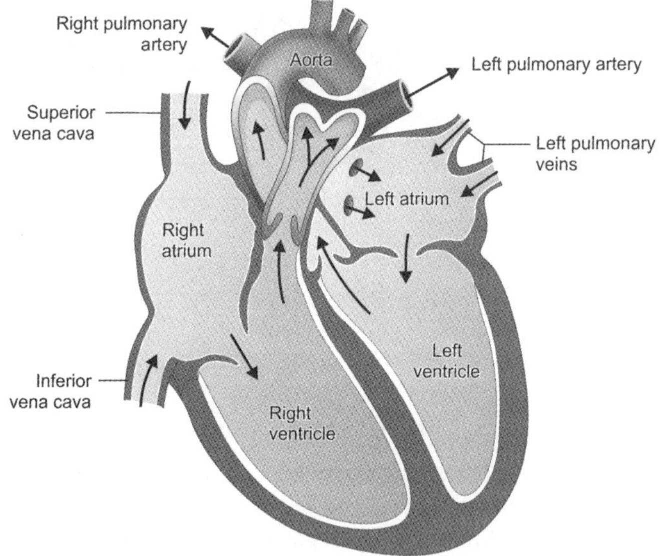

FIG. 3.3 Structure of heart

Valves of the Heart

The valves of the heart play an important role to prevent the backflow of the blood into the chambers.

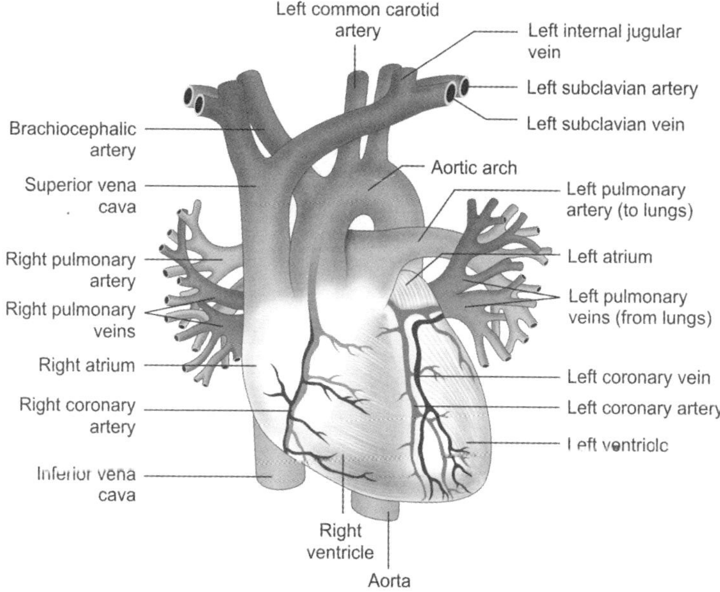

FIG. 3.4 Exterior section of the heart with blood flow and names of different parts of the heart

- *Mitral valve:* Bicuspid valve is situated between the left atrium and ventricle (left side of the heart).
- *Tricuspid valve:* Lies between the right atrium and right ventricle.
- *Semilunar valves:* Lies on the mouth of the pulmonary artery, which arises from the right ventricle and on the mouth of the aorta, which arises from the left ventricle.

Heart Cycle or Cardiac Cycle (Figs. 3.5 and 3.6)

The heart cycle consists of two phases. The first phase is called diastole (relaxation) and the second is systole (contraction).

Diastole

During diastolic phase the ventricles relax and deoxygenated blood flows into the right atrium of heart through the vena cava, and the oxygenated blood from the lungs pours into the left atrium through pulmonary veins. The tricuspid and mitral valves are open in diastolic

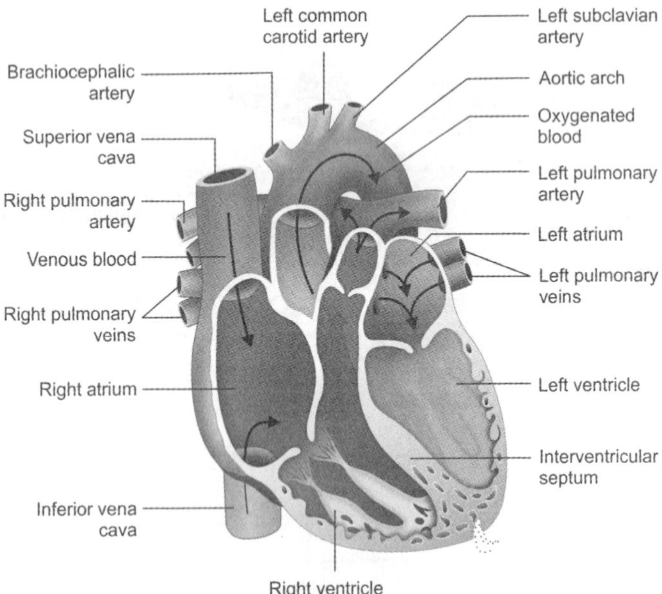

FIG. 3.5 Interior section of the heart with blood flow and names of different parts of the heart

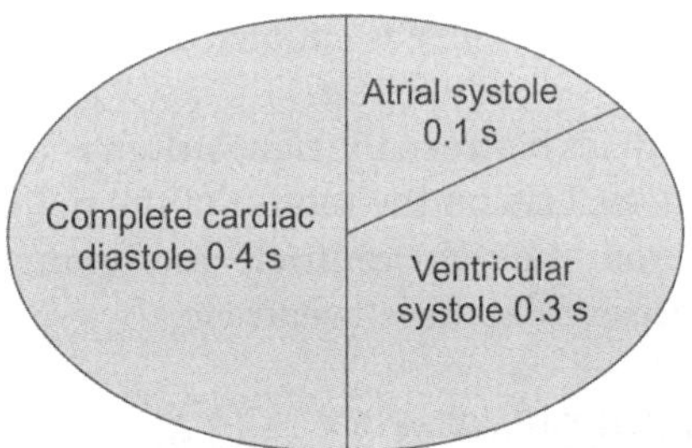

FIG. 3.6 Heart cycle or cardiac circulation

phase and the blood passes from the right and left atria into the ventricles.

Systole

The next phase is systolic phase. During this phase the walls of the ventricle contract and the semilunar valves open, and the blood is pumped into the pulmonary artery and aorta from the right, and left ventricles respectively. The diastole-systole cardiac cycle last about 0.8 seconds and occurs between 70 and 80 times per minute. The cardiac cycle consists of atrial systole—contraction of the atria, ventricular systole—contraction of ventricles, complete cardiac diastole—relaxation of atria and ventricles. Thus, the heart pumps about 70 mL of blood with each contractions.

PULMONARY AND SYSTEMIC CIRCULATION

The circulation of blood through the vessels from the heart to the lungs and then back to the heart again is known as the **pulmonary circulation.** The circulation of blood from the body organs (except the lungs) to the heart and back again is called the **systemic circulation.**

Systemic Circulation (Fig. 3.7)

Deoxygenated blood enters the heart through two largest veins in the body, the superior vena cava and inferior vena cava to the right atrium. The right atrium contracts to force the blood through

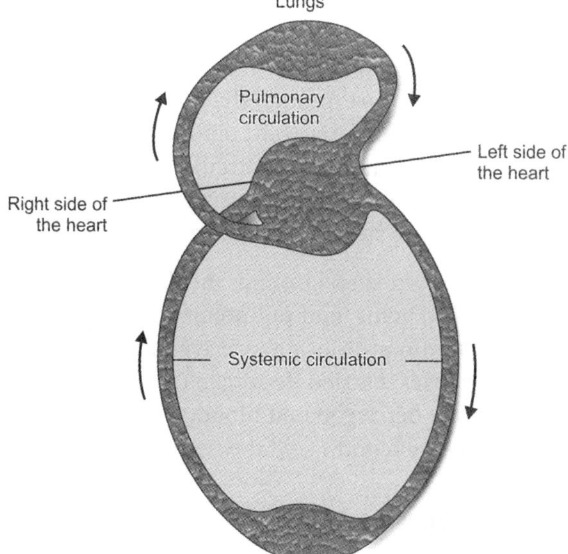

FIG. 3.7 Systemic circulation

tricuspid valve into the right ventricle. As the right ventricle contracts to pump deoxygenated blood to the lungs through pulmonary artery, the tricuspid valve is closed to prevent any blood from pushing back into the right atrium. The pulmonary (semilunar) valve, between the right ventricle and pulmonary artery opens as the blood is pumped into the pulmonary artery.

Similarly, the newly oxygenated blood enters into the left atrium through the pulmonary vein. The walls of the left atrium contract to force blood through the mitral valve into the left ventricle. The left ventricle pumps blood with great force so that the blood is pumped through the aortic valve, into the aorta, which have three branches ascending aorta, arch of aorta and descending aorta, and the blood is pumped to all parts of the body through the arteries. The aortic valve prevents the return of aortic blood to the left ventricle once it has been pumped out.

Pulmonary Circulation

During the contraction of the ventricle, the deoxygenated blood is pumped into the pulmonary artery through the pulmonary (semilunar) valve from the right ventricle. This blood when reaches the capillaries of the lung, the exchange of the carbon dioxide and oxygen occurs, and the blood is purified. The newly purified blood is brought back to the heart through the pulmonary vein to the left atrium. This is called pulmonary circulation. The important point to be noted is that in pulmonary circulation, the arteries carry deoxygenated blood, whereas the veins carry oxygenated blood, which is reverse in the systemic circulation.

Note: The reader should keep in mind, the differences between the systemic arteries and veins, and pulmonary arteries and veins. For instance, the systemic arteries carry oxygenated blood, whereas the pulmonary arteries, carried deoxygenated blood, similarly, the systemic veins carry deoxygenated blood, whereas the pulmonary veins carry oxygenated blood.

Portal Circulation (Flowchart 3.1)

Portal circulation is an important subdivision of the general circulation. Blood from the stomach, pancreas and spleen is collected

FLOWCHART 3.1 Block diagram representing the functioning of the heart and blood circulation

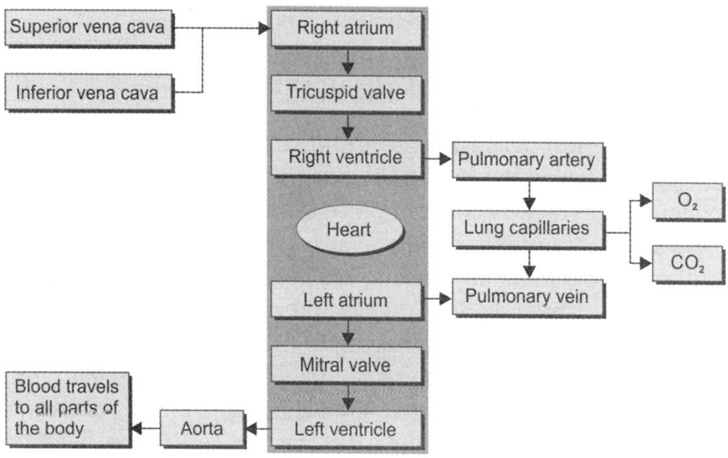

by the portal vein and passed to the liver. Here the capillary network unites with the capillary network of the hepatic artery. This double blood supply is collected by the hepatic vein and passed to the inferior vena cava.

BLOOD PRESSURE

The force exerted by the blood against the arterial walls during the systole and diastole of heart is called blood pressure. The blood pressure is expressed as systolic pressure/diastolic pressure separated by a slash. The normal BP is 120/80, but it may vary due to the influence of age, emotional stress, constriction of blood vessels, etc.

The diastole (dilation) and systole (contraction) cardiac cycle last about 0.9 seconds and occurs between 70 and 80 times per minute (100,000 times a day).

PULSE

The arterial pulse is a wave of increased pressure felt in the arteries when blood is pumped out of the heart. The pulse is most readily felt where an artery passes over a bone and lies near the surface, e.g. the radial pulse at the wrist. The pulse rate is usually described as the number of heart beats per minute. The adult range is between 60 and 80 beats per minute. In children the rate is higher.

ELECTRICAL CONDUCTION OF THE HEART PULSES

An electrical impulse originates from small muscle tissue, in the right atrium called the sinoatrial node (SA node), this is called the pacemaker of the heart. The impulse from the pacemaker radiates to the posterior portion of the interatrial septum (AV node). The AV node sends electrical impulses to the bundle of His, which further divides into right and left branches and carries the impulse to the right and left ventricles, resulting them to contract. Thus, systole of ventricles occurs and the blood is pumped away from the heart. After a short duration, the way of excitation is initiated by the pacemaker again. Electrocardiogram is the instrument to record the electrical impulse of the heart, commonly called as ECG.

Chapter Summary

Two distinct body systems, the cardiovascular system and the lymphatic system are responsible for transportation of products to and from the cells of the body. Since body cells are not always located near the source of the products they require and they are not always near the organs necessary for elimination of waste, a transportation system is required.

The cardiovascular system is compound of the (1)........................ The lymphatic system is composed of lymph glands, lymph vessels and lymph. Only the heart and blood vessels are discussed in this chapter. Blood is considered with the lymphatic system because of the similarity between them.

Vascular System

Three types of vessels carry blood throughout the body. Each differs in structure, depending on its function. These vessels are arteries, capillaries and veins.

Arteries

Arteries carry blood from the heart to (2)....................

The blood is propelled through the arteries by the pumping action of the heart. Consequently, arterial walls are thick and muscular and capable of expanding to accommodate the surge of blood that results when the heart contracts. The expansion of the arterial walls at each heartbeat is referred to as a pulse. Because of the pressure against the arterial walls associated with the pumping action of the heart, a cut or severed artery is a serious condition.

The blood in the arteries (except for the pulmonary artery) contains a high concentration of oxygen (O_2). Such blood is referred to as oxygenated blood. It is characterized by a bright red color. Arteries branch to form smaller vessels called arterioles (little arteries). Arterioles further divided to form the smallest vessels of the circulatory system, the capillaries.

Capillaries

Capillaries are microscopic vessels that join the arterial system with the venous system. Although, seemingly, the most insignificant of the three vessel types because of size (only one blood cell at a time is able to pass through the lumen), they are functionally the most important. The walls of the capillaries are composed of a single layer of (3)....................

The thinness of these walls makes it possible for substances to pass quite readily in and out of vessels. Consequently, the primary function of the vascular system providing cells with vital products is achieved by the capillaries.

It is important to note that the vast number of capillaries makes their combined diameter so great that blood flow through them vary slowly. This allows sufficient time for the exchange of materials to occur between blood and body cells.

Veins

Veins carry blood to the heart from (4)....................

Veins are formed from smaller vessels called venules (little veins), which develop from the union of capillaries. It connects arterioles to venules. This connection provides a gateway for the return of blood to the heart. Since the extensive network of capillaries throughout the body absorb the propelling pressure exerted by the heart. These methods include skeletal muscle contraction (especially in the legs), gravity (in the upper areas of the body), and respiratory activity (in the thoracic area). In addition, valves aid in the return of blood to the heart. Valves are small structures within the vein that prevent the backflow of blood. Valves are especially important in the legs because blood must travel a long distance against the force of gravity in order to reach the heart.

Blood carried in the veins (except for the pulmonary vein) contains a high concentration of carbon dioxide (CO_2). This gas is waste product of cell metabolism and is produced by all cells of the body. When CO_2 is present in blood, the blood takes on characteristic purple color. Such blood is said to be deoxygenated. Deoxygenated blood is continuously transported to the lungs, where the CO_2 is expelled.

Heart

The heart is hollow, muscular organ that pumps blood through the arteries, capillaries and veins. It is enclosed in a fibroserous sac called (5)....................

The heart has three distinct layers of tissue:

1. The endocardium, which is a serous membrane that lines the four chambers of the heart and its valves. It is continuous with the arteries and veins.
2. The myocardium, which is the muscular layer of the heart.
3. The epicardium, which is the outermost layer of the heart.

The heart is divided into four chambers. These chambers are the right atrium, right ventricle, left atrium and left ventricle. The two upper chambers, the atria, collect blood; the two lower chambers, the ventricles, pump blood from the heart. The right side of the heart provides for the oxygenation of blood (pulmonary circulation), and the left side is responsible for the transportation of blood to body cells, which compose all the systems of the body (systemic circulation). The muscular wall dividing the right side of the heart from left is called septum.

Body cells produce waste products during metabolism. These waste products include CO_2, a gas that must be removed or tissue death will occur. The thin-walled capillaries allow CO_2 to enter the blood, where it is transported to the heart by way of two large veins—the superior vena cava, which collects and carry blood from the top portion of the body; and the inferior vena cava, which collects and carry blood from the lower portion of the body. The superior and inferior vena cava deposits the deoxygenated blood into the right upper chamber of the heart, the right atrium. From the right atrium, blood passes through the tricuspid valve to the (6)....................

The tricuspid valve prevents blood from returning to the right atrium during contraction of the ventricle. When the heart contracts, blood leaves the right ventricle by way of the pulmonary artery. The pulmonic semilunar valve (pulmonary valve) in the pulmonary artery restrains blood from passing back into the right ventricle. In the lungs, this artery branches into millions of capillaries, each lying in close proximity to the alveoli. Here CO_2, in the blood is replaced by O_2 that has been drawn into the lungs during inhalation. The blood is now oxygenated and takes on a bright red appearance.

The pulmonary capillaries unite to form the pulmonary veins, which carry blood back to the heart. The right and left pulmonary veins carry oxygenated blood into the left atrium of the heart. The blood passes from the left atrium through the bicuspid valve (also called mitral valve) to the left ventricle. Upon contraction of the heart, the oxygenated blood leaves the left ventricle through the largest artery of the body, the aorta. Within the aorta is a valve called the aortic (7).................... valve, or aortic valve. This valve permits blood to flow in only one direction from the left ventricle to aorta. The aorta branches into many smaller arteries that carry blood to all parts of the body. Some arteries derive their name from the organs or areas of the body that they vascularize the heart muscle, the renal arteries vascularize the kidneys and so forth.

It is important to recognize that the O_2 present in the blood passing through the chambers of the heart cannot be used by myocardium. Instead, an arterial system called the coronary arteries, branches from the aorta and provides the heart muscle with its own blood supply. If flow of the blood in the coronary is diminished, myocardial damage may result. When sever damage occurs, necrosis of muscle tissue results.

Blood Pressure

Each heartbeat is composed of two phases, the contraction phase is called systole, when the blood is forced out of the heart; and a relaxation phase is called (8)....................

Blood pressure measures the force exerted by the blood against the arterial walls during these two phases. Systole indicates the maximum force exerted by the blood against the arterial walls, diastole and the weakest. These are recorded as two figures separated by diagonal line; the systolic pressure is given first, followed by the diastolic pressure. For example, a blood pressure may be recorded as 120/80, where 120 is the systolic pressure and 80 is the diastolic pressure.

Several factors influence the blood pressure, including resistance of blood flow in the blood vessels, the pumping action of the heart, the viscosity or thickness, of the blood, the elastic of the arteries, and the quality of blood in the vascular system. Elevated blood pressure is called hypertension; decreased pressure is called hypotension.

Conduction System of the Heart

Within the heart is a specialized cardiac tissue known as conductive tissue. Its sole function is the initiation and propagation of contraction impulses. The contractive tissue consists of four masses of highly specialized cells:

1. Sinoatrial (SA) node
2. Atrioventricular (AV) node
3. Bundle of His
4. Purkinje fibers.

The SA node, which is located in the upper portion of the right atrium, possesses its own intrinsic rhythm. Without being stimulated by external nerves, it has the ability to initiate and propagate each heartbeat, thereby setting the basic pace for the cardiac rate. For this reason, it is commonly known as pacemaker. Cardiac rate may be altered by impulses from autonomic nervous system. Such an arrangement allows outside influences to accelerate or decelerate of the heartbeat. For example, during a period of physical exertion the heartbeats faster and during a restful interval the rate becomes slower.

Each electrical impulse discharged by the SA node is transmitted to the AV node, causing the aorta to contract. The AV node is located at the base of right atrium. From this point, a tract of conduction fibers called bundle of His, composed of a right and left branch, relays the impulse to the Purkinje fibers. These fibers extend up the walls of the ventricles. The Purkinje fibers transmit the impulse to both the right and left ventricles, causing them to contract. The blood is now forced out of the heart through the pulmonary artery and the aorta. To be precise:

SA node → AV node → Bundle of His → Purkinje fibers

Impulse transmission through the conduction system generates weak electrical currents that can be detected on the surface of the body. These electrical impulses can be recorded on an instrument called (9)....................

The deflection of the needle of the electrocardiograph produces waves of peaks designated by the letters P, Q, R, S, and T, each of which is associated with a specific electrical event. The P wave is the depolarization (contraction) of the atria, and the QRS complex is the depolarization (contraction) of the ventricles. The T wave, which appears a short time later, is the repolarization (recovery) of the ventricles.

Answers

1. Heart, blood vessels and blood
2. Body tissues and organs
3. Endothelial cells
4. Body organs and tissues
5. Pericardium
6. Right ventricle
7. Semilunar
8. Diastole
9. Electrocardiograph

Review Questions

Exercise 1: Answer in One Word

1. Various systems of anatomy and physiology composed of millions of ______________.
2. Cardiovascular system is composed of the heart, blood vessels, and ______________.
3. The lymphatic is composed of lymph glands, lymph vessels, and ______________.
4. ______________ types of vessels carry blood throughout the body.
5. ______________ carry blood from the heart to body tissues and organs.
6. Arterioles (little arteries) are the branches of ______________.
7. ___________ are the smallest vessels of the circulatory system.
8. Capillaries vessels that join the arterial system with the ___________.
9. The walls of the capillaries are composed of a single layer of ___________.
10. ___________ carry blood to the heart from body organs and tissues.
11. Ventricles (little veins), are part of smaller vessels ______________.
12. Veins are formed from smaller vessels are called Venules or ______________.
13. Capillaries connect arterioles to ______________.
14. Union of capillaries carry blood to the ______________.
15. Valves are small structures of the vein that prevent the backflow of ______________.
16. Blood carried in the veins except for the ______________.
17. Blood carried in the veins contains high concentration of ______________.
18. The heart pumps blood through the arteries, capillaries and ______________.
19. Heart is enclosed in a fibroserous sack called the ______________.
20. The heart has three layers of tissue: endocardium, myocardium and ______________.
21. The heart is divided into ______________ four chambers.
22. The four chambers of heart include: right atrium, right ventricle, left atrium, ______________.
23. The ______________ divides the right side of the heart from the left side.
24. Body cells produce waste product during ______________.
25. The superior and inferior vena cava deposits the deoxygenated blood ______________.

26. Blood from the right atrium, passes through the tricuspid valve to ______________.
27. When heart contracts, blood leaves the right ventricle by way of ______________.
28. Each heartbeat is composed of two phases, systolic and ______________.
29. Contraction phase, or ______________, the blood is forced out of the heart, ______________.
30. Elevated blood pressure is called ______________.
31. Decreased blood pressure is called ______________.
32. BP may be recorded as 120/80; 120 is the systolic pressure, and 80 ______________.
33. Within the heart is a specialized cardiac tissue known as ______________.
34. The conductive tissue consists of four masses of highly ______________.
35. Cardiac rate may be altered by impulses from the autonomic ______________.
36. The AV node is located at the base of the ______________.
37. Electrical impulses discharged by the SA node is transmitted to the ______________.
38. The AV node is located at the base of the ______________.
39. Bundle of His, relays impulse to the ______________.
40. SA node → ______________ → Bundle of His → Purkinje fibers.

Exercise 2: Complete the Following

1. The cardiovascular system includes the ______________, ______________, ______________ and ______________.
2. The external layer of the sac-like membrane covering the heart is called ______________.
3. The heart is divided into ______________ chambers.
4. The valves of the heart prevent a ______________ of blood into the atria.
5. Arteries carry ______________ blood from the heart throughout the body and ______________ transport it back to the heart.
6. The four blood types are ______________, ______________, ______________ and ______________.
7. ______________ veins are the only veins carrying oxygenated blood.
8. The ______________ is the largest artery in the body.
9. The three branches of the aorta are the ______________, ______________ and ______________.
10. The ______________ drains into the right atrium.

Exercise 3: Match the Following

1. Cardiosclerosis	A. Pacemaker
2. Atrium	B. Contraction of the heart
3. Systole	C. A lower heart chamber
4. Sinoatrial node	D. Hardening of heart tissues and vessels
5. Diastole	E. Inflammation of the heart muscle
6. Ventricle	F. Bluish skin color caused by reduced amounts of hemoglobin in the blood
7. Pulmonary value	G. Relaxation of heart
8. Myocarditis	H. Inflammation of the veins
9. Phlebitis	I. Valve between the heart and lungs
10. Cyanosis	J. An upper chamber of the heart

Answers

Exercise 1

1. Cells
2. Blood
3. Lymph
4. Three types
5. Arteries
6. Arteries
7. Capillaries
8. Venous system
9. Endothelial cells
10. Veins
11. Veins
12. Little veins
13. Venules
14. Heart
15. Blood
16. Pulmonary vein
17. Carbon dioxide
18. Veins
19. Pericardium
20. Epicardium
21. Four
22. Left ventricle
23. Septum
24. Metabolism
25. In right atrium
26. Right ventricle
27. Pulmonary artery
28. Diastole
29. Systolic
30. Hypertension
31. Hypotension
32. Diastolic pressure
33. Conductive tissue
34. Specialized cells
35. Nervous system
36. Right atrium
37. AV node
38. Right atrium
39. Purkinje fibers
40. AV node

Exercise 2

1. Heart, blood, arteries, veins
2. Pericardium
3. Four
4. Backflow
5. Oxygenated, veins
6. A, B, O, AB
7. Pulmonary
8. Aorta
9. Ascending aorta, aortic arch, descending aorta
10. Inferior vena cava

Exercise 3

1. D
2. J
3. B
4. A
5. G
6. C
7. I
8. E
9. H
10. F

Blood and Lymphatic System

On completion of this chapter, the student will be able to:

- Recognize the composition of blood and their functions
- List the components of blood plasma and their functions
- Describe the blood clotting mechanism
- List different blood groups and explain their compatibility and incompatibility
- Explain the functions of lymph
- Describe various lymphatic organs and their functions

INTRODUCTION

Blood and lymph are the specialized liquid tissues of the body; each is composed of cells that are suspended in a liquid medium. Both these tissues play a vital role in defending the body against infection. They also act as the transportation system for body cells, since they are movable throughout the entire body.

BLOOD

The blood is red and viscid, alkaline in reaction and it is divided into a fluid part and a solid part as follows:

Fluid Part

Plasma, which is straw-colored fluid and contains essential substances.

Solid Part

The solid part of the blood is composed of three major blood cells (Fig. 4.1):

1. Red blood cells (erythrocytes)
2. White blood cells (leukocytes)
3. Platelets (thrombocytes).

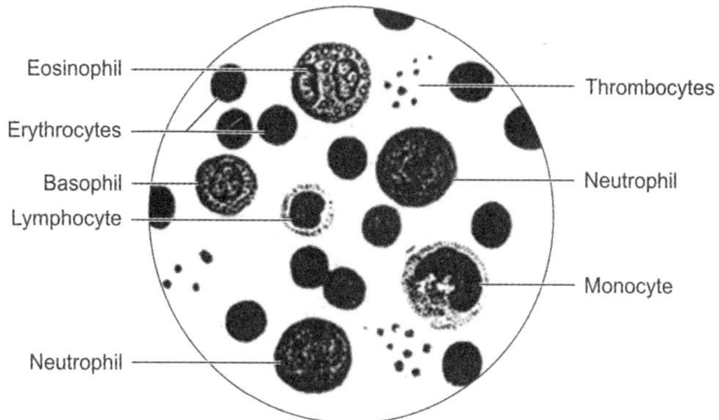

FIG. 4.1 Blood cell

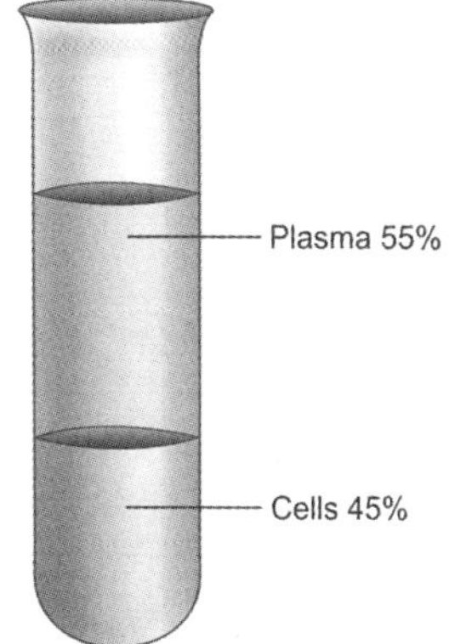

FIG. 4.2 Blood in the test tube shows the percentage composition of plasma and cells

Plasma accounts for about 55% and blood cells accounts for about 45% of the total blood volume (Fig. 4.2).

Functions of the Blood

The main functions of the blood are to:

- Convey oxygen to the tissues by means of hemoglobin in the red blood cells
- Remove waste products from the tissue
- Carry nutrients to all parts of the body
- Carry hormones or chemical messengers of the body

- Aid in defense of the body by phagocytic action
- Participate in the circulation of lymphocytes required for immune response
- Carry antibodies to the sites of infection.

PLASMA

Plasma is the liquid portion of the blood in which the corpuscles are suspended. It is composed of about 92% water and solid materials, which are mainly proteins with lesser amounts of sugar, wastes, salts, hormones and other substances. The four major proteins presents in the plasma are:

1. Albumin
2. Globulin
3. Fibrinogen
4. Prothrombin.

Plasma makes it possible for the chemical communication between all the body cells by carrying these products to different parts of the body.

Albumin and globulin are the serum proteins that help to maintain the proper water content of the blood by holding water in the blood, opposing its tendency to leak out into the tissue spaces, which would cause edema (swelling). The globulin portion of plasma contains antibodies, which can fight off foreign antigens. There are three different kinds of globulins in plasma. They are called alpha, beta and gamma, and they are distinguished by the process of electrophoresis. Immunoglobulins are a specific type of gamma-globulin, which are capable of acting as antibodies. Examples of immunoglobulin antibodies are immunoglobulin G (IgG) and immunoglobulin A (IgA). When free of corpuscles, plasma is thin and colorless. The fibrinogen helps in clotting of blood.

Blood serum is a product of blood plasma. It differs from plasma in that serum does not contain fibrinogen. This can be represented as follows:

Plasma - Fibrinogen = Serum

Composition

The composition of the plasma is as follows:

- Water 90–92%

- Plasma proteins 60 g/L
  - Albumin 35–50 g/L
  - Globulin 20–37 g/L
  - Fibrinogen 2–4 g/L
  - Prothrombin 100–150 mg/L
- Mineral salts
- Nutrient materials
- Organic waste products
- Hormones
- Enzymes
- Antibodies and antitoxins
- Gases.

ERYTHROCYTES (RED BLOOD CELLS)

Erythrocytes are formed in the red bone marrow of the spongy bones that are at the ends of the long bones. The development of red blood cells is called erythropoiesis. During their development, red blood cells (RBCs) develop a special compound called hemoglobin, which is rich in iron-containing pigment, that gives the erythrocyte its red color. It is the hemoglobin in the erythrocytes that enable the cell to carry oxygen all through the body. The combination of oxygen and hemoglobin (oxyhemoglobin) produces the bright red color of blood. Normally, 13–18 g/100 mL of hemoglobin is present in male and 12–16 g/100 mL hemoglobin is present in female.

The average life of the erythrocytes is about 120 days in the circulating bloodstream. After this time, the worn-out erythrocytes are destroyed by the cells of spleen, liver and bone marrow. These cells called macrophages, set the hemoglobin free from the erythrocyte and break the hemoglobin down into its heme and globin portions. The heme decomposes into bilirubin and iron. Iron is used to form new red cells or is stored in the spleen, liver and bone marrow for later use. Bilirubin is carried to the liver and excreted through the intestine with bile.

The process of breakdown of the worn-out cells is called hemolysis, which is carried out by the cells of the reticuloendothelial system. These cells are called phagocytic, i.e. capable of engulfing and destroying foreign bodies such as microorganisms and worn erythrocytes.

LEUKOCYTES (WHITE BLOOD CELLS)

The leukocytes play a vital role in the body's immune system by protecting it against the invasion by bacteria and other foreign substances. It also plays a vital role in tissue repair, but this activity is still not fully understood.

White blood cells (WBCs) can be classified into two categories, the granulocytes (with granules in the cytoplasm) and agranulocytes (without granules). Each of these categories can be further subdivided as follows:

1 Granulocytes:
   - Neutrophils
   - Eosinophils
   - Basophils.
2 Agranulocytes:
   - Monocytes
   - Lymphocytes.

Granulocytes

Granulocytes are the most numerous leukocytes (about 60%). The granulocytes are formed in the red bone marrow from stem cells, which give rise to myeloblasts. Myeloblasts differentiate into:

- Neutrophils
- Eosinophils
- Basophils.

These names were derived from the dye used to stain blood smears in the laboratory.

Neutrophils

They compose 57% of the leukocytes. The neutrophils are motile and highly phagocytic. They fight disease by engulfing and swallowing up germs. They also increase in a number of pyrogenic (fever-producing) infections and in some types of leukemia.

Eosinophils

It protects body by releasing many substances that are capable of detoxifying foreign protein and other material. Eosinophils are increased in allergic conditions and parasitic infections. They are also capable of destroying antigen/antibody complexes.

Basophils

The exact functions are not known. It releases histamines and heparin in the area of damaged tissues. Histamines causes inflammatory reaction, ultimately increasing the blood flow. Therefore, additional neutrophils or phagocytes are brought to the damaged area.

Agranulocytes

Agranulocyte cells contain single large nucleus and therefore they are called mononuclear cells. These form 33% of the leukocytes. It is composed of:

- Lymphocytes
- Monocytes.

Lymphocytes

They play a vital role in the immune system of the body. They are capable of making antibodies, which can neutralize and destroy foreign antigens (bacteria and viruses) that may enter the body. The harmful invader is called antigen; the defense provided by the body is called the antibody. This reaction is called antigen-antibody reaction.

Monocytes

Monocytes provide protection to the body, in the same manner as neutrophils, by phagocytes. They dispose dead and dying cells, and other debris by engulfing and swallowing the cells.

Thrombocytes (Platelets)

The thrombocytes are the smallest elements within the blood. Platelets are formed in the red bone marrow from giant multinucleated cells called megakaryocytes. The main function of platelets is to help in the clotting mechanism of the blood.

BLOOD CLOTTING MECHANISM

Blood clotting or coagulation is a complicated process involving many different chemical reactions as follows:

- Prothrombin activator (thromboplastin) is released when there is a break in the tissue or at the site of injury or when platelets rupture.
- The thromboplastin acts on prothrombin and converts prothrombin into thrombin.
- The thrombin acting on the fibrinogen converts it into fibrin, which is insoluble, which trap red blood cells to form the clot.

The period of time, taken by fibrin to form the blood clot is known as the coagulation time. Normally, it will be less than 15 minutes. The time taken for the platelets to plug up a small puncture of the skin is called bleeding time and it is normally less than 8 minutes.

BLOOD GROUP

Blood is divided into four groups namely A, B, AB and O based on the presence or absence of blood antigens in the RBCs. The presence of the antigen and antibodies for the four different types of blood group, and the possible donor are given in Table 4.1.

Besides grouping by classifying A and B antigen, there are many other antigens located on the surface of the RBC. One of these is called the rhesus (Rh) factor (named because it was first found in the blood of a rhesus monkey). The term Rh-positive refers to a person who is born with Rh antigen on his/her red blood cells, and the Rh-negative person does not have the Rh antigen.

TABLE 4.1 Blood groups

Blood group	*Antigen present*	*Antibody present*	*Can receive blood from*	*Can donate blood to*
A	A	Anti-B	A and O groups	A and AB groups
B	B	Anti-A	B and O groups	B and AB groups
AB	A and B	No antibody present	A, B, O, AB (universal recipients)	AB group only
O	No antigen present	Both Anti-A and Anti-B	O	A, B, AB, and O groups (universal donors)

LYMPHATIC SYSTEM

The lymphatic system consists of lymph a tissue fluid, which is found all over the body through a network of transporting structure called lymph vessels, lymph nodes and the spleen, thymus and tonsils. Other noncellular constituents of lymph are water, salts, sugar and wastes of metabolism, such as urea and creatinine. The primary functions of the lymphatic system are:

- To drain fluid from tissue spaces and return it to the blood
- Transporting materials to body cells
- Carrying waste products from body tissues back to the bloodstream
- To convey lipids or fats, away from the digestive organs
- To control infection by providing lymphocytes and monocytes, which are used to defend against infections caused by microorganisms.

Lymph originates from the blood plasma. As blood circulates through the capillaries, some of the plasma steps out of these thin-walled vessels. This fluid, now called interstitial or tissue fluid, resembles plasma, except it contains less protein. When the fluid enters into the capillaries, it is called lymph. Lymph capillaries are thin-walled tubes, same like blood capillaries. These capillaries carry lymph from the tissue space to the large lymphatic vessels and finally to lymph nodes, which serve as depositories for cellular debris. The lymph nodes are present all over the body (Fig. 4.3). As lymph passes through the nodes it is filtered and replenished with lymphocytes, globulins and antibodies. Bacteria and debris are engulfed by macrophages that line the nodes.

The thoracic duct acts as the major duct to drain the lymph from all parts of body except the right chest and arm, which drains into the left subclavian vein. Whereas the lymph vessels of the right chest and arm join the right lymphatic duct, which drains into the right subclavian vein. Thus, the lymph is recycled into the circulating blood in order to begin the cycle, once again, throughout the body.

Lymph Nodes (Fig. 4.3 and Table 4.2)

The lymph node is bean-shaped and has afferent (away from lymph node) lymphatics at the convex border and efferent (towards the lymph node) lymphatics at the hilum. Each lymph node has a capsule, an outer cortex containing mostly lymphatic nodules and an inner

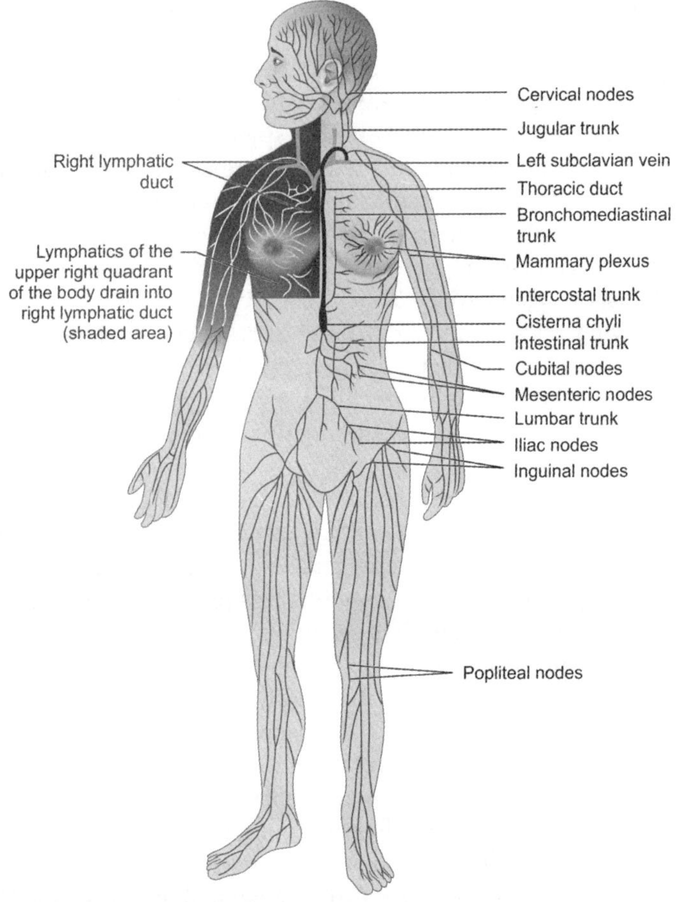

FIG. 4.3 Lymph nodes and their location

TABLE 4.2 Lymph nodes and their locations

Lymph nodes	Location
Superficial and deep cervical nodes	Neck
Parotid, submandibular, mastoid and occipital nodes	Head
Bronchomediastinal, bronchopulmonary and tracheobronchial nodes	Thorax
Gastric, hepatic, splenic, mesenteric and lumbar	Abdomen
Axillary nodes	Axilla
Inguinal nodes	Groin

medulla containing lymphatic sinuses. Lymph nodes are placed along the lymphatics. When a part of the body is infected and inflamed, the lymph nodes drain, hence that part become enlarged and palpable.

Related Lymphatic Organs

The organs composed of lymphatic tissue are:

- Spleen
- Thymus
- Tonsils.

Spleen

Spleen is the biggest lymphatic organ. It is located in the left upper quadrant of the abdomen, adjacent to the stomach. The main functions of the spleen are:

- Destruction of old RBC, by which bilirubin is formed and added to the bloodstream.
- Filtration of microorganisms and other foreign materials from the blood
- Production of antibodies and immunity, chiefly by leukocytes
- Storage of blood, especially RBC; Blood is released by the spleen when the body needs it
- Production of blood cells such as lymphocytes and monocytes
- Stimulates the production of blood cells from the bone marrow.

Thymus

Thymus is located in the mediastinum, posterior to the breastbone and between the lungs. It plays a vital role in the body's immunologic system. It produces special lymphocytes called T cells, which migrate to the site of antigens and to destroy the antigen by the process of phagocytosis. Other types of lymphocytes are called B cells, these cells are produced in the bone marrow and they destroy antigen by producing antibody.

Tonsils

Three sets of tonsils, the palatine, pharyngeal and lingual tonsils, contain T and B lymphocytes, which protect against infection at the entrance of the digestive and respiratory tracts.

IMMUNITY

The study of the body's defense mechanism against the foreign organisms is called immunology. Immunity is a capacity to resist all types of organisms and toxins. Natural immunity is one's own ability to fight against disease. Acquired immunity is the protection against invasive organisms to which the body does not have natural immunity. Vaccination is a process of injecting antibodies against the foreign organisms and then remain in the body to protect against subsequent infection. Many diseases can be prevented by artificial immunization. For example:

- Poliomyelitis
- Smallpox
- Tetanus
- Tuberculosis
- Typhoid fever
- Diphtheria
- Measles
- Hepatitis B.

Acquired active immunity involves two major disease fighters, B-cell lymphocytes (humoral immunity) and T-cell lymphocytes (cell-mediated immunity). B-cells originate from bone marrow stem cells and migrate to lymph nodes and other lymphoid tissue. When a B cell is confronted with a specific type of antigen, it transforms into an antibody-producing cell called plasma cell. The antibodies that are made by plasma cell are immunoglobulins, such as immunoglobin M (IgM), IgG, immunoglobin D (IgD), immunoglobin E (IgE) and IgA. Immunoglobulins travel to the site of an infection to react with and neutralize antigens.

T-cell lymphocytes originate from stem cells in the bone marrow and are processed in the thymus gland where they are acted upon by thymic hormones. Then they migrate to lymph nodes and lymphoid organs. When an antigen encounters a T cell, the T-cell multiplies rapidly and can engulf, and digest the antigen (bacterium, virus, cancer cell or fungus) T cell also react to foreign tissues, such as skin grafts and transplanted organs.

Some T cells are cytotoxic or killer (called T8 cells), whereas other T-cells produce chemicals (interferon's and interleukins) that destroy cells or bacteria. One special class of T cells, called helper cells or T4 cells, stimulates antibody production. CD4+ T cells (CD4+ is the name of the protein on the cell) are attacked by the human immunodeficiency virus (HIV) in acquired immunodeficiency syndrome (AIDS). Suppressor cells are other T cells that regulate the amount of antibody produced by inhibiting the activity of the B-cell lymphocytes.

Chapter Summary

Blood and lymph are specialized tissues of the body. Each composed of cells that are suspended in a liquid medium. Both of these tissues play a vital role in defending the body against infection. Since blood and lymph have the ability to move throughout the entire body, they provide a transportation system for body cells. They transport nourishment, water, vitamins, electrolytes (sodium, potassium, and calcium), immune substances, heat and oxygen to all parts of the body. Conveyance of waste products to appropriate body organs for removal and distribution from the endocrine glands to numerous organs are some of the other vital functions performed by blood and lymph.

Blood

Blood is composed of liquid medium called plasma and a solid portion that consists of three major blood cells (1)....................

All blood cells develop from an undifferentiated cell, the hemocytoblast, also called stem cell. The maturation of the different blood cells is called hematopoiesis. The immature forms are in the bone marrow; the mature forms circulate in the peripheral blood. The composition of whole blood is detailed below:

- Whole blood = Liquid portion + Solid portion
- Plasma + Erythrocytes + Leukocytes + Thrombocytes (platelets).

Plasma accounts for about 55% and blood cells account for about 45% of the blood volume.

Erythrocytes

Erythrocytes are the most numerous circulating blood cells. They are formed in the (2).................... of the spongy bones of the skull, ribs, sternum, vertebrae, pelvis and at the ends of long bones of the arms and legs. Red blood cell development is called erythropoiesis. During erythropoiesis, red cells develop a specialized compound called hemoglobin, which is an iron-containing pigment that gives the erythrocyte its red color. Hemoglobin carries O_2 to body tissues, where it is exchanged for CO_2. The fact that there are millions of hemoglobin molecules in each of the trillions of red blood cells can help to appreciate the magnitude of the job that is accomplished by erythrocytes. The size of the red cell and its nucleus decreased during erythropoiesis. Just prior to maturity, the nucleus is extruded from the cell, leaving behind a small vestige of nuclear material (DNA). This DNA disappears and the new mature erythrocyte enters the circulatory system.

The mature erythrocyte appears as a smooth, biconcave structure with the cytoplasm filled with hemoglobin. It is thin in the center where nucleus was extruded, while the peripheral of the cell is thicker.

Erythrocytes live about 120 days and then rupture, releasing hemoglobin and cell fragments. The hemoglobin breaks down into hemosiderin, a compound that contains iron and several bile pigments. Most of the hemosiderin returns to the bone marrow and is reused to manufacture new blood cells. The bile pigments are eventually excreted by the liver.

Leukocytes

The chief function of the leukocyte is protection of the body against invasion by bacteria and other foreign substances. Their amoebic nature permits them to leave the bloodstream in order to search for and destroy harmful substances. Leukocytes also play a role in tissue repair, but this activity is still not fully understood. Leukocytes are classified into two categories, i.e. (3)....................

Granulocytes

Granulocytes are formed in the red bone marrow from stem cells, which give rise to myeloblasts. Myeloblasts differentiate into neutrophils, eosinophils and basophils. These names are derived from a polychromatic dye used to stain blood smears in the laboratory. The dye imparts specific colors to the granules of each of these cell types: eosinophils take up the acid dye eosin; basophils stain with a basic, or alkaline, dye and neutrophils stain with both the acid and basic dyes and hence are 'neutral' in their staining preference. In addition to the presence of granules, these cells are further characterized by a nucleus that is composed of several lobes in their mature form; hence these cells are also called polymorphonuclear cells.

The neutrophil is a type of the circulating white cells. It is very motile and highly phagocytic. Permitting it to ingest and devour bacteria and other particulate matter. In some functions, it is not common to find that one neutrophil has ingested as many as 20 bacteria. The eosinophils and basophils, although capable of phagocytosis, rarely display this activity. Eosinophils protect the body by releasing many substances that are capable of detoxifying foreign protein and other material especially of a chemical nature. They also are capable of destroying antigen/antibody complexes. Their number usually increased during allergic reactions.

Basophils release histamines and heparin in the area of damaged tissue. Histamines initiate the inflammation reaction, which increases blood flow. Therefore, additional neutrophils for phagocytosis are brought to the damaged area.

Agranulocytes

Agranulocyte include both monocytes and lymphocytes. These cells are characterized by the absence of granules in their cytoplasm. In addition, they both have a single large nucleus and are therefore called mononuclear cells. Agranulocytes develop from reticuloendothelial cells, the same cells that give rise to both erythrocytes and granulocytes. Nevertheless, in early development, monocytes and lymphocytes migrate from the bone marrow and enter the lymphatic system, where they undergo change and maturation. Some of these changes still are not fully understood.

Monocytes

Monocytes provide protection to the body in much the same manner as neutrophils, that is, they engage in phagocytosis. Monocytes migrate into tissue become macrophages. In this form, they are able to consume large numbers of bacteria or other invaders. They can phagocytize as many as 40 or 50 bacteria before they die.

Lymphocytes

On the other hand, lymphocytes provide protection through immunologic activity. An immune response is the body's ability to distinguish foreign material as harmful and invasive and then neutralize, eliminate or metabolize it, thereby rendering it harmless. The harmful invader is called antigen; the defense provided by the body is called antibody.

The immunologic response can be divided into two categories—humoral immunity and cellular immunity.

Humoral Immunity

Humoral immunity is provided by a specialized type of lymphocytes called (4)..................... It involves the production of a substance called antibody, which seeks out and renders harmless the invading substance called an antigen. As a general rule, the antigen-antibody reaction is specific, that is, the antibody reacts only with the antigen that induces its formation. For example, if the body has developed anti-polio antibodies in response to the presence of polio antigens (a situation that occurs after the administration of polio vaccine), these anti-polio antibodies provide no protection against any other antigen except polio. In order to produce antibodies, certain B-cells are activated in the presence of antigen to become plasma cells. Plasma cells synthesize and export antibodies. Some activated B-cells do not develop into plasma cells but remain as 'memory cells.' These cells stay in the lymphoid tissue. In the event of a future encounter by the same antigen, the memory cells immediately produce the plasma cells that are capable of manufacturing a specific antibody. It is believed that each plasma cell can manufacture specific antibodies at a rate of 2,000 per second for about 4–5 days.

The other type of protection provided by lymphocytes is cellular immunity. This immunity is a function of T-lymphocytes, also called T-cells. It matures in the thymus gland, hence the designation T-cells. When they encounter an antigen, T-cell become sensitized and changes into 'killer cells'. They produce a lymphotoxin or cytotoxin that damages or ruptures the cell membranes of the antigen. T-cells also aid in the production of interferon induces noninfected cells that have been invaded by viruses or other antigen. Interferon induces noninfected cells to form an antiviral protein that inhibits viral multiplication within the cell.

Thrombocytes

The smallest formed elements within the blood are thrombocytes or platelets. They are known as platelets because of their small plate-like appearance. Their chief function is to initiate (5)............... when injury occurs.

Blood clotting is not a single reaction, but rather a chain of interlinked reactions. At least 13 separate steps are involved, but this complex reaction can be described as essentially three major reactions.

Thromboplastin is either released by traumatized tissue at the site of injury or formed when platelets rupture. The action of thromboplastin causes prothrombin, a blood protein, to convert to thrombin. Eventually, thrombin converts soluble blood protein fibrinogen, to fibrin, an insoluble protein. Fibrin forms a meshwork in which blood cells become entangled. This jelly-like mass of protein and blood cells is a blood clot. The following shows the formation of a clot:

- Prothrombin to thromboplastin → Thrombin
- Fibrinogen (soluble) to thrombin → Fibrin (insoluble).

Plasma

Plasma is the liquid portion of blood in which the corpuscles are suspended. It is composed of about 92% water and contains the plasma protein (albumins, globulins and fibrinogen), gases, nutrients, salts, hormones and excretory products. Plasma makes possible the chemical communication between all blood cells by carrying these products to different parts of the body. When free of corpuscles, plasma is thin and colorless or has faint yellow tinge. Blood serum is a product of blood plasma. It differs from plasma in that serum does not contain fibrinogen. This signifying as follows:

Plasma - fibrinogen = (6) ....

When blood sample placed in a test tube and permitted to clot, the resulting clear fluid that remains after the removal of the clot from the test tube is serum. The formation of the clot has removed fibrinogen from the plasma.

Blood Groups

Human blood is divided into (7)..................... based on the presence or absence of blood antigens on the surface of the red blood cells. These four groups are A, B, AB and O. Type A blood has A antigen; type B blood B antigen; type AB blood has both A and B antigens; and type O has neither A nor B antigens. In each of these four blood groups, the plasma does not contain the antibody against the antigen that is present on the red cells. Rather, the plasma contains opposite antibodies. For example, A blood contains A antigen on the surface of the red cells; therefore, its plasma contains B antibodies. B blood contains B antigen on the surface of the red blood cells; therefore, its plasma contains A antibodies.

Lymphatic System

The lymphatic system consists of lymph, a network of transporting structure called lymph vessels, lymph nodes and the spleen, thymus, and tonsils. The primary function of the lymphatic system is to drain fluid from tissue spaces and return it to the blood. Other functions provided by the lymphatic system include transporting materials (nutrients, hormones and oxygen) to the body cells and carrying waste products from body tissues back to the bloodstream. It also conveys lipids or fats, away from the digestive organs. Finally, it helps in the control of infection by providing (8)....................., which are used to defend against infections caused by microorganisms.

Lymph originates from blood plasma. As whole blood circulates through the capillaries, some of the plasma seeps out of these thin-walled vessels. This fluid, now called interstitial or tissue, fluid, resembles plasma, except it contains less protein. Interstitial fluid nourishes and cleanses the body tissue through which it circulates. It also collects cellular debris, bacteria and particulate matter. Eventually, interstitial fluid enters into blind-ended vessels called lymph capillaries. Once it enters a capillary is called lymph. Lymph passes from the capillaries to large vessels and finally to lymph nodes, which serve as depositories for cellular debris. As lymph passes through the nodes it is filtered and replenished with lymphocytes, globulins and antibodies. Bacteria and debris are phagocytized by macrophages that line the nodes. At times, the number of bacteria entering a node is so great that the node enlarges and becomes tender.

Lymph vessels from the right chest and arm join the right lymphatic duct. The duct drains into the right subclavian vein, a major vessel in the cardiovascular system. Lymph from all other parts of the body enters the thoracic duct, which drains into the left subclavian vein. In this fashion, lymph is redeposited into the circulating blood in order to begin the cycle, once again, throughout the body. Three organs are associated with lymphatic system—spleen, thymus gland and tonsils. Similar to the lymph nodes, the spleen acts as a filter for lymph. Phagocytic cells within the lining of the spleen remove cellular debris, bacterial, parasites, and other infectious agents, thereby cleansing the lymph. The spleen also functions in the destruction of old (9)..................... and serves as a repository for healthy blood cells, to be put into circulation when needed. The thymus gland is located in the mediastinum, the upper part of the chest. It partially controls the immune system. The thymus changes lymphocytes to T-cells, which provide cellular immunity. Three sets of tonsils, palatine, pharyngeal and lingual tonsils, contain T- and B-lymphocytes. They guard against infection at the entrance of the digestive and respiratory tracts.
add after this

Answers

1. Red blood cells (erythrocytes), white blood cells (leukocytes) and platelets (thrombocytes)
2. Red bone marrow (myeloid tissue)
3. Granulocytes (those with granules in the cytoplasm) and agranulocytes (those without granules)
4. B cells or B lymphocytes
5. Blood clotting
6. Serum
7. Four groups
8. Lymphocytes and monocytes
9. Red blood cells

Review Questions

Exercise 1: Answer in One Word

1. Blood and lymph are specialized ____________.
2. Blood and lymph tissues defend the blood against ____________.
3. The maturation of the different blood cells is called ____________.
4. The immature blood cell forms are found in the bone marrow; ____________.
5. The mature blood cell forms circulate in the ____________.
6. Whole blood = Liquid portion + ____________.
7. Plasma accounts about 55% and blood cells account about ____________.
8. Most of the circulating blood cells are ____________.
9. Erythrocytes are formed in the ____________.
10. Red blood cell development is called ____________.
11. The size of the red cell and its nucleus decreases during ____________.
12. DNA resembles a fine, lacy net, giving this cell its name as ____________.
13. Erythrocytes live about 120 days and then rupture, releasing ____________.
14. Hemosiderin, a compound that contains iron, and several bile ____________.
15. The bile pigments are eventually excreted by the ____________.
16. Protects against invasion by bacteria and other foreign substances ____________.
17. Leukocytes are classified into the granulocytes and ____________.
18. Granulocytes are further classified as neutrophils, eosinophils, and ____________.
19. Agranulocytes are further classified as monocytes and ____________.
20. The neutrophil is the most numerous of the circulating ____________.
21. Monocytes migrate into tissue to become ____________.
22. Monocytes can phagocytes as many as 40 or 50 bacteria or other ____________.
23. The harmful invader is called the ____________.
24. The defense provided to antigen by the body is called the ____________.
25. The humoral immune includes the production of a substance called ____________.
26. This immunity is a function of T-lymphocytes, also called ____________.
27. T-cells mature in the ____________.
28. The smallest formed elements within the blood are platelets or ____________.

29. Thrombocytes chief function is to initiate blood clotting when __________.
30. Thromboplastin is released by traumatized tissue at the site of __________.
31. Thromboplastin are formed when platelets __________.
32. Prothrombin, a blood protein, converts to __________.
33. Fibrin forms a meshwork in which blood cells become __________.
34. Plasma is the liquid of the blood in which the corpuscles are __________.
35. Plasma is composed of about 92% __________.
36. Blood serum is the product of blood __________.
37. Plasma minus fibrinogen __________.
38. The names of four blood groups __________.
39. Type A blood has __________.
40. Type AB blood, both and __________.
41. Type O has neither __________.
42. __________ system conveys lipids/fats, away from the digestive organs.
43. Lymphocytes and monocytes, used to defend against __________.
44. Lymph originates from __________.
45. __________ fluid nourishes and cleanses the body tissues.
46. Eventually, interstitial fluid enters into blind-ended vessels called __________.
47. Interstitial fluids once it enters a capillary it is called __________.
48. Bacteria and debris are phagocytized by macrophages that line the __________.
49. Like the lymph nodes, the spleen acts as a filter for __________.
50. The thymus changes lymphocytes to T-cells, which provide cellular __________.

Exercise 2: Complete the Following

1. The three major types of blood vessels are __________, __________ and __________.
2. Arteries carry __________ blood from the heart throughout the body and __________ transport it back to the heart.
3. Erythrocytes contain an iron-containing pigment called __________.
4. Lack of iron in erythrocytes results in __________.
5. Leukocytes are divided into two groups, __________ and __________.

6. The lymphatic system plays roles in the ________________ and ________________ systems.
7. Five areas where lymph glands are located are ________________, ________________, ________________, ________________ and ________________.
8. The largest structure of lymphoid system is the ________________.
9. There are ________________ pairs of tonsils.
10. The important functions played by the tonsils in the immune system is ________________.

Exercise 3: Match the Following

1. Spleen	A. Hardening of walls of a vessel
2. Complement	B. Decrease of leukocytes
3. Thymus	C. T-cells
4. Lymphatic vessels	D. Decrease of granulocytes
5. Lymph nodes	E. Palate
6. Leukocytopenia	F. Decrease of erythrocytes
7. Pyrogens	G. Hypersensitivity
8. Tonsils	H. Production of granulocytes
9. Cisterna chyli	I. Storage sac
10. Granulocytopenia	J. Gland-like
11. Null cells	K. Fire-like chemicals
12. Erythropenia	L. Filters
13. Allergy	M. Protein group
14. Angiosclerosis	N. Natural killer
15. Granulocytopoiesis	O. Beaded appearance

Answers

Exercise 1

1. Tissues of the body
2. Infection
3. Hematopoiesis
4. Bone marrow
5. Peripheral blood
6. Solid portion
7. 45%
8. Erythrocytes
9. Red bone marrow
10. Erythropoiesis
11. Erythropoiesis
12. Reticulocyte
13. Hemoglobin
14. Pigments
15. Liver
16. Leukocytes
17. Agranulocytes
18. Basophils

19. Lymphocytes
20. White blood cells
21. Macrophages
22. Invaders
23. Antigen
24. Antibody
25. Antibody
26. T-cells
27. Thymus gland
28. Thrombocytes
29. Injury occurs
30. Injury
31. Rupture
32. Thrombin
33. Enlarged
34. Suspended
35. Water
36. Plasma
37. Serum
38. A, B, AB, and O
39. A antigen
40. A and B antigens
41. A nor B antigens
42. Lymphatic
43. Infection
44. Blood plasma
45. Interstitial fluid
46. Lymph capillaries
47. Lymph
48. Nodes
49. Lymph
50. Immunity

Exercise 2

1. Arteries, capillaries, veins
2. Oxygenated, veins
3. Hemoglobin
4. Anemia
5. Granulocytes and agranulocytes
6. Cardiovascular, immune
7. Lower jaw, neck, axilla, groin, knee (or any other known areas)
8. Spleen
9. Three
10. Filters out bacteria and foreign matter

Exercise 3

1. J
2. M
3. C
4. O
5. L
6. B.
7. K
8. E
9. I
10. D
11 N
12. F
13. G
14. A
15. H

5

CHAPTER

Nervous System

On completion of this chapter, the student will be able to:

- Explain the divisions of the nervous system
- List the organs of the central nervous system and their functions
- List and identify the major structures and functions of the brain, and spinal cord
- Elucidate the peripheral nervous system and their divisions
- Name the 12 pairs of cranial nerves and their functions

INTRODUCTION

The nervous system is one of the most complex of all human body systems. This system communicates between the various parts of the body. More than 10 billion nerve cells are operating all over the body. Some of the important and day-to-day activities such as speaking, moving, hearing, tasting, seeing, thinking, emotions, secreting hormones, responding to dangerous situations such as pain, heat, cold, touch, etc. are composed of small number of many activities, which are controlled by the nervous system.

Microscopic nerve cells collected into bundles are called nerves, which carry electrical message all over the body. External stimuli, as well as internal chemicals such as acetylcholine activates the cell membranes of nerve cells so as to release stored electrical energy within the cells. This energy when released and passed through the length of the nerve cells are called nerve impulses. Thus, the external receptor such as sense organs (eye, ear, tongue, skin, nose) as well as internal receptors in muscles and blood vessels receive, and transmit these impulses to the complex network of the nerve cells in the brain and the spinal cord. Within the central part of the nervous system impulses are recognized, interpreted and finally relayed to other nerve cells, which extends to all parts of the body, such as muscles, glands and internal organs.

The nervous system is made up of innumerable number of nerve cells called neurons and it is the basic unit of the nervous system. A neuron is an individual nerve cell, a microscopic structure through which impulses are passed along the path of the nerve cell in a definite manner and direction. The nerve cells collectively form the gray matter of the brain, and the nerve fibers are grouped together to form the white matter.

A bundle of nerve fibers is a nerve, bound together by connective tissue and the interbranching of nerves is known as plexus. Nerves are classified into two types, namely sensory or afferent nerves and motor or efferent nerves (Fig. 5.1).

STRUCTURE OF NERVOUS SYSTEM

The nervous system may be divided into two main portions namely, the central nervous system (CNS) consisting of brain and spinal cord. The peripheral nervous system or autonomic nervous system consist of spinal nerves between the CNS, muscles and various organs.

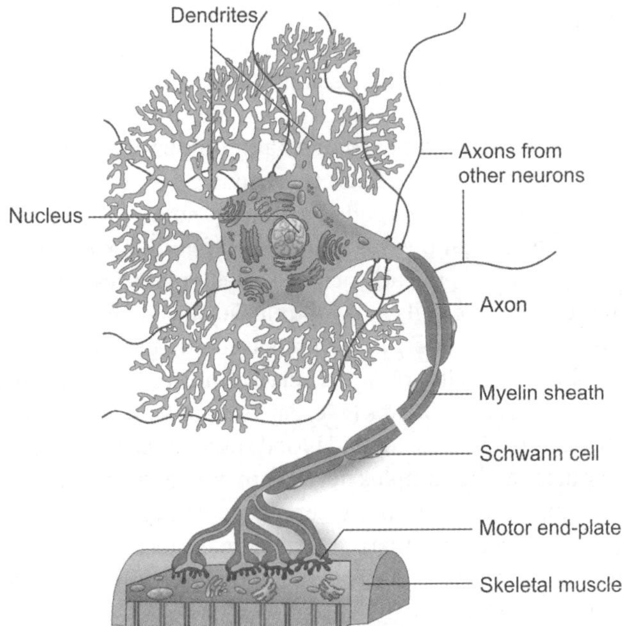

FIG. 5.1 A motor or efferent neuron

FLOWCHART 5.1 Structure of nervous system

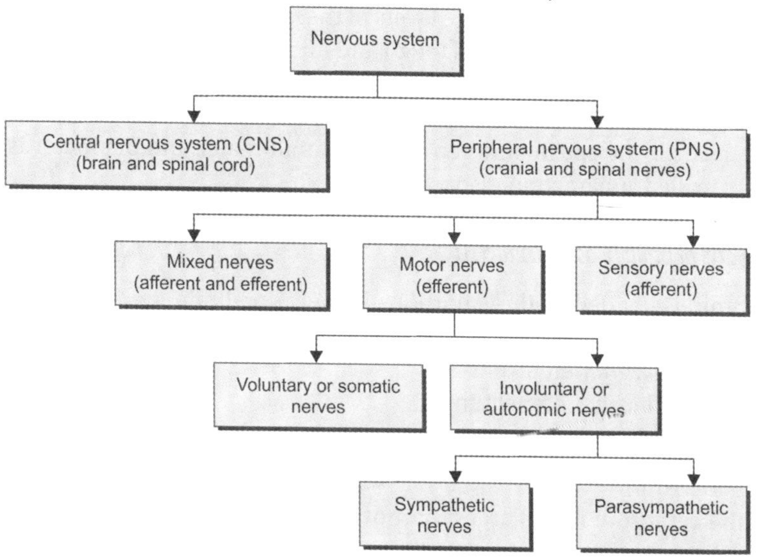

The peripheral nervous system is further divided into two nervous systems, such as somatic nerves (voluntary) and autonomic nerves (involuntary). The autonomic nerves are further branched into sympathetic and parasympathetic nerves (Flowchart 5.1).

CENTRAL NERVOUS SYSTEM

The CNS controls voluntary muscles and the nerves supplied to the limbs, etc. The main parts of the CNS are brain and spinal cord.

Brain

The brain is the major part of CNS. The brain is composed of billions of neurons and nerve endings. It looks like a giant wrinkled walnut crammed inside the skull. It integrates almost every physical and mental activity of the body. This organ is also the center for memory, emotion, thought, judgment, reasoning and consciousness.

The brain is covered by a three-layer membrane collectively called meninges, to protect the delicate nerve tissue, to secrete cerebro-spinal fluid, which protect the spinal cord from any concussion and to carry the blood vessels to the brain. Approximately, the weight of the brain is 1.3 kg. The three layers of the meninges are:

1. *Dura mater:* Dense and tough and lines the skull
2. *Arachnoid mater:* Fine middle layer
3. *Pia mater:* Inner layer covering the fissures of the brain and spinal cord. The space between the arachnoid mater and pia mater is called subarachnoid space.

Parts of Brain (Figs. 5.2 and 5.3)

Brain is divided as three portions namely, forebrain, midbrain and hind brain.

1. *Forebrain:* Cerebrum
2. *Hindbrain:* Cerebellum
3. *Midbrain/Brainstem:* Pons varolii and medulla oblongata.

Cerebrum

The cerebrum is the largest part of the brain, which is divided into right and left cerebral hemispheres connected by corpus callosum. Each lobe is covered by outer covering of gray matter known as the cortex and an inner part made up of white matter. Each cerebral hemisphere has frontal, parietal, temporal and occipital lobes. It is arranged in folds to form elevated portion known as convolutions

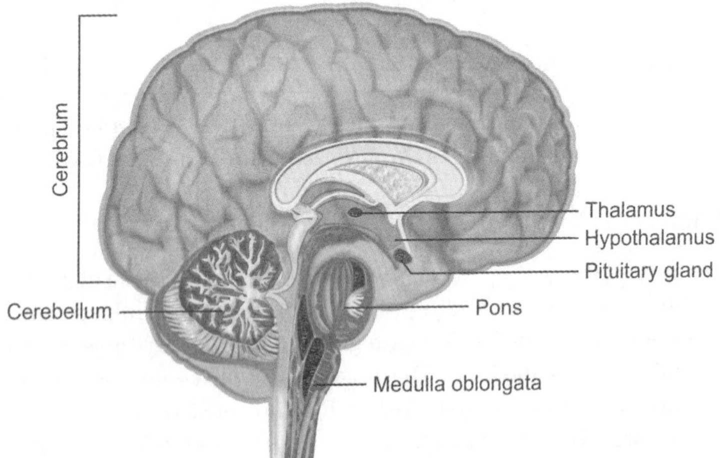

FIG. 5.2 Parts of brain

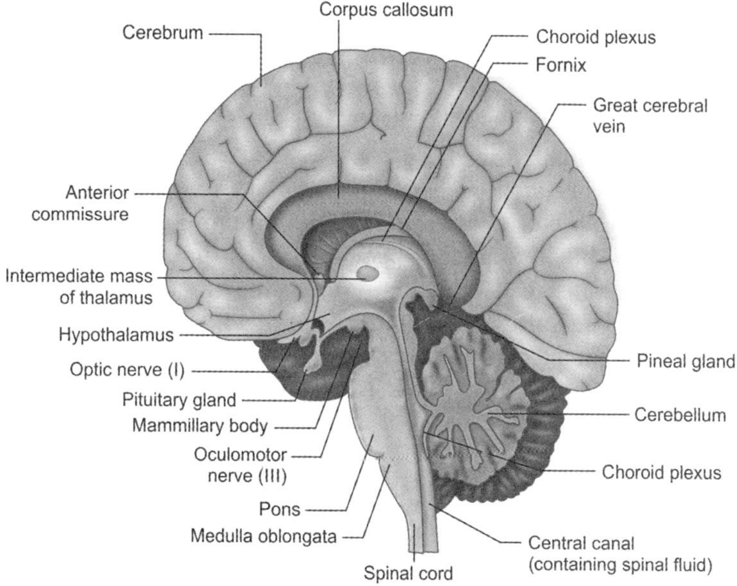

FIG. 5.3 Cross-section of brain

or gyri and depressions known as fissures or sulcus. These divide the cerebrum into lobes such as frontal, temporal parietal and occipital lobes. The cerebral cortex has important functional areas such as motor areas in frontal lobe, general sensory and gustatory areas in parietal lobe, olfactory and auditory areas in temporal lobe, and visual area in occipital lobe.

The main functions of cerebrum are memory, association, judgment, discrimination and thought. In addition to that sensory impulses and motor impulses are registered and controlled. The spaces or canals in the middle region of the cerebrum are called ventricles, which contain a watery fluid flowing throughout the brain and spinal cord called cerebrospinal fluid (CSF). The CSF can be withdrawn for diagnosis and relief of pressure from the brain. This is called spinal puncture or lumbar puncture.

Cerebrospinal Fluid

The CSF is a clear, slightly alkaline fluid, consisting of water, mineral salts, glucose, protein, creatinine and urea. Its specific gravity is 1.005. The main functions of the CSF are:

- To protect brain and spinal cord from any shock, and acts as a cushion
- To maintain uniform pressure around these delicate structures
- To keep the brain and spinal cord moist.

Cerebellum (Small Brain)

Cerebellum is located beneath the posterior part of the cerebrum. The internal structure and functional organization of the cerebellum is complex, but the general principle of its function are easily understood. The main function of the cerebellum is to maintain the balance, posture and co-ordination of voluntary movements and muscle tone. To perform this task it requires information and it receives this from the motor area of the cerebral cortex, and sensory receptors, namely vestibular and auditory receptors, visual receptors, proprio receptors (detecting sensation from within the body, e.g. as to the position of its parts, tactile touch), and visceral receptors.

The brainstem is composed of midbrain, pons varolii and medulla oblongata. The midbrain forms the upper part of the brainstem. The reflex areas of sight and hearing, and from its base, to continue below through the pons and medulla oblongata to the spinal cord.

Pons

The pons is the part of the brain, which literally means 'Bridge'. It lies between midbrain and medulla oblongata. Trigeminal, abducent, facial and vestibulocochlear nerves arise from it. It is part of the brain containing nerve fibers, which connect the cerebellum and cerebrum with the rest of the brain.

Medulla Oblongata

Medulla oblongata is located at the base of the brain, which connects the spinal cord and the brain. Nerve tracts crossover in medulla oblongata. Hence, the nerves that control the movement of left side of the body are found in the right of the cerebrum and vice versa. In addition, it contains vital centers, which control the rate and depth of breathing, rate of heartbeat, swallowing, and vomiting.

Thalamus and Hypothalamus

The thalamus is a large mass of gray matter, which is situated below the cerebrum. Thalamus is predominantly a sensory relay station, with incoming fibers from the spinal cord and brainstem, and onwards to the cerebral cortex. Lesions of the thalamus may cause pain, often continuous and of a burning nature, in the opposite side of the body.

The hypothalamus is composed of a number of nuclei and is the areas below the thalamus, at the base of the brain. The hypothalamus has neural connections to the posterior lobe of the pituitary gland (hypophysis) and vascular connections (known as portal hypophyseal vessels) to the anterior lobe of that gland.

Functions of Hypothalamus

The functions of hypothalamus are:

- Synthesis of vasopressin
- Control of anterior pituitary secretion
- Control of appetite
- Control of thirst
- Regulation of body temperature
- Emotional feeling and expression
- Sexual behavior
- Control of cardiac rhythms.

Spinal Cord

Spinal cord is a major part of the CNS, which lies in the vertebral canal. It extends from the medulla oblongata to second lumbar vertebra within the vertebral column. It ends as the cauda equina (horse tail), a fan of nerve fibers found below the second lumbar vertebra of the spinal column. The spinal cord is 45 cm long and 2 cm thick. It has two wider parts, namely the cervical and lumbar enlargement from where the nerves of limbs originate. These nerves are called spinal nerves.

Bones protect both the brain and the spinal cord against injury. The brain is enclosed within the skull and the spinal cord is enclosed within the vertebral column. In addition, both the brain and the spinal cord receive limited protection from a set of three coverings called meninges.

The outermost coat, the dura mater is tough and fibrous. Immediately beneath the dura mater is the cavity called subdural space. The next layer of meninges is the arachnoid mater. The space beneath the arachnoid mater is called subarachnoid space, which is filled with cerebrospinal fluid, which provides additional protection for the brain and spinal cord by acting as shock absorbers. The inner most layer, the pia mater contains numerous blood vessels and lymphatics, which provides nourishment for the underlying tissues.

Functions of Spinal Cord

The functions of spinal cord are to relay impulses:

- In and out at the same level
- Up and down to other levels of the cord
- To and from the brain.

PERIPHERAL NERVOUS SYSTEM (FIG. 5.4 AND TABLE 5.1)

The peripheral nervous system (PNS) consists of cranial and spinal nerves. The PNS includes 12 pairs of cranial nerves, emerging from the base of the skull, and 31 pairs of spinal nerves, emerging from the spinal cord. All of these nerves consist of fibers that may be either sensory or motor or a mixture of both. Sensory or afferent nerves, carry impulses from the tissues to the brain for interpretation and

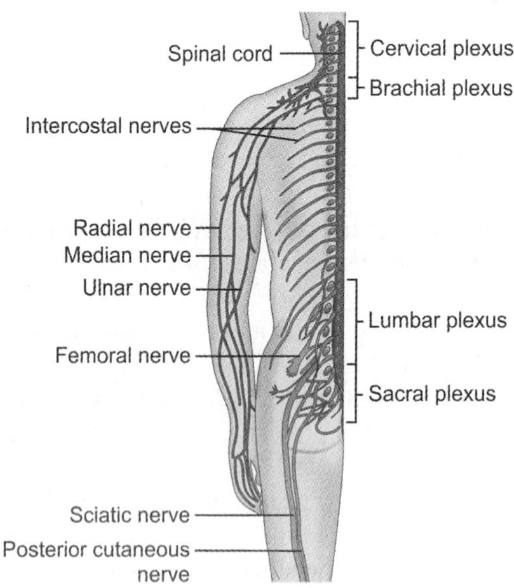

FIG. 5.4 Peripheral parts of nervous system

TABLE 5.1 Names of cranial nerves and their functions

Position of cranial nerve	Name of the cranial nerve	Functions
I	Olfactory	Sensory nerves of smell from the nose
II	Optic	Sensory nerves of sight from the eye
III	Oculomotor	Motor nerves to the various muscles of eye
IV	Trochlear	Motor nerves to the various muscles of the eyeball
V	Trigeminal	Has three branches—sensory nerves from the skin of the head and face, membrane of the mouth and nose, and teeth and motor supplying the muscles of mastication (chewing)
VI	Abducent	Motor to one muscle of the eyeball
VII	Facial	• Sensory nerves of taste from the front part of the tongue • Motor nerves to the muscles of expression and the scalp
VIII	Auditory/Acoustic/ Vestibulocochlear	Sensory nerve of hearing and balance
IX	Glossopharyngeal	Sensory nerve of taste from back part of tongue
X	Vagus	Sensory from many of the internal organs of the thorax and abdomen and blood vessels
XI	Spinal accessory	Motor joining the vagus to supply the larynx and pharynx, and motor to the muscles of the neck
XII	Hypoglossal	Motor to the muscles of the tongue

give rise to sensations such as cold, heat, pain, etc. Motor or efferent nerves carry impulses away from the brain and spinal cord, to the tissues. Nerves composed of both sensory and motor fibers are called mixed nerves. An example of this is facial nerve, as it transmits the taste through the tongue and it supplies facial muscles impulses for smiling or masticating, etc.

Spinal Nerves

There are 31 pairs of spinal nerves namely, eight cranial, 12 thoracic, five lumbar, five sacral, one coccygeal. Each spinal nerve is attached to the spinal cord by an anterior and a posterior root and divides into an anterior and a posterior ramus. The anterior root consists of motor fibers. The posterior root consists of a sensory fiber and has a posterior root (spinal) ganglion. The anterior ramus supplies the skin and muscles of the front, and sides of the trunk and the limbs. The posterior ramus supplies the skin and muscles of the back of the trunk. Each spinal nerve consists of sensory and motor fiber. A nerve fiber branches and terminates in nerve endings, e.g. of sensory nerve endings, free nerve endings for pain, Meissner's corpuscles for touch, Pacinian corpuscles for pressure, Krause end organs for cold, Ruffini end organs for warmth, and muscle spindles for proprioception (sensitivity), e.g. for motor nerve endings, motor end plates on a muscle fiber. The PNS is divided into two specialized nerves such as somatic nerves and autonomic nerves.

Somatic Nerves

The somatic nerves are under the direct control of the individual. It innervates the extremities and the body wall, including skeletal muscles and the skin. It is under the conscious control and therefore it is voluntary, e.g. voluntary activity include walking, talking, etc.

Autonomic Nerves (Fig. 5.5)

The autonomic nerves comprise the sympathetic and parasympathetic nerves, producing actions that balance one another. The sympathetic and parasympathetic nerves function quite opposite to each other. The sympathetic nerves produce vasoconstriction, increase heart rate, elevate blood pressure and depress gastrointestinal activity. While parasympathetic nerves decrease blood pressure, dilate the pupil, slower heart rate, etc. The autonomic functions are evident in fight or flight situations. In either way the blood flow increases in skeletal muscles to prepare the individual to either fight or run away from a threatening situation.

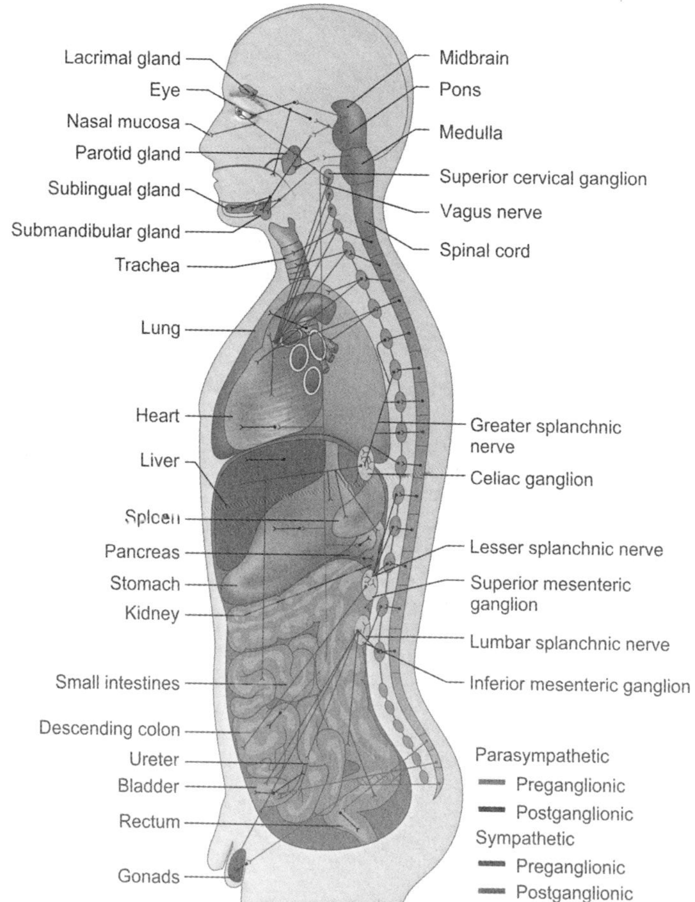

FIG. 5.5 Autonomic nervous system—comprising names of different parts of nerves of the body

Cranial Nerves

There are 12 pairs of cranial nerves connecting with the brainstem at different levels; some of them are motor nerves, some sensory and some mixed nerves (*refer* Table 5.1 and Fig. 5.6).

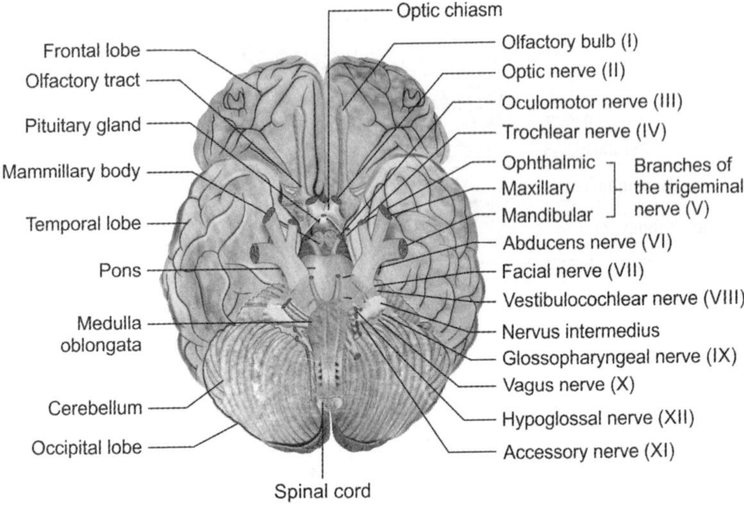

FIG. 5.6 Cross-section of brain with cranial nerves

Chapter Summary

The nervous system is most vital, but at the same time the most complicated system of the body. Along with the endocrine system, it controls many bodily activities. The nervous system senses changes in both internal and external environments, interprets these changes and then coordinates appropriate responses that are designed to maintain homeostasis, which is a state of equilibrium in the internal environment.

Divisions of Nervous System

The nervous system has two major divisions—(1)...................., which includes all other nervous tissue of the body found outside of the central nervous system (CNS).

The peripheral nervous system (PNS) includes 12 pairs of cranial nerves which emerge from the base of the skull and 31 pairs of spinal nerves which emerge from the spinal cord. All of these nerves consist of fibers that may be either sensory or motor, or a mixture of both sensory and motor fibers.

Sensory Nerves

Receive impulses from the (2).................. such as the eyes, ears, nose, tongue, skin and then transmit the impulses to the CNS. Because they conduct impulses toward a specific site—the central nervous system-they are also known afferent nerves.

Motor Nerves

Conduct impulses away from the CNS; thus, they are known as efferent nerves. These impulses travel to muscles and other body organs, causing them to respond in some manner. Nerves composed of both sensory and motor fibers are called mixed nerves. An example of a mixed nerve is the facial nerve. When it supplies the facial muscles with impulses for smiling or frowning, the facial nerve is functioning as a motor nerve. But when the tongue transmits a taste impulse to the brain through this nerve, it is responding in sensory capacity.

Functionally, the PNS is divided into two specialized systems—the somatic nervous system (SNS) and the autonomic nervous system (ANS). The somatic component is under the direct control of the individual. It innervates (supplies with nerves) the extremities and the body wall, including skeletal muscles and skin. Since the SNS produces movement only in the skeletal muscles, it is under conscious control of the organism and is therefore voluntary. Examples of voluntary activity include walking, talking and playing games. In contrast, the autonomic component conveys impulses to glands, smooth muscles and cardiac muscles. This division is therefore considered involuntary since it operates without conscious control. Examples of autonomic activity include digestion, heart contraction, and vasoconstriction.

The ANS is further specialized into two subdivisions: (3) ....

To a large extent, these subdivisions function in opposing the action of each other, although in certain instances, they may exhibit independent action. In general, sympathetic nerve fibers produce vasoconstriction, increased heart rate, elevated blood pressure and depressed gastrointestinal activity, while the parasympathetic system generally conveys impulses to bring about vasodilation, a slower heart rate, a decrease in blood pressure, a return to normal gastrointestinal activity. These autonomic functions are evident in 'fight or flight' situations. Blood flow increases in skeletal muscles to prepare the individual to either fight or run away from a threatening situation. When the danger passes, more blood is directed to the internal organs.

Nervous Tissue

In spite of its complexity, the nervous system is composed of only two principal types of nerve cells, (4).................... Neurons, the functional cells of the nervous system are responsible for impulse conduction. All neural circuits are composed of neuron chains. In contrast to neurons, neuroglia does not transmit impulses. Neuroglia is specialized nervous tissue that functions as connective tissue supporting and binding neurons. During infection, neuroglia is capable of performing certain phagocytic activities.

Neurons

Neurons consist of three major structures:

1. Dendrites, which are branching cytoplasmic projections that receive impulses and transmit them to the cell body.
2. Cell body, which contains the cell nucleus.
3. Axon, which is a long single projection that transmits the impulse from the cell body.

Many axons in both the PNS and CNS are covered with a white lipoid sheath called myelin. This wrapping acts as an electrical insulator that reduces the possibility of an impulse stimulating adjacent nerves. In addition, myelin accelerates impulses through the axon. The presence of myelin on an axon in the brain and spinal cord gives a white appearance to these structures, and they make up what is called white matter of the CNS. Unmyelinated fibers, dendrites and nerve cell bodies make up the gray matter.

On peripheral nerves, a thin cellular membrane called neurolemma or neurolemmal sheath, wraps around the myelin sheath. The neurolemmal sheath permits a damaged axon to regenerate. Since neurolemma is not found in the CNS, several nerves in the CNS cannot regenerate thus, nerve function is permanently lost unless alternate pathways are established. Neurons are not continuous with one another. Instead, a small space, known as synapse, is found between the axon of one neuron and the dendrite or cell body of another. In order for the impulse to travel along a nerve path, it must be transmitted at the synapse. This transmission is facilitated by certain chemical substances called neurotransmitters.

Neuroglia

The term neuroglia literally means nerve glue. It was once believed that neuroglia served only supporting role for neurons. But it is now known that different shaped neuroglia cells perform many other functions. Astrocytes, as their name suggests, are star-shaped neuroglia and are believed to be involved in the transfer of substances from the blood to the brain. Oligodendrocytes are cells with only a few processes. They are believed to help in the development of myelin on neurons of the CNS. Microglia, the smallest of the neuroglia, possesses phagocytic properties and may become very active during times of infection.

Brain

The brain is one of the largest organs of the body and the most complex in structure and function. It integrates almost every physical and mental activity of the body. The organ is also the center for memory, emotion, thought, judgment, reasoning and consciousness. The brain is composed of four major sections, i.e. (5)....................

The cerebrum is the largest and upper portion of the brain. It consists of two hemispheres divided by a deep longitudinal fissure or groove. The fissure does not completely separate the hemispheres. A structure called corpus callosum joins them medially on their inferior surfaces. Each hemisphere is further divided into five lobes. Four of these lobes are named for the bones that lie directly above them. The fifth lobe of the cerebrum is hidden from view and can only be seen upon dissection.

Numerous folds or convulsions, called gyri, are found on the cerebral surface. These are separated by furrows or fissures called sulci. A thin layer of gray matter, the cerebral cortex, which is composed of millions of cell bodies, covers the entire cerebrum and is responsible for its gray color. The residue of the cerebrum is composed primarily of white matter (myelinated axons). Major functions of the cerebrum include sensory perception and interpretation, muscular movement and the emotional aspects of behavior and memory.

The cerebrum is the largest part of the brain, occupies the back portion of the brain. It is attached to the brain stem. When the cerebrum initiates muscular movement, the cerebellum coordinates and refines the movement. The cerebellum also aids in maintaining equilibrium and balance of the body.

The diencephalon or interbrain is composed of many smaller structures, two of which are the thalamus and hypothalamus. All sensory stimuli except olfactory are received by the thalamus. Here they are processed and transmitted to the proper area of the cerebral cortex. In addition, impulses from the cerebrum are received by the thalamus and relayed to different nerves. Beneath the thalamus is a small structure called (6)....................

Its chief function is the integration of autonomic nerve impulses and the regulation of certain endocrine functions.

The brain stem completes the last major section of the brain. It is composed of three structures, i.e. medulla oblongata, pons and the midbrain (mesencephalon). In general, the brainstem serves as a pathway for impulse conduction between brain and spinal cord. The brainstem also serves as the origin of 10 of 12 pairs of cranial nerves. The brainstem is the center that controls respiration, blood pressure, and heart rate.

Spinal Cord

The spinal cord conveys to the brain sensory impulses from different parts of the body and also transmits motor impulses from the brain to all (7)....................

The sensory nerve tracts are also called ascending tracts, since the direction of the impulse is upward. Conversely, motor nerve tracts that relay motor impulses to muscles and organs are called descending tract, since they carry impulses in a downward direction. A cross-section of the spinal cord reveals an inner gray area composed of cell bodies and dendrites, with a white outer area composed of myelinated tissue of the ascending and descending tracts. The entire spinal cord is located within the spinal cavity of the vertebral column. About 31 pairs of spinal nerves exit from between the intervertebral spaces almost throughout the entire length of the spinal column. Unlike the cranial nerves, which have specific names, the spinal nerves are known by the region of the vertebral column from which they exit.

Meninges

Bones protect the brain and spinal cord against injury. The brain is enclosed within the skull and spinal cord is enclosed within the vertebral column. In addition, both brain and spinal cord receive limited protection from a set of three coverings called (8)..................... The outermost coats, the dura mater, is tough and fibrous. Immediately beneath the dura mater is a cavity called subdural space. It is filled with serous fluid. The next layer of the meninges is the arachnoid. As its name suggests, the arachnoid has a spider-web appearance. A subarachnoid space, which is filled with cerebrospinal fluid, provides additional protection for the brain and spinal cord by acting as a shock absorber. The innermost layer, the pia mater, contains numerous blood vessels and lymphatics, which provide nourishment for the underlying tissues.

Cerebrospinal fluid circulates around the spinal cord and the brain and through spaces called ventricles. These ventricles are located within the inner portion of the brain. This clear, colorless fluid contains proteins, glucose, urea, salts and some white blood cells. As it circulates, this fluid provides nutritive substances to the central nervous system. It also acts as a shock absorber for the delicate structures of the central nervous system. Normally, cerebrospinal fluid is absorbed as rapidly as it is formed. Any interference with absorption results in hydrocephalus.

Answers

1. Central nervous system (CNS), which is composed of the brain and spinal cord, and the peripheral nervous system (PNS)
2. Sense organs
3. Sympathetic and parasympathetic divisions
4. Neurons and neuroglia
5. Cerebrum, cerebellum, diencephalon (interbrain) and brain stem
6. Hypothalamus
7. Muscles and organs
8. Meninges

Review Questions

Exercise 1: Answer in One Word

1. The central nervous system (CNS), is composed of the brain and ________.
2. The PNS -12 pairs of cranial nerves emerge from the base of the ________.
3. 31 pairs of the spinal nerves, emerge from the ________.
4. Sensory nerves receive impulses from the ________.
5. The eyes, ears, nose, tongue, and skin, transmit the impulses to the ________.
6. Sensory nerves are also known as ________.
7. Motor nerves conduct impulses away from CNS, thus, they are known as ________.
8. Sensory and motor fibers are called ________.
9. PNS is divided into two specialized systems: the (SNS) and the ________.
10. The somatic component is under the direct control of the ________.
11. Involuntary operates without ________.
12. Which activity includes walking, talking, and playing any game?
13. The ANS is divided into two subdivisions: the sympathetic and ________.
14. Sympathetic nerve fibers produce ________.
15. What increases heart rate and elevated blood pressure?
16. The nervous system is composed of two types of nerve cells, neurons and ________.
17. Neurons are responsible for impulse ________.
18. Neuroglia can perform certain phagocytic activities during ________.
19. Cell body, which contains the cell is ________.
20. Axon, which transmits impulses from the ________.
21. Axons in the PNS & CNS are covered with a white, lipoid sheath called ________.
22. Unmyelinated fibers, dendrites and nerve cell bodies make up the ________.
23. A small space between neurons is known as a ________.
24. The term neuroglia means nerve ________.
25. Name the organ for memory, emotion, thought, judgment, reasoning.
26. The cerebrum, cerebellum, diencephalon and brain stem belong to ________.
27. The cerebrum is the largest and uppermost portion of the ________.

28. Numerous folds, or convolutions, called are ________.
29. Gyri is found in the________.
30. Gyri folds are separated by furrows or fissures called ________.
31. The second largest part of the brain is the ________.
32. The cerebellum occupies the back portion of the________.
33. What is attached to the brain stem?
34. What aids in maintaining equilibrium and balance of the body?
35. All sensory stimuli, except olfactory, are received by the ________.
36. Beneath the thalamus is a small structure called the ________.
37. The medulla oblongata, the pons, and the midbrain belong to ________.
38. The impulse conduction pathway between the brain and the spinal cord is ________.
39. The brain stem is the center that controls respiration, blood pressure, and ________.
40. The entire spinal cord is located within the spinal cavity of the ________.
41. ____ pairs of spinal nerves exit from between the intervertebral spaces.
42. What protects both the brain and the spinal cord against injury?
43. The brain is enclosed within the ________.
44. The spinal cord is enclosed within the ________.
45. Immediately beneath the dura mater is a cavity called the subdural ________.
46. Cerebrospinal fluid circulates around the spinal cord and ________.
47. Spinal cord and brain circulate through spaces called ________.
48. Ventricles are located within the inner place of the ________.
49. What provides nutritive to the central nervous system?
50. Any interference with the absorption of cerebrospinal fluid results in ________.

Exercise 2: Complete the Following

1. The nervous system is divided into the __________ and __________.
2. Thread-like dendrites and axons are also called __________.
3. The three meningeal membranes are the __________, __________ and __________.
4. The brainstem consists of the __________, __________ and __________.
5. The four lobes of the cerebrum are the __________, __________, __________ and __________.
6. __________ is found inside the spinal cord.
7. There are __________ pairs of spinal nerves along the spinal cord.

8. The peripheral nervous system includes the ______________ system, the __________________ nerves and the __________________ nerves.
9. There are __________________ pairs of cranial nerves.
10. The first cranial nerve, for the sense of smell, is the __________________ nerve.
11. The second cranial nerve, the ________________ is the nerve of vision.
12. ______________ is the eight cranial nerve, which maintains the balance and equilibrium.
13. The nerve, which controls the muscles of the tongue, and functions in speech and swallowing is ________________.
14. _________________ nerve is the longest of the cranial nerves, which has extensive distribution over the pharynx, larynx, trachea, esophagus, etc. and stimulates the secretion of hydrochloric acid for the process of digestion.
15. The autonomic nervous system has two divisions: __________________ and __________________.

Exercise 3: Match the Following

1. Long nerve cell processes that carry impulses from the cell body	A. Subarachnoid
2. Numerous short nerve cell processes that conduct nerve impulses toward the cell body	B. Vagus
3. Neurons concerned with muscle or gland action	C. Sulcus
4. Peripheral neurons that conduct afferent impulses from the sense organs to the spinal cord	D. Synapse
5. Region of connection between process of two adjacent neurons for transmission of impulses	E. Oculomotor
6. Peripheral nerve endings	F. Dendrites
7. Space between the pia mater and the arachnoid	G. Terminal twigs
8. Space between the dura mater and arachnoid	H. Axon
9. Centrally body of the cerebellum, shaped like a worm	I. Subdural
10. A furrow or groove, separating folds of the brain	J. Plexus

11.	Second cranial nerve, which innervates the retina of the eye	K.	Sensory neurons
12.	Third cranial nerve, which innervates the eye muscles and the sphincter of the pupil and ciliary processes	L.	Optic
13.	Interlacing network of spinal nerves	M.	Vermis
14.	Nerve that originates in the spinal cord and innervates the diaphragm	N.	Motor neurons
15.	A so-called wandering nerve, both motor and sensory, with an extensive distribution, with some gastric, pyloric, hepatic and celiac branches	O.	Phrenic

Answers

Exercise 1

1. Spinal cord
2. Skull
3. Spinal cord
4. Sense organs
5. CNS.
6. Afferent nerves
7. Efferent nerves
8. Mixed nerves
9. (ANS)
10. Individual
11. Conscious
12. Voluntary
13. Parasympathetic
14. Vasoconstriction
15. Vasoconstriction
16. Neuroglia.
17. Conduction
18. Infection
19. Nucleus
20. Cell body
21. Myelin
22. Gray matter
23. Synapse
24. Glue
25. Brain
26. Brain
27. Brain
28. Gyri
29. Cerebral surface
30. Sulci
31. Cerebellum
32. Brain
33. Cerebellum
34. Cerebellum
35. Thalamus
36. Hypothalamus
37. Brain stem
38. Brain stem
39. Heart rate
40. Vertebral column
41. Thirty-one
42. Bones
43. Skull
44. Vertebral column
45. Space
46. Brain
47. Ventricles
48. Brain
49. Cerebrospinal fluid
50. Hydrocephalus

Exercise 2

1. Central, peripheral
2. Nerve fibers
3. Dura mater, arachnoid, pia mater
4. Medulla oblongata, pons, midbrain
5. Frontal, temporal, parietal, occipital
6. Cerebrospinal fluid
7. 31
8. Autonomic, cranial, spinal
9. 12
10. Olfactory
11. Optic
12. Auditory
13. Hypoglossal
14. Vagus
15. Sympathetic, parasympathetic

Exercise 3

1. H
2. F
3. N
4. K
5. D
6. G
7. A
8. I
9. M
10. C
11. L
12. E
13. J
14. O
15. B

6

CHAPTER

Digestive System

On completion of this chapter, the student will be able to:

- Explain the main functions of the digestive system
- Identify and name the organs of digestive system
- Identify and name the accessory organs of the digestive system
- Explain the process of digestion
- Elucidate metabolism

INTRODUCTION

The digestive system is one of the important systems of the body, through which the energy is supplied externally as food, which is converted into the required chemicals for the nutrition of the cells, tissues, etc. The digestive system is also called alimentary or gastrointestinal system.

Food is one of the essential needs of the body and good health depends on proper nutrition. There are six essential nutrients with which the body must be constantly supplied. They are proteins, vitamins, carbohydrates, mineral salts, fats and water. When food is ingested, the digestive system plays a vital role in the conversion process of complex food substances such as proteins to simple amino acids, complex sugars to simple sugars (glucose) and large fat molecules are broken down to fatty acids and glycerol, which can be absorbed by the cells as nutrients. Finally, the unwanted materials are eliminated through the anus.

DEFINITION

Digestion can be defined as the complete process of changing the chemical and physical compositions of food in order to facilitate assimilation of the nourishing ingredients of food by cells of the body. The primary functions of the organs of the digestive system can be explained simply in three stages:

1. *Digestion:* Breaking down of the complex food materials mechanically or chemically into simpler amino acids, glucose, fatty acids and triglycerides, as it travels through the gastrointestinal (GI) tract (passageway).
2. *Absorption:* Absorption of the digested food into the bloodstream by entering into the walls of small intestine.
3. *Elimination:* The third and final function of the digestive system is to eliminate the solid waste materials, which are unable to be absorbed into the bloodstream. This process is called defecation.

ORGANS OF DIGESTIVE SYSTEM (FIGS. 6.1 AND 6.2)

The organs of the digestive system are:

- Oral or buccal cavity or mouth:
  - Lips
  - Cheeks
  - Palate
  - Uvula
  - Tongue

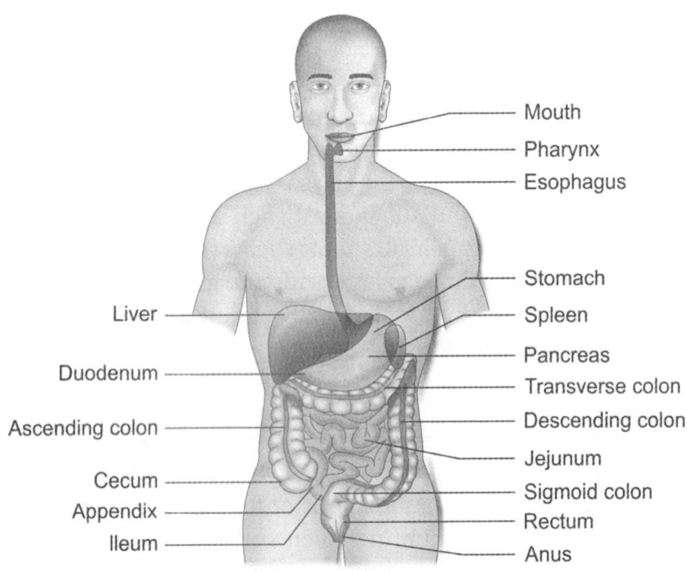

FIG. 6.1 Organs of the digestive system

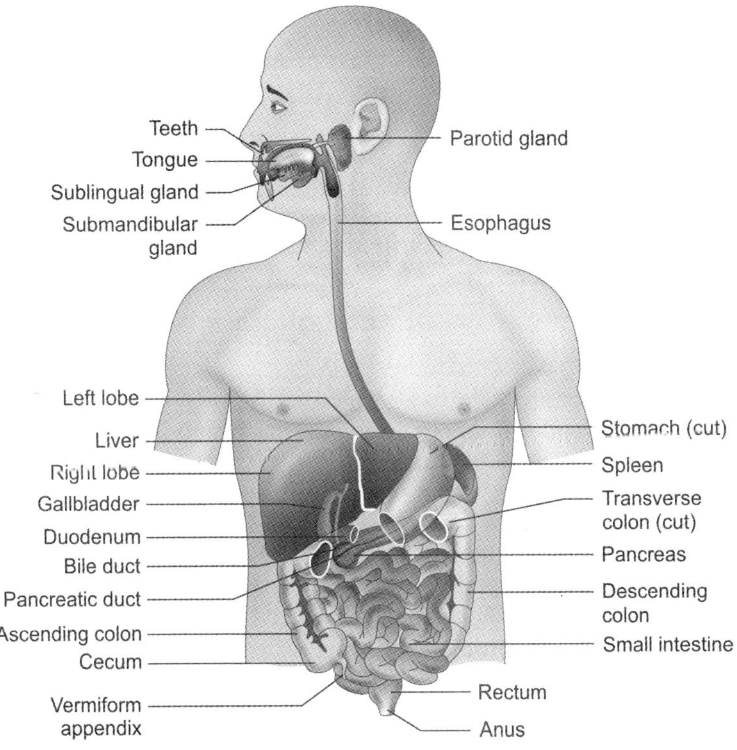

FIG. 6.2 Parts of the digestive system

  - Teeth
  - Gums
  - Tonsils
  - Epiglottis
  - Salivary glands.
- Pharynx
- Esophagus
- Gastrointestinal tract:
  - Stomach
  - Small intestine
  - Large intestine
  - Colon
  - Rectum
  - Anus.

Oral Cavity (Fig. 6.3)

The GI tract is a continuous tubular passageway that begins at the oral cavity or mouth.

Lips

Lips form an opening for the oral cavity. The lips are a highly muscular, vascular and motile organ, which also serves as the organ for speech.

Cheeks

Cheeks are the walls of the oval-shaped cavity. It acts as the temporary reservoir for food substances during the mastication process.

Palate

Palate forms the bottom and roof of the mouth (oral cavity). There are two palates, viz. hard palate forms the anterior portion of roof of oral cavity and the muscular soft palate lies in its posterior portion and it separates the mouth from the pharynx.

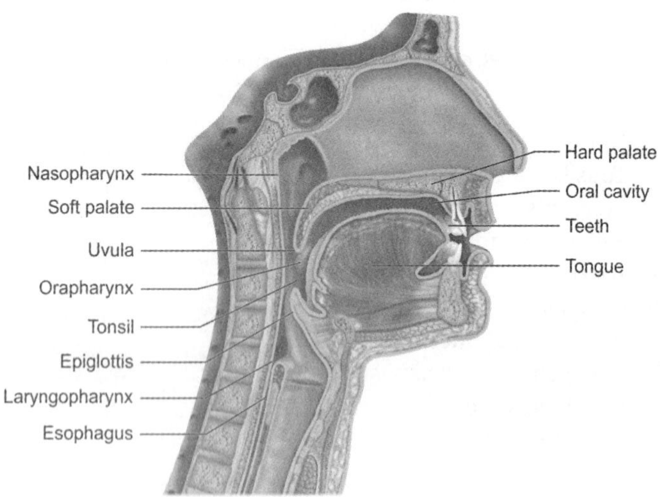

FIG. 6.3 Cross-section of the oral cavity

Uvula

A small V-shaped soft tissue hanging from the soft palate. The main function of the uvula is producing sounds and speech, while the other is to guide the downward movement of the food after chewing into the pharynx.

Tongue

Tongue extends across the floor of mouth. Tongue acts as a sense, speech and digestive organ. The main functions of the tongue are to move the food around during mastication (chewing), deglutition (swallowing), speech production and determination of taste. The surface of the tongue is covered by small projections called papillae, which contain cells, called taste buds, which are sensitive to the chemical reaction. These taste buds respond to the brain through the seventh cranial nerve (facial nerve) and ninth cranial nerve (glossopharyngeal nerve) to determine the taste and nature of the substance in contact.

Teeth (Fig. 6.4)

Teeth are situated in the front of the oral cavity. They play an important role in the initial stages of digestion. A tooth consists of a crown, which is above the gum and a root, which is embedded in the body tooth socket. The outmost protective layer of the crown is called enamel. It is a dense, hard white substance. The dentine is the root, covered by a protective and supportive layer called cementum. A periodontal membrane surrounds the cementum and holds the tooth in its place of the tooth socket. Below the dentine, the pulp is present, which contains blood vessels, nerve endings, connective tissue and lymph vessels.

For an adult, normally there will be 16 pairs (32 teeth) of teeth situated at the upper and lower jaw. The teeth located in the front of the oral cavity are called incisors, which cut and tear the food into smaller pieces. The teeth located in the rear of the oral cavity are called molars, they further crush and grind the food into finer particles. The following are the names of the teeth of one half of either lower or upper jaw. Thereby, four times of the eight teeth collectively form 32 permanent teeth in any adult:

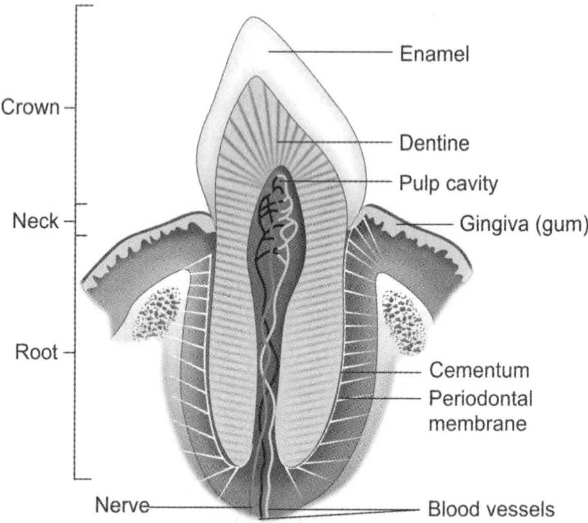

FIG. 6.4 Parts of tooth—crown, neck and root

1. Central incisor.
2. Lateral incisor.
3. Canine.
4. First bicuspid.
5. Second bicuspid.
6. First molar.
7. Second molar.
8. Third molar or wisdom tooth.

In general, there will be two incisors (1 and 2), one canine (3), two premolars (4 and 5), three molars (6–8).

Gums

The gums are made of pink fleshy tissue and are surrounded by the sockets in which the teeth are planted.

Tonsils

The tonsils are the organs made up of lymphatic tissue. They are situated in depressions of the mucous membranes in the wall of the pharynx. They act as filters to protect the body from the invasion of microorganisms and produce lymphocytes, which are white blood cells able to fight diseases.

Epiglottis

A small flap of tissue that covers the trachea. It acts as a gatekeeper to prevent the inflow of food through the trachea (windpipe) and allows all food to be channeled to stomach through the esophagus.

Salivary Glands (Fig. 6.5)

There are three pairs of salivary glands situated in the oral cavity. They are parotid gland in the posterior part of the oral cavity; submaxillary gland under the maxillary bone or beneath the jaw and sublingual gland below the tongue on either side in the mouth. Narrow ducts carry the saliva into the oral cavity. The salivary glands are exocrine glands producing saliva, which contain digestive enzymes. The saliva

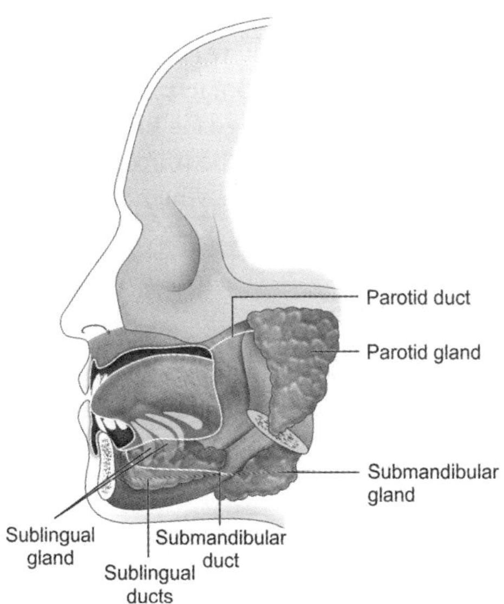

FIG. 6.5 Salivary glands comprising names of different ducts and glands

is released when the food is smelt or during the thought of the food. It contains 90% of water and the enzyme ptyalin, which begins the digestion of carbohydrates. It also contains a thick slippery lubricant called mucin and small amount of calcium salts.

Pharynx

The pharynx is a muscular membrane. It is the common passage for air and food. The walls of the pharynx are composed of muscles arranged in thin overlapping sheets, these form the constrictor muscles, which contract during the act of swallowing. The pharynx is divided into three major sections:

1. Nasopharynx—behind the nose and throat.
2. Oropharynx—behind the mouth.
3. Laryngopharynx—part of the throat above the larynx.

It is further divided into two tubes, one leads to lungs called trachea (windpipe) and other leads to stomach called esophagus.

Esophagus

The esophagus is a tube-like structure called food pipe, which extends from the laryngopharynx to the stomach. It is about 9–10 inches long. The main function of the esophagus is to move the food from the pharynx cavity to the stomach by the process called peristalsis. It is progressive, wave-like contractions, which propel the food through the system.

Gastrointestinal Tract (Fig. 6.6)

The stomach, small intestine and large intestine together form the GI tract.

Stomach

The stomach is an elastic sac-like structure located in the abdominal cavity, below the diaphragm, which separates the abdominal and thoracic cavity. It is a muscular organ and its shape and size vary according to the amount and type of its contents.

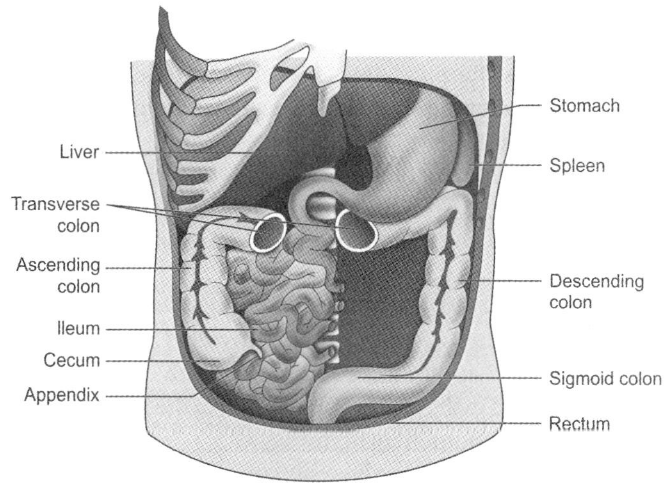

FIG. 6.6 Organs of the abdominal region with names of different parts

Parts of stomach

The stomach is divided into three parts:

1. Fundus (the upper part).
2. Body (the middle part).
3. Antrum (the end part).

The openings of the stomach are governed by the sphincters, the cardiac sphincter between the esophagus and fundus (the upper part of the stomach) preventing the backflow of the food into the esophagus and the pyloric sphincter between the antrum (the end part of stomach) and the small intestine. Within the stomach, there is considerable number of folds called rugae. These rugae appear when stomach is empty and when it is full, it disappears and the inner wall becomes smooth. The stomach is lined by mucous membrane, which secretes mucus that protects the stomach walls and food from the acid secretions. The interior wall of the stomach is composed of mucous membrane and contains the glands that secrete hydrochloric acid (HCl) and gastric juices.

Gastric juice is a clear and slightly acidic fluid, containing HCl, enzymes, minerals and salts. A total quantity of 1½–2 L is secreted every day. The three enzymes play an important role in digestion, by converting food into nourishing ingredients absorbed by the cells of the body.

Beginning the chemical digestion, pepsin reduces proteins to peptones and polypeptides; a further stage of protein digestion takes place in the small intestine.

Rennin converts the soluble milk proteins caseinogens to the insoluble form, casein, which is then reduced to peptones by pepsin.

Gastric lipase is an enzyme produced in small amounts, and it begins the digestion of fats.

The intrinsic factor (protein compound) is necessary for the absorption of vitamin B_{12}. Vitamin B_{12} is also called antianemic factor. It is present in food and is absorbed through the walls of the small intestine and stored in the liver until required in the red bone marrow for the normal development of erythrocytes.

Food entering into the cardiosphincter is mixed with the gastric secretions such as gastric juice, HCl and mucus by churning. Once the food is mixed with gastric juices and HCl, it forms semicreamy fluid called chyme. When it is sufficiently digested, the chyme leaves the stomach through the pyloric sphincter to enter into the small intestine.

Functions of stomach

- Physical digestion
- Changing solid food into semisolid
- Chemical digestion begins here.

Small Intestine

The small intestine is the continuation of the GI tract from the pyloric sphincter to the large intestine. It is about 20′long and has three parts:

1. *Duodenum:* Upper most division about 1 foot long.
2. *Jejunum:* The second part of the intestine which is about 8 feet long.
3. *Ileum:* The third part of the intestine, which is about 11 feet long.

Layers of small intestine

The small intestine has four layers:

1. An outer serous layer.
2. Muscular middle layer.

3. Submucous layer.
4. Innermost mucous membrane layer.

The functions of the small intestine are completion of digestion of food and to absorb the essential nutrients (end products) of digestion.

The secretion of the acid chyme in the duodenum distends the intestinal wall and causes the mucosa to secrete mucus and intestinal juice, which contain the enzyme enterokinase. At the same time the hormones such as secretin and cholecystokinin are secreted and stimulate the pancreas to secrete the fluid containing sodium bicarbonate that reacts with the acid in the chyme and neutralize it. This process prevents the ulceration of duodenum.

Cholecystokinin causes the pancreas to secrete digestive enzymes, i.e. amylase for digesting carbohydrates, trypsinogen and chymotrypsionogen for digesting proteins, lipase for digesting fats. Cholecystokinin also stimulates the gallbladder to empty bile, (which is essential for the digestion of fats) into duodenum through thc bile duct and the ampula of vater.

In the walls of the entire small intestine, there are tiny projects called villi. Through the tiny capillaries in villi, the nutrients such as monosaccharides and amino acids are absorbed into the bloodstream, in addition to this, iron, vitamins and calcium, any fluids that are ingested, and almost all the secretion of the alimentary tract are also reabsorbed, which is approximately 8 L a day. Only about 800 mL is passed to the large intestine.

Functions of small intestine

- Complete physical and chemical digestion
- Secreting digestive juice, which contain enzymes
- Provides a large surface area for absorption of food
- Passes waste material to large intestine by peristalsis
- Protection by screening bacteria.

Large Intestine

The large intestine is a continuation of the gastrointestinal tract and is attached to ileum of the small intestine and ends at the sigmoid colon. The large intestine is divided into two major divisions cecum and colon. The large intestine has four layers, they are serous, muscular, submucous and mucous layers.

The cecum or the first part of the large intestine is about 5–7 cm (2–3 inches) long and it is connected to the ileum by ileocecal sphincter. The vermiform appendix suspends from the cecum. The appendix is the only organ which has no anatomy.

Colon is about 5 feet long and has three divisions

1. *Ascending colon*: Extending from the cecum to the lower border of the liver.
2. *Transverse colon*: Extending the ascending colon and passing horizontally to the left towards the spleen.
3. *Descending colon*: Extending from the transverse colon and being downwards and bending in the S-shape, at the distal end to form the sigmoid colon.

The major function of large intestine is to receive the waste products from the small intestine after the digestion and store them until these are released from the body. The water in the waste products is absorbed here and the solid feces (stools) are formed.

Functions of large intestine:

- Absorption of water from the fecal matter
- Secretion of mucus
- Passes the fecal by mass peristalsis into rectum
- Rectum expels the fecal known as defecation.

Rectum

The rectum extends from the sigmoid colon and it ends in the lower opening of the GI tract called anus. It serves as a storage area for the waste products.

Anus

The anus is the end part of the GI tract. It has internal and external sphincters or muscles, which are closed, except during the process of defecation.

ACCESSORY ORGANS OF DIGESTION (FIG. 6.7)

The important accessory organs of the digestive system are:

- Liver
- Pancreas
- Gallbladder.

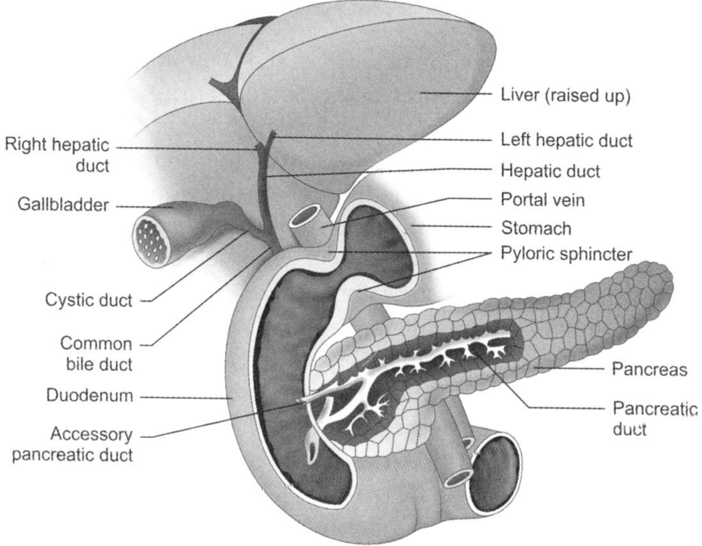

FIG. 6.7 Liver, gallbladder, pancreas, and duodenum with associated names of blood vessels and ducts

Liver

The liver is the largest gland in the body and weighs around 1–1.5 kg. It lies under the diaphragm on the right-hand side of the abdomen. It has a large right lobe and a small left lobe. The vital functions of the liver are:

- Produces bile, which is used in the small intestine to break and absorb fats
- Removes glucose (sugar) from blood, which it synthesizes and stores as glycogen
- Stores vitamins such as B12, A, D, E and K
- Removal of poisons from the blood
- Destroys old erythrocytes and releases bilirubin
- Produces various blood proteins, such as prothrombin and fibrinogen, which helps in the clotting of blood.

The liver substance consists of hepatic lobules, which are composed of hepatic cells arranged as sheets called hepatic laminae. Between the laminae are hepatic sinusoids. Blood enters the sinusoids from hepatic artery and portal vein and leaves by hepatic veins, which join the inferior vena cava.

Bile

Bile is the external secretion of the liver and is produced in a diluted form, which is then concentrated by gallbladder to a greenish viscous fluid. It is composed of water, salts, bile pigments and mucus. Bile salts play an important role in assisting the digestive action of pancreatic enzymes and in aiding the absorption of fat and fat-soluble vitamins from the small intestine. Bile pigments are derived from the breakdown of hemoglobin of worn-out red blood cells and give the bile its characteristic color. If there is an obstruction to the excretion of bile, it accumulates in the blood, giving the skin and mucous membrane a yellow color (jaundice). At the same time they appear in the urine, which turns into dark brown.

Bile is continuously released from the liver, travels down to the hepatic duct, cystic duct and gallbladder where it is stored and concentrated for later use.

Gallbladder

The gallbladder is a small pear-shaped organ situated below (underneath) the liver and acts as reservoir for the bile from the liver and to concentrate it. It is capable of storing 60 mL of bile. The hepatic duct connects the liver and gallbladder through which the bile is passed and stored in the gallbladder. It has three layers:

1. An outer serous peritoneal coat.
2. A middle muscular layer.
3. An inner lining of mucous membrane continuous to the lining of the bile ducts. This membrane secretes mucin and absorbs water and electrolytes thus concentrating the bile.

Gallbladder is connected to the duodenum by cystic duct with which the hepatic duct becomes the common bile duct. Whenever any fatty substance is identified in the duodenum, hormone cholecystokinin is released and when it reaches the gallbladder, the bladder contracts, to release bile through the cystic duct into the common bile duct, which joins the pancreatic duct before entering into the duodenum.

Pancreas

The pancreas is a leaf-like structure situated behind the stomach between the loop of duodenum and spleen. It acts as both endocrine and exocrine gland. In the digestive system, it provides digestive juices that pass through the pancreatic duct, thus it becomes an exocrine gland and also releases hormones directly into the bloodstream and functions as endocrine or ductless gland. The exocrine part secretes three enzymes:

1. Trypsin: Acts on protein
2. Amylase: Acts on maltose
3. Lipase: Acts on fat. The endocrine part of the pancreas is related to islets of Langerhans, whose β-cells secrete the hormone insulin and α-cells secrete the hormone glucagon, which regulate the blood sugar level.

Functions of Pancreas

Exocrine pancreatic juice contains three enzymes:

1. *Trypsin:* Acts on protein.
2. *Amylase:* Acts on maltose.
3. *Lipase:* Acts on fats.

Endocrine secretes insulin, necessary for metabolism of glucose and fat.

METABOLISM

Metabolism is the chemical reaction, which occurs in the whole body. It is divided into two major processes, i.e. anabolism and catabolism.

Anabolism is building or synthesis of new compound and this process is energy-consuming. Catabolism is the breaking down of large molecules to smaller units to release energy and heat. In healthy adults, there will be a balance between anabolism and catabolism, which is called energy balance. Both processes occur continuously and simultaneously in regulating chemical reactions in series.

Chapter Summary

The digestive system has mainly two purposes; one is to prepare the food that one eats for absorption by millions of body cells and to eliminate waste materials from the body.

When food is digested, it is in a form that cannot reach the cells because of its inability to pass through the intestinal mucosa into bloodstream. Hence, the consumed food must be altered physically and chemically as well. Therefore, digestion can be defined as the complete process of changing the chemical and physical composition of food in order to facilitate assimilation of the nourishing ingredients of food by the cells of the body.

The organs of the gastrointestinal (GI) system form a tube that begins at the mouth and terminates at the anus. This tube is referred to as the alimentary canal or the digestive tract.

Mouth (Oral Cavity, Buccal Cavity)

The GI tract is a continuous tubular passageway that begins at the (1)....................

The structures within the oral cavity are the cheeks (bucca) and the tongue and its muscles, which extend across the floor of the mouth. The main functions of the tongue are manipulation of food during the chewing process, deglutition (swallowing), speech production and determination of taste. The surface of the tongue has rough elevations, these elevations are taste buds. These sense organs are called papillae and are capable of perceiving a variety of flavors found in the foods, such as sweetness, bitterness, sourness and saltiness.

Teeth

The teeth are found in the oral cavity and play a vital role in the initial stages of digestion. The teeth are located in the front of the oral cavity, the incisors and cuspids, cut and tear the food into small pieces. The teeth that are in the rear of the oral cavity are called molars, which crush and grind the food into finer particles. Teeth are covered by hard (2).................... that gives them a white and smooth appearance. Beneath the enamel is the dentine is the main structure of the tooth. Dentin is surrounded by thin layer of modified bone called cementum. In the innermost of the tooth is the pulp, which stores the nerves and blood vessels of the tooth. The teeth are imbedded in pink fleshy tissue known (3)....................

Two other structures hard and soft palates are located within the mouth. The hard palate lies in the anterior portion of the roof of the oral cavity, while the soft palate lies in its posterior portion. The soft palate forms a partition between the mouth and the nasopharynx and is continuous with the hard palate. The entire oral cavity is lined with (4).................... as the rest of the digestive tract.

After the food is chewed, it is formed into a round, sticky mass called bolus. The bolus is pushed by tongue from the mouth into the pharynx (throat). Its downward movement is guided into the pharynx by the soft, fleshy V-shaped tissue called uvula. The uvula hangs from the superior roof of the oral cavity. The pharynx is a muscular tube, which is divided into three important sections:

1. **Nasopharynx:** It is the part of the throat behind the nose
2. **Oropharynx:** It is the part of the throat behind the mouth
3. **Laryngopharynx:** It is the part of the throat above the larynx. The laryngopharynx is further divided into two tubes—one that leads to the lungs, called trachea and one that leads to the stomach, called esophagus.

A small flap of tissue, the epiglottis, covers the trachea. The main function of the epiglottis is preventing food from entering the trachea, thus allowing all food to be channeled to the stomach through the esophagus.

Stomach

The stomach is a sac-like structure located in the (5)..................... cavity directly below the diaphragm. It is continuous with the esophagus. Thus, food continues its descent down the stomach. The stomach mixes the undigested food with gastric juices to further break it down for digestion. Within the stomach, there is a considerable number of folds called (6)....................

The rugae appear only when the stomach is empty. As the stomach fills, the interior walls become smooth. The interior lining of the stomach is composed of mucous membranes and contains the glands that secrete hydrochloride (HCl) and gastric juices. Once the food or bolus is mixed with gastric juices and HCl, it forms a semicreamy fluid called chyme.

There are two valves in the stomach. The first valve is called (7)..................... and is located at the top of the stomach. It connects the esophagus to the stomach. The second valve is called (8)..................... and is located at the base of the stomach. It connects the stomach to the small intestine. Both valves are composed of a round band of muscles called sphincters, which contract and expand to allow food to enter and leave the stomach.

Small Intestine

The small intestine is approximately 2.5 cm (1 inch) in diameter and is a continuation of the GI tract about 21 feet tube. The small intestine consists three parts:

1. The duodenum, the uppermost division, which is about 25.4 cm (10 inch) long.
2. The jejunum, which is approximately 8 feet long.
3. The ileum, which is about 12 feet long. Most of the absorption of food takes place in the ileum by tiny finger-like projections called villi. Inside the villi is a network of fine capillaries, veins and arteries. This network allows the absorption of food into the bloodstream.

There are also many other intestinal digestive glands located in the mucous membrane lining of the small intestine. These microscopic glands secrete additional digestive juices.

The (9) .... produce digestive secretions, and these secretions are added to the chyme at the beginning of the small intestine. With the exception of some forms of fat, water and waste products, all of the food ingested into the body is absorbed through the walls of the small intestine.

Colon

The colon is a continuous of the GI tract and it is attached to the ileum by the ileocecal valve. This valve is composed of sphincter muscles that serve to close the ileum at the point at which the small intestine connected to the colon. The large intestine has an average diameter of 6.35 cm (2½ inch) and is approximately 5 feet long. It is divided into two major divisions: (10)....................

The cecum is the first 5 or 7.6 cm (2 or 3 inch) of the large intestine. Attached to the cecum is a worm-like projection, the vermiform appendix, which performs no function in the digestive system. The colon consists of the following parts:

- The ascending colon, which extends from the cecum to the lower border of the liver (hepatic flexure)
- The transverse colon, which passes horizontally across the abdomen to the left toward the spleen (splenic fixture)
- The descending colon, which continues down to form the sigmoid colon

- The rectum, which serves as a storage area for the waste products of digestion, leads to the orifice called anus and it is kept closed by internal and external sphincters or muscles except during the process of defecation (elimination of feces).

Accessory Organs of Digestion

Liver

The liver is the largest glandular organ in the body and weighs approximately 3–4 pounds. It is located beneath the (11)....................

Diaphragm

Diaphragm is the right upper quadrant (RUQ) of the abdominal cavity. The liver performs so many vital functions that people cannot survive without it. Some important functions of the liver include the following:

- Produces bile, which is used in the small intestine to emulsify and absorb fats
- Removes glucose (sugar) from blood, which it synthesizes and stores as glycogen (starch)
- Stores vitamins, such as B_{12}, A, D, E and K
- Breaks down or transforms some toxic products into less harmful compounds
- Maintains normal levels of glucose in the blood
- Destroys old erythrocytes and releases bilirubin
- Produces various blood proteins, such as prothrombin and fibrogenic, which aid in the clotting of blood.

Pancreas

The pancreas is an elongated, somewhat flattened organ that lies posterior and slightly inferior to the stomach. The pancreas acts as both (12)....................

In the digestive system, it provides digestive juices that pass through the pancreatic duct, thereby giving it its exocrine function. These enzyme juices help in the digestive process. The pancreatic duct extends along the gland and enters the duodenum in the company of the bile duct from the liver. By secreting digestive juices through a duct, the pancreas functions as an exocrine gland in the GI system. But in the endocrine system, the pancreas releases hormones directly into the blood stream and functions as an endocrine or ductless gland. The endocrine function of the pancreas is related to the islets of (13)..................... whose β-cells secrete the hormone insulin and α-cells secrete the hormone glucagon, which regulate blood sugar levels.

Gallbladder

The gallbladder serves as a storage area for bile. During the process of digestion, when there is a need for some bile, the gallbladder releases it into the duodenum through the (14).....................

Bile is also drained from the liver through the hepatic ducts. The hepatic ducts connect with the cystic duct from the gallbladder, forming the common bile duct.

Answers

1. Oral cavity or mouth
2. Enamel
3. Gums or gingiva
4. Mucous membranes
5. Abdominal
6. Rugae
7. Cardiac valve or cardiac sphincter
8. Pyloric valve or pyloric sphincter
9. Pancreas and liver
10. Cecum and the colon
11. Cecum and the colon
12. An endocrine gland and an exocrine gland
13. Langerhans
14. Common bile duct

Review Questions

Exercise 1: Answer in One Word

1. The consumed food must be altered not only physically but also ___________.
2. Gastrointestinal (GI) system forms a tube that begins at the mouth and terminates at the ___________.
3. The gastrointestinal (GI) tube is referred to as the alimentary canal or ___________.
4. Gastrointestinal (GI) measures in adults approximately ___________.
5. The structures within the oral cavity are the cheeks, or bucca, and the ___________.
6. The surface of the tongue has rough elevations; these elevations are taste ___________.
7. Buds are sense organs called ___________.
8. The teeth are found in the ___________ cavity.
9. Teeth are covered by hard enamel, that gives a ___________ and ___________ appearance.
10. Dentin is surrounded by a thin layer of modified bone called ___________.
11. Pulp, which stores the nerves and blood vessels of the ___________.
12. The entire oral cavity, like the rest of the digestive tract, is lined with ___________.
13. After the food is chewed, it is formed into a round, sticky mass called a ___________.
14. The uvula hangs from the superior root of the ___________.
15. The pharynx is divided into 3 sections-nasopharynx, oropharynx and ___________.
16. A small flap of tissue, that covers the trachea is called ___________.
17. The main function of the epiglottis is to prevent food from entering the ___________.
18. Trachea, allowing all food to be channeled to the stomach through the ___________.
19. Within the stomach, there are a considerable number of folds, called ___________.
20. The rugae appear only when the stomach is ___________.
21. Food mixed with gastric juices and HCl forms a semicreamy fluid called ___________.
22. There are ___________ valves in the stomach.
23. The cardiac valve is also known as the cardiac ___________.

23. Pyloric valve, or pyloric sphincter connects the stomach to the __________.
24. How many parts the small intestine consists __________.
25. The small intestine consists of the duodenum, jejunum and __________.
26. The duodenum is 10 inches long, the jejunum is 8 feet long and the ileum is __________.
27. The pancreas and liver produce a secretion called __________ secretion.
28. Digestive secretions are added to the chyme at the beginning of the __________.
29. The ileocecal valve closes the ileum at the small intestine and is connected to the __________.
30. The large intestine has an average of approximately __________ feet long.
31. The cecum is the first 2–3 inches of the __________.
32. The colon consists of an ascending colon, a transverse colon and __________.
33. The ascending colon extends from the cecum to the lower border of the __________.
34. The descending colon, which continuous down to form the __________.
35. Which organ is the largest glandular organ in the body.
36. Which is used in the small intestines to emulsify and absorb fats?
37. What breaks down some toxic products into less harmful compounds?
38. What maintains normal levels of glucose in the blood?
39. What destroys old erythrocytes and releases bilirubin?
40. Liver produces prothrombin and fibrinogen, which aid in the clotting of __________.
41. The pancreas acts as both an endocrine gland and an __________.
42. Digestive juices that pass through the pancreas duct, giving its __________.
43. What enzymatic juices aid in the digestive process?
44. How the pancreatic duct enters the duodenum in the company of the bile?
45. Beta cells secrete the __________.
46. Alpha cells secrete the __________.
47. Beta cells and Alpha cells regulate blood __________.
48. What serves as a storage area for bile __________.
49. The gallbladder releases bile into the duodenum through the common __________.
50. Bile is drained from the liver through the __________.

Exercise 2: Complete the Following

1. The wave-like movement of the intestines is called ___________.
2. The ___________ serves a dual purpose in the respiratory and gastrointestinal systems.
3. The stomach is divided into ___________, ___________ and ___________.
4. The three divisions of the small intestine are the ___________, ___________ and ___________.
5. The colon is divided into ___________ sections.
6. The accessory organs of the digestive system are ___________, ___________ and ___________.
7. The ___________ both an exocrine and endocrine gland.
8. The largest gland in the body is ___________.
9. ___________ stores the bile.
10. The four types of the teeth are ___________, ___________, ___________ and ___________.
11. The thin lubricating, serous fluid secreted by the salivary glands is called ___________.
12. Two hormones secreted by the islets of Langerhans are ___________ and ___________.
13. The two main functions of the tongue in digestive system are ___________ and ___________.
14. Most of the water absorption of the body take place in the ___________.
15. The last segment of the large intestine is ___________.

Exercise 3: Match the Following

1. Rigid body structure in the roof of the mouth	A. Chyme
2. Musculomembranous tube from pharynx to stomach	B. Lesser curvature
3. Lower left margin of the surface of the stomach	C. Uvula
4. Upper right margin of the surface of stomach	D. Greater curvature
5. Very hard substance that covers the exposed part of the tooth	E. Sphincter
6. Semifluid material produced by gastric digestion of food	F. Hard palate
7. Any one of the four front teeth of either jaw	G. Molars

8. Broad teeth used in grinding food H. Enamel
9. Pendulum of the soft palate I. Esophagus
10. Ring-like muscles that contract to close an opening J. Incisor

Answers

Exercise 1

1. Chemically
2. Anus
3. Digestive tract
4. 30 feet
5. Tongue
6. Buds
7. Papillae
8. Oral
9. White and smooth
10. Cemented
11. Tooth
12. Mucous membrane
13. Bolus
14. Oral cavity
15. Laryngopharynx
16. Epiglottis
17. Trachea
18. Esophagus
19. Rugae
20. Empty
21. Chyme
22. Two
23. Small intestine
24. Three parts
25. Ileum
26. 12 feet long
27. Digestive
28. Small intestine
29. Colon
30. 5
31. Large intestine
32. Descending colon
33. Liver
34. Sigmoid colon
35. Liver
36. Bile
37. Liver
38. Liver
39. Liver
40. Blood
41. Exocrine gland
42. Exocrine function
43. Digestive juices
44. Bile duct
45. Hormone insulin
46. Hormone glucogen
47. Sugar levels
48. Gallbladder
49. Bile duct
50. Hepatic ducts

Exercise 2

1. Peristalsis
2. Pharynx
3. Fundus, body, pylorus
4. Duodenum, jejunum, ileum
5. Four
6. Liver, pancreas and gallbladder
7. Pancreas

8. Liver
9. Gallbladder
10. Incisors, canines, premolars, molars
11. Saliva
12. Insulin, glucagons
13. Keeps food between teeth during chewing, aids in swallowing
14. Large intestine
15. Rectum

Exercise 3

1. F
2. I
3. B
4. D
5. H
6. A
7. J
8. G
9. C
10. E

Endocrine System

On completion of this chapter, the student will be able to:

- Understand endocrine and exocrine systems and differences between them
- List the glands of the endocrine system
- Describe the functions of hormones released by each gland
- Identify and discuss about the diseases caused by the hyper- or hyposecretion of the endocrine hormones

INTRODUCTION

The endocrine system is composed of endocrine glands that release hormones, a chemical substance, which regulate the basic metabolic activities of the body, for example, the growth hormone regulates the growth of bones. Glands, which secrete their hormones directly into the bloodstream rather than into ducts leading to the exterior of the body are called endocrine glands, in short, they are ductless glands. The glands, which transport hormones through ducts are called exocrine glands, e.g. lacrimal glands, sweat glands and mammary glands.

HORMONES (FIG. 7.1)

A chemical substance produced by the cells and transported through bloodstream to the cells and organs on which it has to act. Hormones are secreted in minute, but effective quantities. In structure, they are either steroids or proteins. Most of the hormones are excreted by the pituitary gland, liver and kidneys.

DIFFERENT ENDOCRINE GLANDS PRESENT IN HUMAN BODY (FIG. 7.2)

Different endocrine glands present in the human body are as follows:

- Thyroid gland
- Parathyroid gland (4 glands)

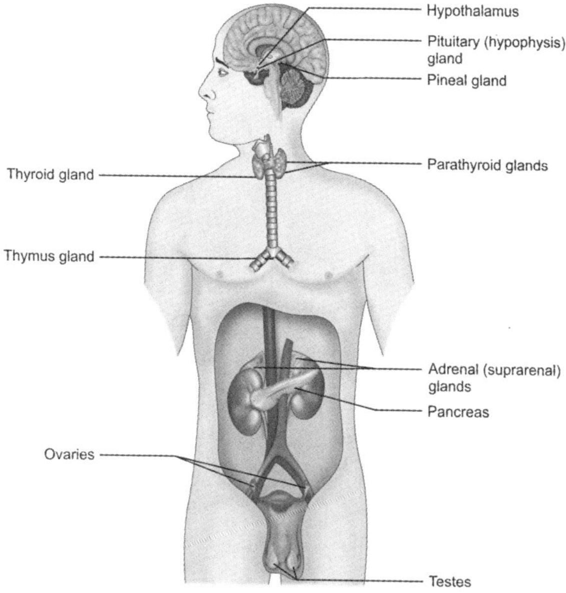

FIG. 7.1 Endocrine system with location of glands that produce hormones

- Adrenal gland (1 pair)
- Pancreas
- Pituitary gland
- Ovaries in female (1 pair)
- Testes in male (1 pair)
- Pineal gland
- Thymus gland.

Thyroid Gland

The thyroid gland is the largest gland of the endocrine system. It is an H-shaped organ located in the neck just below the larynx. This gland is composed of two fairly large lobes left and right lobes, that are separated by a tissue called isthmus. The major function of the thyroid gland is to produce, store and release two hormones—thyroxine (T_4) and triiodothyronine (T_3). Recent research indicate that a new hormone by name calcitonin is also secreted by thyroid gland.

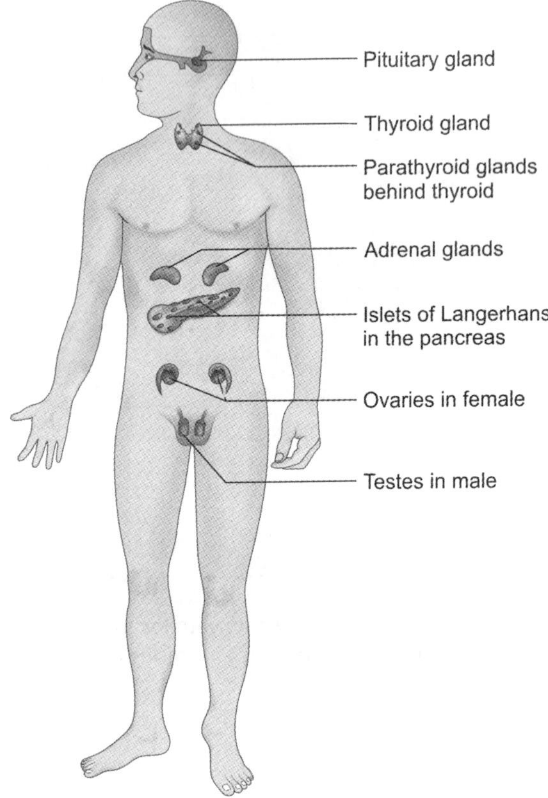

FIG. 7.2 Endocrine glands of human body with their names and location

Hormones Secreted by Thyroid Gland and their Functions

Thyroxine and Triiodothyronine

- Increase the oxygen consumption and metabolism of all cells
- Increase the rate of fat utilization
- Both work with the growth hormone to stimulate the nervous system.

Calcitonin

Regulates the calcium level in blood, when the calcium level is high, it inhibits the production of calcium by the bones.

Hyposecretion of Thyroid Hormone

The condition of hyposecretion of the thyroid is called hypothyroidism. In infants, the condition of hypothyroidism is called Cretinism. It may lead to mental retardation, impaired growth, low body temperatures and abnormal bone formation. When hypothyroidism is developed in adults it is known myxedema. The indication of this disease are edema, low level of T_3 and T_4, mental retardation, weight gain and sluggishness.

Hypersecretion of Thyroid Hormone

The condition of hypersecretion of the thyroid is called hyperthyroidism. The most common disorders of this condition are Graves' disease and toxic goiter.

Graves' disease is marked by elevated metabolic rate, abnormal weight loss, excess perspiration, muscular weakness and emotional instability. In severe conditions, the eye may protrude, because of edematous swelling in the tissue behind the eye called exophthalmos.

Toxic goiter: When the thyroid stimulating hormone (TSH) of the pituitary gland secretes more, the thyroid cells are likely to enlarge and secrete extra amounts of hormones.

Parathyroid Glands

The parathyroid glands are four small oval bodies, located on the posterior surface (behind) of the thyroid gland. It secretes only one hormone called parathyroid hormone (PTH). This hormone is also known parathormone. The functions of the PTH are:

- Regulates the calcium metabolism by influencing three types of organs—bones, intestine, and kidneys
- Mobilizes calcium from bones into the bloodstream, where the calcium is necessary for proper functioning of body tissues, especially muscles
- Enhances the absorption of calcium and phosphates from food in the intestine
- Causes kidneys to conserve blood calcium and to increase the excretion of phosphates in urine.

Hyposecretion of Parathyroid Hormone

The hyposecretion of the PTH hormone is called hypoparathyroidism. It can be caused by some injury or surgical removal of the parathyroid gland or accidentally during thyroid surgery. Hypoparathyroidism is characterized by—calcium being unable to enter into the bloodstream from bones, which leads to nerve and muscle weakness, spasm of muscles, which is called tetany.

Hypersecretion of Parathyroid Hormone

The hypersecretion of the PTH is called hyperparathyroidism. Usually, it is caused by the benign tumor of the parathyroid gland. Excessive secretion of the PTH hormone will cause:

- Calcium to leave the bones and to enter into the bloodstream, this condition is called hypercalcemia
- Demineralization of bones making them highly prone to fracture or deformity. This condition is called osteitis fibrosa
- Tendency to develop kidney stones due to hypercalcemia.

Adrenal Glands

The adrenal glands are two small glands situated on top of each kidney. It is also called suprarenal glands. Each gland consists of two parts, an outer portion called adrenal cortex and inner portion called adrenal medulla. These two parts of each adrenal gland secretes different endocrine hormones. The adrenal cortex secretes hormones called steroids and medulla secretes hormones called catecholamine. The adrenal cortex secretes three types of steroid hormones, they are:

1. ***Mineralocorticoids:*** The most important mineralocorticoid hormone is called aldosterone. This hormone regulates the kidneys to conserve sodium and to excrete potassium. It also promotes water conservation and reduces urine output.
2. ***Glucocorticoids:*** The most important glucocorticoids is cortisol. It helps to regulate the metabolism of sugars, fats and proteins within all body cells.
3. ***Gonadocorticoids:*** The most important gonadocorticoids are androgens, estrogens and progesterone. These are

male and female hormones, which maintain, secondary sex characteristics. These hormones are also produced in the ovaries and testes.

The adrenal medulla secretes two types of hormones epinephrine and norepinephrine (adrenaline and noradrenaline), which are closely related hormones. Both epinephrine and norepinephrine are called sympathomimetic agents, as they function on the sympathetic nervous system. They help the body to respond to crisis situations.

Addison's disease is characterized by the hyposecretion of cortical hormones of adrenal cortex, which results, when the adrenal cortex is destroyed by atrophy of adrenals.

Cushing's disease: Hyperfunctioning of the adrenal cortex with increased glucocorticoid secretion. It is characterized by moon-like fullness of the face, hypertension, high blood sugar, excess deposition of fat at the back of thoracic region, excess hair growth in unusual places (hirsutism) especially in females.

Pancreas

The pancreas is located behind the stomach in the bed of duodenum. It functions as both endocrine and exocrine gland. The specialized cells in the pancreas, which produce hormones are called islets of Langerhans. There are two kinds of main cells in the islets α-cells produce glucagon and constitute about 25% of the islets and β-cells produce insulin and constitute about 75% of the islets cells. Both the hormones, glucagon and insulin play an important role in the proper metabolism of sugars and starches in the body.

Hyposecretion of Insulin

The hyposecretion of the insulin is called diabetes mellitus. It is the most common pancreatic disorder. It is recognized to exist in two forms the insulin-dependent form caused by failure of the β-cells to produce insulin and noninsulin dependent form, caused by the insufficient insulin production to facilitate the oxidation of the glucose.

Hypersecretion of Insulin

Hypersecretion of insulin condition is known as hyperinsulinism. It may be caused by tumor in the pancreas. By excessive secretion of the insulin, excess glucose is drawn out of the bloodstream, resulting in hypoglycemia.

Pituitary Gland

The pituitary gland is a small, pea-sized gland located at the base of the brain. It is also known master gland as it regulates many body activities and stimulates other glands to secrete their own specific hormones.

The pituitary gland consists of three distinct parts—anterior lobe (adenohypophysis or pars distalis), middle lobe (pars intermedia) and posterior lobe (neurohypophysis or pars nervosa). All these lobes secrete many hormones (Fig. 7.3), they are:

1. ***Anterior lobe of pituitary (adenohypophysis):*** Table 7.1.

TABLE 7.1 Hormones secreted by anterior lobe of pituitary and their actions

Hormone	Action
Growth hormone (GH)	Acts on bone tissues to stimulate bone and body growth
Thyroid-stimulating hormones (TSH)	Controls the stimulation and secretion of thyroid hormones
Prolactin	Promotes growth of breasts tissue during the puberty period of the female and stimulates milk production after the childbirth
Adrenocorticotropic hormone (ACTH)	Stimulates the secretions by adrenal cortex especially corticoids
Gonadotropic hormones	There are many gonadotrophic hormones, which influence the growth and hormone secretion of the ovaries in females and testes in males
Follicle-stimulating hormone (FSH)	Stimulates the growth of eggs in the ovaries, secretions of the estrogen in the females and stimulates the production of sperm cells in testes (in males)
Luteinizing hormone (LH)	Induces the secretion of the progesterone for ovaries in females and promotes the secretion of sex hormones in both males and females

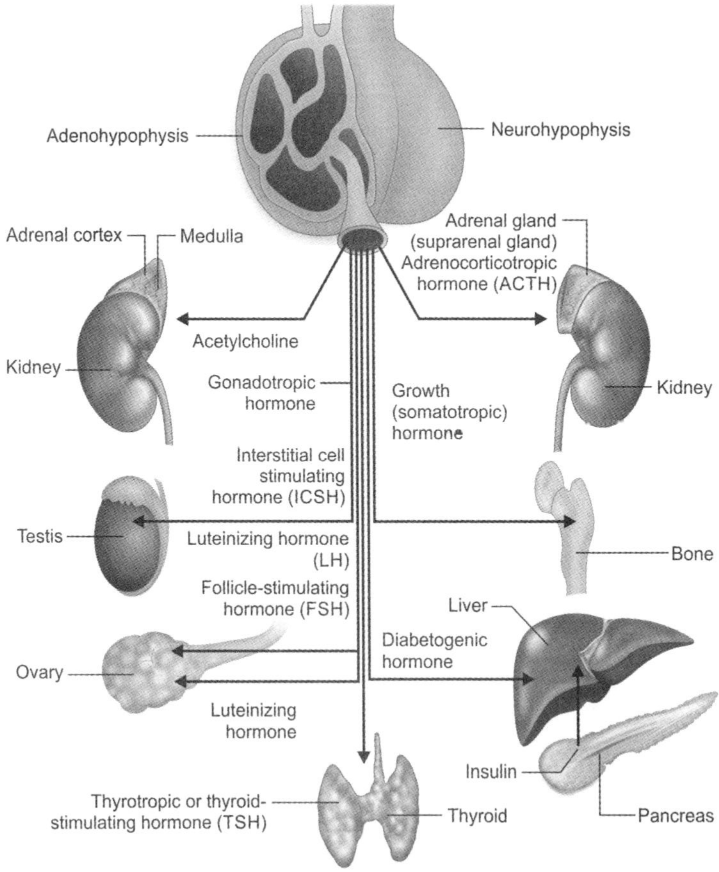

FIG. 7.3 Hormones of pituitary gland—direct and indirect effect on target organs

2. ***Middle lobe of pituitary (pars intermedia):*** It secrets melanocyte stimulating hormone (MSH).
3. ***Posterior lobe of pituitary (neurohypophysis):*** Table 7.2.

Diseases Related to Hypo- and Hypersecretions of Pituitary Glands

Anterior Pituitary Gland

- ***Gigantism:*** Hyperfunctioning of the anterior pituitary gland before leading to abnormal overgrowth of body.

TABLE 7.2 Hormones secreted by posterior lobe of pituitary and their actions

Hormone	Action
Antidiuretic hormone (ADH)	This hormone is also known as vasopressin; it stimulates the reabsorption of water by the kidney and can also increase the blood pressure by constricting the arterioles
Oxytocin	Stimulates the contraction of uterus during labor and milk secretion after childbirth

- ***Acromegaly:*** Hyperfunctioning of the anterior pituitary gland, leads to abnormal enlargements of extremities. Hypersecretion of the growth hormone (GH) causes abnormally large growth of the bones in the hands, feet, face and jaw.
- ***Dwarfism:*** This is due to the hyposecretion of growth hormone. It is a congenital disorder characterized by bones remaining small and underdeveloped.
- ***Panhypopituitarism:*** Hyposecretion of all hormones secreted by anterior pituitary gland. It largely affects the functions of the target glands such as adrenals, testes, ovaries and thyroid.

Posterior Pituitary Gland

- ***Inappropriate antidiuretic hormone (IADH):*** Hypersecretion of ADH. This condition is characterized by excessive retention of water in the body.
- ***Diabetes insipidus:*** Hyposecretion of ADH. Clinical symptoms include polyuria and polydipsia.

Pineal Gland (Body)

The pineal gland is pinecone-shaped gland attached to the posterior part of the third ventricle of the brain. The exact functioning of the gland is not found out so far. However, it is believed that it secretes melatonin hormone, which plays a vital role in inhibiting the activities of ovaries.

Ovaries

The ovaries are two small glands located in lower abdominal region of the female. The ovaries produce the female sex cells called ovum, as well as hormones, which are responsible for female sexual characteristics and regulation of the menstrual cycle.

The hormones secreted by the ovaries are estrogen and progesterone. Estrogen is responsible for the development and maintenance of secondary sex characteristics. Progesterone is responsible for the preparation and maintenance of the uterus during pregnancy.

Testes

The testes are two small, ovoid gland suspended from the inguinal region of the male by the spermatic cord and surrounded by the scrotal sac. The testes produce male sex cells spermatozoa, as well as the male hormone called testosterone. It regulates the growth and maintenance of secondary sexual characteristics in the male.

Chapter Summary

The functions of endocrine system and nervous system are closely related and work together to maintain homeostasis (the state of equilibrium in the internal environment of the body) and also regulate the basic metabolic activities of the body. The endocrine system is essentially a chemical communication system and is composed of (1) ...., which are responsible for secretion of hormones. Included in the endocrine system are number of ductless glands located in various parts of the body. These glands are called endocrine glands because they release their secretions directly into blood vessels that run through the glands. They are not to be confused with exocrine glands, such as the seat and oil glands of the skin, which release their secretions externally through ducts.

Pituitary Gland

The pituitary gland or hypophysis is known as the master gland, because it regulates many body activities and stimulates other glands to secret their own specific hormones. The gland consists of two portions-(2) ....

Thyroid Gland

The thyroid gland is the largest gland of the endocrine system. It is an H-shaped organ located in the neck just below the larynx. This gland is composed of two large lobes that are separated by a strip of tissue called isthmus. The function of the thyroid gland is to produce, store and release (3) .... and T4 regulate metabolism and are responsible for a person's energy level. They increase the rate of oxygen consumption and thus the rate at which carbohydrates are used, and proteins are broken down. They also increase the rate at which fats are utilized. In addition, both hormones work with the grown hormone (GH) and stimulate activity in the nervous system.

Parathyroid Glands

The parathyroid glands consist of four separate glands located on the posterior surface of the lobes of the thyroid gland. The only hormone known to be secreted by the parathyroid gland is a protein called (4) .... PTH helps to regulate the metabolism of calcium by influencing three types of organs—bones, intestine and kidneys.

Parathyroid hormone (PTH) seems to stimulate the formation of new bone cells (osteoblasts). As a result of this increased activity, calcium and phosphates are released from the bone and the blood concentrations of these substances increase. Hence, the calcium that is necessary for the proper functioning of the body tissues is present in the bloodstream. About the same time, PTH enhances the absorption of calcium and phosphates from foods in the intestine, and this action also produces a rise in the blood levels of calcium and phosphates. PTH causes the kidneys to conserve blood calcium and to increase the excretion of phosphates in the urine.

Adrenal Glands

The adrenal glands are paired structures located to the superior to the kidneys. Because of their location on top of the kidneys, the adrenal glands are also known as suprarenal glands. Each adrenal gland is structurally and functionally differentiated into two sections—the other adrenal cortex, which makes up the bulk of the gland and the inter adrenal medulla. Although, these regions are not sharply divided, they represent distinct glands that secret different hormones. Steroids are secreted by the cortex. Cells of the adrenal medulla secrete two closely related hormones, (5) ....

The hormones of the adrenal cortex are all steroids (corticosteroids) and are essential to life. In fact, in the absence of cortical secretions, a person usually dies within a week unless extensive electrolyte therapy (sodium, potassium and calcium levels are carefully controlled) is provided.

The cortex is subdivided into three zones. Each zone has a different cellular arrangement and secretes different groups of hormones, which are given below:

Mineralocorticoids

Mineralocorticoids help to regulate water and mineral salts (also known electrolytes) that are retained in the body. One of the mineralocorticoids of major importance in human is aldosterone. Similar to all of the hormones of the adrenal cortex aldosterone is a steroid. This hormone acts mainly through the kidneys to maintain the homeostasis of sodium and potassium. More specifically, aldosterone causes the kidneys to conserve sodium and excrete potassium. At the same time, it promotes water conservation and reduces urine output.

Glucocorticoids

Glucocorticoids influence the metabolism of carbohydrates, fats and protein. The glucocorticoid with the greatest activity is cortisol. It helps to regulate the concentration of glucose in the blood, protecting against low blood sugar between meals. Another effect of cortisol is to stimulate the breakdown of fats in adipose tissue and release fatty acids into the blood. The increase in the fatty acids are caused for many cells to use relatively less glucose.

Gonadocorticoids (Sex Hormones)

Gonadocorticoids (sex hormones) affect sex characteristics. Although, the sex hormones are primarily male type (adrenal androgens), small quantities of female hormones (adrenal estrogens and progesterone) are also present. The normal functions of these hormones are not clear, but they may supplement the supply of sex hormones from the gonads and stimulate early development of the reproductive organs. Also, there is some evidence that the adrenal androgens play role in controlling the female sex drive.

Epinephrine (adrenaline and norepinephrine (noradrenaline) are closely related hormones secreted by the adrenal medulla. The effects of the medullary hormones resemble those of the sympathetic nervous system. The adrenal medulla, as the rest of the sympathetic nervous system, is not essential to the life, but is important to the ability of the organism to meet emergencies.

Pancreas (Islets of Langerhans)

The pancreas lies inferior to the stomach in a bend of the duodenum. It functions both as an exocrine and endocrine gland. A large pancreatic duct runs through the gland carrying enzymes and other exocrine digestive secretions from the pancreas to the small intestine. The pancreas has the groups of cells called Islets of Langerhans, which produce endocrine secretions. There are two kinds of main cells in the islets—α-cells produce glucagon and constitute about 25% of the islet cells. Both of these hormones, glucagon and insulin, play an important role in the proper metabolism of sugars and starches in the body.

Pineal Gland

The pineal gland is a pine cone-shaped gland and is attached to the posterior part of the third ventricle of the brain. There is evidence that it secretes melatonin hormone (however, the exact functions of this gland are not known). It is believed that melatonin may inhibit the activities of the ovaries. When melatonin production is high, ovulation is blocked and there may be a delay in puberty development. The pineal gland starts to degenerate at about 7 years of age; in the adult, it consists mostly of fibrous tissue.

Answers

1. Endocrine glands
2. An anterior lobe (adenohypophysis) and a posterior lobe (neurohypophysis)
3. Thyroxine (T4) and triiodothyronine (T3)
4. Parathyroid hormone (PTH) or parathormone
5. Epinephrine (adrenaline) and nor-epinephrine (noradrenaline)

Review Questions

Exercise 1 Answer in One Word

1. What glands are responsible for the secretions of hormones?
2. An endocrine system is a number of ____ located in various parts of the body.
3. Endocrine glands release their secretions directly into____________.
4. Exocrine glands release their secretions externally through ____________.
5. The sweat and oil glands of the skin, that release their secretions belong to____________.
6. The pituitary gland, or hypophysis, is located at the base of the____________.
7. Which gland is known as the "master gland"?
8. The pituitary gland consists of ________three distinct portions.
9. Anterior lobe, middle lobe and posterior lobe belong to____________.
10. Which is the largest gland of the endocrine system?
11. What is an H-shaped organ located in the neck just below the larynx?
12. The two large lobes of thyroid gland are separated by a strip of tissue called____________.
13. Which hormone stimulates bone and body growth?
14. Which hormone promotes the growth of breast tissue?
15. Which hormone stimulates milk production after birth?
16. Which hormone stimulates secretions by the adrenal cortex, cortisol?
17. Which hormone causes contraction of the uterus during labor and childbirth?
18. Thyroxin and triiodothyronine, the major thyroid hormones belong to ____________.
19. How many separate glands of the parathyroid glands consist?
20. Parathyroid hormone (PTH), or parathormone PTH is the only hormone of ____________.
21. PTH seems to stimulate the formation of new____________.
22. PTH enhances the absorption of calcium and phosphates from foods in the____________.
23. The adrenal glands are paired structures located superior to the____________.
24. How many sections are each adrenal gland functionally differentiated into?

25. The two sections of the adrenal gland are the outer adrenal cortex and the inner_____________.
26. Steroids are secreted by the_____________.
27. Cells of the adrenal medulla secrete two hormones, epinephrine and_____________.
28. The hormones of the adrenal cortex are all steroids and are essential to_____________.
29. Histologically, how many zones is the cortex subdivided into?
30. Mineralocorticoids which help to regulate water and_____________.
31. Mineral salts (also called electrolytes) that are retained in the_____________.
32. Glucocorticoids influence the metabolism of carbohydrates, fats and _____________.
33. Gonadocorticoids (sex hormones), which affect what characteristics _____________.
34. Epinephrine and norepinephrine are two hormones secreted by the adrenal _____________.
35. The effects of the medullary hormones resemble those of the sympathetic_____________.
36. The pancreas lies inferior to the stomach in a bend of the_____________.
37. The pancreas functions both as an exocrine and_____________.
38. The pancreas has groups of cells called islets of Langerhans, which produce_____________.
39. The pineal gland is attached to the posterior part of the third ventricle of the_____________.
40. At what age does the pineal gland start to degenerate?

Exercise 2: Complete the Following

1. Endocrine gland secretions are called _____________.
2. The endocrine system is made up of _____________ glands of internal secretion.
3. The two parts of the pituitary gland are the _____________ and _____________ lobes.
4. The islands (islets) of Langerhans in the pancreas secrete _____________ and _____________.
5. Two little cap-like glands on top of the kidneys are the _____________ gland.
6. The two distinct parts of the adrenals whose functions differ are the _____________ and _____________.

7. The ________________ of the adrenal gland secretes epinephrine and norepinephrine.
8. The ________________ lobe of the pituitary gland secretes an antidiuretic hormone that stimulates water reabsorption by tubules of the kidneys.
9. The pineal gland secretion is ________________.
10. The essential element of the thyroid hormone is ________________.

Exercise 3: Match the Following

1. Melatonin	A. Male hormone producing secondary sex characteristics
2. Oxytocin	B. Hormone secreted by the islands of Langerhans, which increases blood glucose
3. Prolactin	C. Adrenal cortex hormones concerned with fat, protein and carbohydrate metabolism
4. Glucagons	D. Thyroid hormone that helps to regulate calcium levels in the blood
5. Calcitonin	E. Hormone secreted by the posterior lobe of the pituitary gland that stimulates uterine contractions
6. Testosterone	F. Hormone that reduces glucose in the blood
7. Glucocorticoids	G. A skin lightening hormone of the pineal gland
8. Parathyroid hormone	H. Hormone secreted by the adrenal medulla that helps the body to meet stresses by stimulating the sympathetic nervous system
9. Epinephrine	I. Hormone regulating calcium and phosphorus in blood and bone
10. Insulin	J. Hormone responsible for development of breast in pregnancy

Answers

Exercise 1

1. Endocrine glands
2. Ductless glands
3. Blood vessels
4. Ducts
5. Exocrine glands
6. Brain

7. Pituitary gland
8. Three
9. Pituitary gland
10. Thyroid gland
11. Thyroid gland
12. An isthmus
13. Growth hormone
14. Prolactin
15. Prolactin
16. Adrenocorticotropic
17. Oxytocin
18. Thyroid gland
19. Four
20. Parathyroid gland
21. Bone cells
22. Intestine
23. Kidneys
24. Two sections
25. Adrenal medulla
26. Cortex
27. Norepinephrine
28. Life
29. Three zones
30. Mineral salts
31. Body
32. Proteins
33. Sexual
34. Medulla
35. Nervous system
36. Duodenum
37. Endocrine gland
38. Endocrine secretions
39. Brain
40. About 7 years

Exercise 2

1. Hormones
2. Ductless
3. Anterior, posterior
4. Insulin, glucagons and pancreatic polypeptide
5. Adrenal
6. Cortex, medulla
7. Medulla
8. Posterior
9. Melatonin
10. Iodine

Exercise 3

1. G
2. E
3. J
4. B
5. D
6. A
7. C
8. I
9. H
10. F

Respiratory System

On completion of this chapter, the student will be able to:

- List the major organs of the respiratory system
- Describe briefly the functions of the respiratory organs
- Explain the divisions of the lung
- Elucidate the mechanism of respiration-inspiration/expiration

INTRODUCTION

The essential features of respiratory system are the exchange of oxygen from atmosphere to the tissues and carbon dioxide from the tissue to the outer air. With the cooperation of the cardiovascular system, it supplies oxygen to the tissues of the body and takes away carbon dioxide. There are two phases in the respiration—external respiration and internal respiration.

EXTERNAL AND INTERNAL RESPIRATION

External Respiration

External respiration is an exchange of oxygen and carbon dioxide between the lungs and capillaries.

Internal Respiration

Internal respiration is an exchange of gas (oxygen and carbon dioxide) between individual body cells and tiny capillaries.

During external respiration, the air inhaled contains 21% of oxygen, during exhalation the air contains 16% carbon dioxide.

PARTS OF THE RESPIRATORY SYSTEM (FIGS. 8.1 AND 8.2)

Nose

Air enters through the nose and passes through nasal cavities (turbinates), which are lined with mucous membranes and fine hairs,

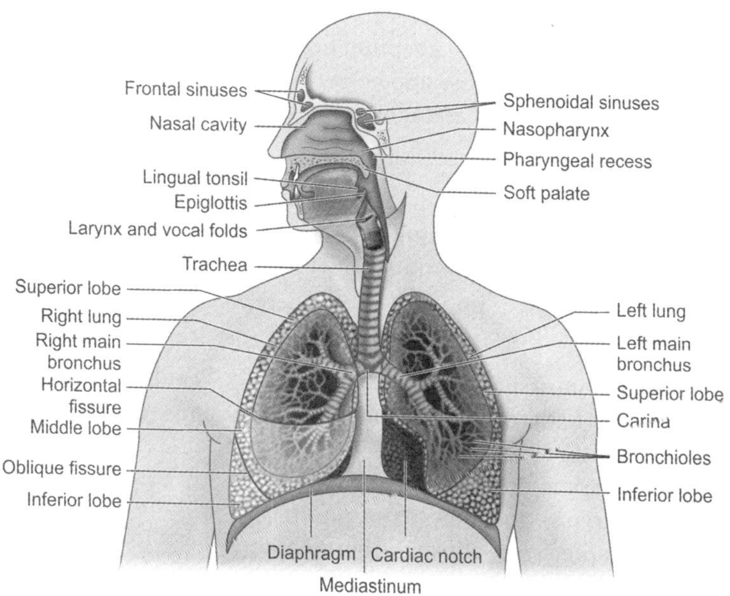

FIG. 8.1 Cross-section with names of different parts of respiratory system

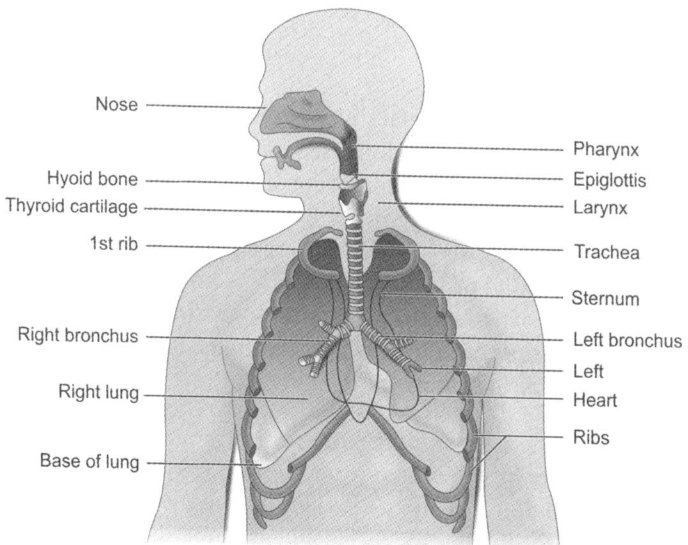

FIG. 8.2 Important parts of organs of respiratory system

which help in filtering the dust as well as to warm and moisten the air. The nose is subdivided by a septum into two cavities. These are lined above by olfactory mucosa and below by the respiratory mucosa and skin. The nose also acts as a sense organ to smell.

Paranasal Sinuses

Paranasal sinuses are hollow, air-containing cavities within the cranium, which helps to produce the tune quality of sound.

Pharynx

Pharynx is a muscular tube, and it is about 12.7 cm long. Pharynx is common for both respiratory and digestive systems. There are three sections:

1. Nasopharynx—posterior to the nose
2. Oropharynx—posterior to the mouth
3. Laryngopharynx—above the larynx.

The collection of lymphatic tissue known as adenoids or pharyngeal tonsil is located in the nasopharynx. Another type of lymphatic tissue known as tonsil is located in the oropharynx, which helps to filter and invade the bacteria present in the air and food.

Larynx

Larynx is located under the laryngopharynx in front of the neck. It is the prominent part of the windpipe, and it is made up of sections of cartilage interspersed by membrane and ligaments. The largest cartilage is the thyroid cartilage (Adam's apple) attached to the top of which is the epiglottis. The vocal cords are situated in larynx and are responsible for sound production (speech) or promotion. The cords are actually folds of tissues. Air passing through the glottis and across the cords produces vibrations, which can be changed into sounds and varied by muscle actions.

Epiglottis

Epiglottis is a leaf, like structure present above the larynx and acts similar to a lid for the larynx, by closing and not allowing the food particles into the larynx, while eating.

Trachea (Windpipe)

The trachea is a windpipe, which is of 12 cm long and 2.5 cm in diameter, which extends from the larynx downwards in front of the esophagus and it divides to form the two main (principal) bronchi and crosses the arch of aorta. The trachea is composed of 16–20 C-shaped rings of hyaline cartilage by fibrous tissue, which helps to keep the windpipe permanently open. The trachea is lined with ciliated epithelium.

Bronchi

The end of the trachea is divided into two small pipes called bronchi (left and right). The left and right bronchi passes to the corresponding sides of the lungs. The bronchi is divided into small branches called bronchioles, which ends with air sacs called alveoli, which resemble a balloon-like structure. The capillary structure (bed) lies close to the alveoli. The internal respiration (exchange of oxygen and carbon dioxide) is carried out between the alveoli and capillaries. The structure of bronchi is similar to the trachea and is lined with ciliated epithelium.

Lungs

The lungs are two roughly cone-shaped organs, situated in the right and left side of thoracic cavity protected by ribs, almost filling the thoracic cavity. The two lungs are separated by the heart and great vessels lying in the mediastinum. The base of the lungs lies on the diaphragm. Lungs are covered by pleural cavity containing pleural fluid, which helps to glide smoothly over the pleura during the respiration, which helps in breathing. Mediastinum is the space between the two pleural sacs (lungs).

Each lung is divided into lobes. The right lung has three lobes and the left has two lobes. The lobes are further divided into lobules, which are bound together by loose connective tissue. Each lobule has bronchioles, which are divided and subdivided becoming finer until they end in small dilated air sacs or alveoli. The overall lung tissue is elastic and spongy in order to carry out its respiratory functions.

Diaphragm

Diaphragm is a large muscular partition, which lies between chest cavity and abdominal cavity. By contracting and relaxing the diaphragm produces the needed pressure differential for respiration.

MECHANISM OF EXTERNAL RESPIRATION (FLOWCHART 8.1)

Inspiration

Inhaling oxygen into the lungs is called inspiration. During inspiration the diaphragm is forced down, the sternum and ribs move forward and outward respectively, thus increasing the space of thoracic

FLOWCHART 8.1 Block diagram representing the mechanism of respiration

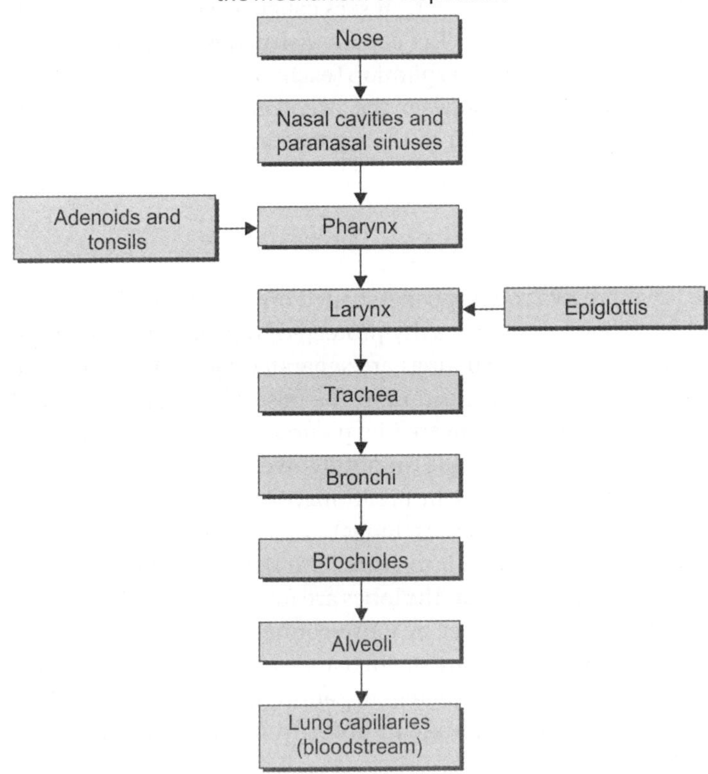

cavity and the lungs enlarge. Being elastic, the lungs expand to fill-up with oxygen 20% and carbon dioxide 0.04% and nitrogen 79% and water vapor depending on degree of humidity in the increased space.

In the alveoli, the basic part of the lung, the oxygen from the inspired air is able to pass through the thin alveolar-capillary membrane and is taken up by the hemoglobin (Hb) in the red cells of the blood. This highly oxygenated blood is passed back to the heart through the pulmonary veins to be pumped around the body.

Expiration

Exhaling carbon dioxide from the lungs is called expiration. During expiration, the diaphragm regains its dome shape and sternum and ribs relax, thus the size of the thorax return to its normal size after the expansion during inspiration and the carbon dioxide (4%), oxygen (16%) and nitrogen (79%) present in the lungs are expelled.

The process of inspiration and expiration is called ventilation. Normal rate of ventilation in adults is 14–18 breaths per minute. In children this rate is more, up to 40 breaths per minute.

Process of Internal or Tissue Respiration (Fig. 8.3)

The well-oxygenated blood is circulated through the arteries and arterioles of the body. When it reaches the capillaries it moves very

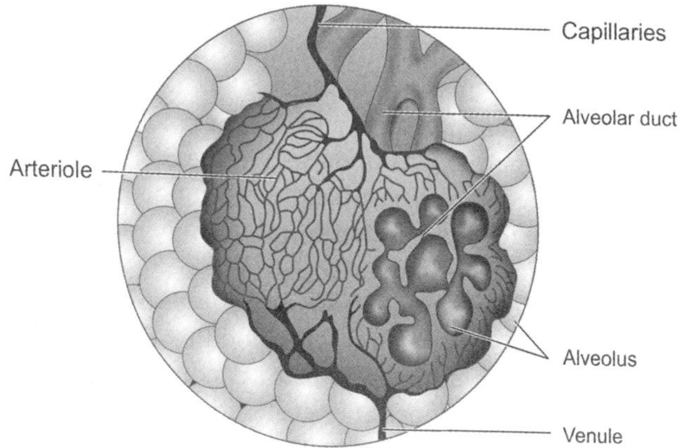

FIG. 8.3 Mechanism of internal or tissue respiration

slowly, the tissue cells take oxygen from the Hb and exchanges it with carbon dioxide, the waste product of metabolism (carbon dioxide) is returned through the venous system to the heart and back to the lungs.

VITAL CAPACITY

The volume of air that can be passed through the lungs is called vital capacity. For men, the normal vital capacity is 4–5 L and for women 3–4 L. The instrument used to measure the vital capacity is spirometer.

FACTORS INFLUENCING THE RESPIRATORY SYSTEM

Normal rhythmic respiration continues even when a person is unconscious or asleep. This rhythm is maintained by a part of the brain referred to as the respiratory center, in the medulla oblongata. One part of the respiratory center facilitates inspiration and is called the inspiratory center. The other part, which facilitates expiration is called expiratory center. The alternating activity of the inspiratory and expiratory centers brings about alternate inspiration and expiration. This alternate activity of the two centers is brought about by:

1. A third part of the respiratory center known as pneumotaxic center
2. Reflexes arising from the lung because of the stretching of the lungs during inspiration.

The factors that influence the respiration are the carbon dioxide content of the blood. If it is raised above the normal level, it can stimulate respiration by acting on the respiratory center directly and through reflexes, producing an increase in both depth and rate. Hypoxia is a partial lack of oxygen in the blood and anoxia is a total lack of oxygen. Both stimulate respiration. The pH of blood is also another factor influencing respiration. Acidosis stimulates respiration and alkalosis inhibits it.

At high altitudes where the atmospheric pressure is low, less amount of oxygen is taken up by the blood resulting in hypoxia. Sudden transfer to high altitudes result in a condition called mountain sickness. Continued residence at high altitudes brings about certain compensatory changes in the mechanism of oxygen carriage referred to acclimatization. The important changes are:

- The subjects begin to breath in a greater quantity of air by increasing both the rate and depth of respiration
- The red blood cell (RBC) count is increased by the red bone marrow producing more RBC so that the Hb content also increases and more oxygen can be carried.

Chapter Summary

Respiratory system deals with two main simultaneous activities: (1) .... The first operation, external respiration, refers to the exchange of oxygen (O_2), between the organism and the external environment. In this operation, oxygen-rich air from the environment is brought into the lungs during inspiration (inhalation) and carbon dioxide (CO_2) is removed from the body during expiration (exhalation). More familiarly, external respiration is called lung breathing.

Internal Respiration

The second operation, internal respiration refers to the exchange of O_2, and CO_2 at the cellular level. Oxygen contained in the red blood cells is exchanged for the waste CO_2 in the tissues. This exchange is also called tissue breathing. Just as the organism as a whole requires the exchange of gases to maintain life, each individual cell must also exchange gases for the metabolic process. Ultimately, CO_2 will be transferred to the lungs to be expelled.

Structures Associated with Breathing

During the breathing process, air from the environment is drawn into the nose and passes through the nasal cavity (turbinate) to the pharynx (throat). The pharynx is a muscular tube that constitutes the first major section of the air passage to the (2) .... It is about 5 inches long and consists of three sections:

1. The nasopharynx, posterior to the nose.
2. The oropharynx, posterior to the mouth.
3. The laryngopharynx, above the larynx.

Within the nasopharynx is a collection of lymphatic tissue known as adenoids or pharyngeal tonsils. Another collection of lymphatic tissue called palatine tonsils or more commonly tonsils, is located in the (3) ....

Beneath the laryngopharynx is the larynx (voice box). This structure is responsible for sound production or phonation. A leaf-shaped flap on top of the larynx, the epiglottis, seals off the air passage to the lungs during swallowing to ensure that foods or liquids do not obstruct the flow of air to the lungs.

The extension of the air passage tube beneath the larynx is the trachea. It is composed of smooth muscles embedded with C-shaped cartilage rings. These rings provide the necessary rigidity to keep the air passage open at all times. The trachea divides into two branches called bronchi (singular form, bronchus). One bronchus leads to the right lung and the other to the left lung. Similar to the trachea, the bronchi contain C-shaped cartilage rings. Without them, the trachea or bronchi may possibly collapse and endanger life.

Each bronchus divides into two branches called bronchioles (little bronchi), which terminate in air sac called (alveolus). An alveolus resembles a small (4) .... because it expands and contracts with flow and outflow of air. Capillary beds of the circulatory system lie adjacent to the thin tissue membranes of the alveoli. CO_2 passed from the blood within the pulmonary capillaries into the alveolar spaces, while O_2 from the alveoli passes into the blood. After the blood becomes oxygenated, it returns to the heart where it is pumped to all the body tissues. At the tissue level, O_2 from the blood is exchanged for tissue CO_2. This exchange of gases is called (5) .... The lungs are divided into lobes—three lobes in the right lung and two lobes in the left lung. The space between the right and left lungs is called mediastinum. It contains the heart, aorta, esophagus and the bronchi.

A double fold serous membrane, pleura, surrounds lungs. The innermost layer lying next to the lung is the visceral pleura; the outmost layer is the parietal pleura. These two membranes provide for a potential space, the pleural cavity. This cavity small amount of lubricating fluid that permits the visceral pleura to glide smoothly over the parietal pleura during respiration.

The ability of the lungs to fill with air and to expel air depends on a pressure differential between the atmosphere and the chest cavity. A large muscular partition, the (6) .... lies between the chest cavity and abdominal cavity. By contracting and relaxing, the diaphragm produced the needed pressure differential for respiration. When the diaphragm contracts, it partially descends into abdominal cavity, decreasing the pressure within the chest. This allows air to enter the lungs. When the diaphragm relaxes, it slowly re-enters the thoracic cavity. This increases the pressure within, and air slowly passes from the lungs. The intercostals muscles assist the diaphragms in changing the volume of thoracic cavity. As the diaphragm contracts, the intercostals muscles elevate the (7) .... Both of these activities result in enlarging the thoracic cavity. Consequently, the air from the environment passes into the lungs. The reverse activity causes the air to pass from the lungs the environment.

Answers

1. External respiration
2. Lungs
3. Oropharynx
4. Balloon
5. Internal respiration
6. Diaphragm
7. Rib cage

Review Questions

Exercise 1: Answer in One Word

1. Respiratory operation have two activities: the exchange of oxygen (O_2) and __________.
2. The first operation external respiration refers to the exchange of__________.
3. The oxygen-rich air is brought into the lungs during__________.
4. The CO_2 is removed from the body during__________.
5. Internal respiration, refers to the exchange of O_2 and CO_2 at what level?
6. Where oxygen contained in the red blood cell is exchanged for the waste carbon dioxide?
7. What purpose each individual cell must also exchange gases for the__________.
8. During the breathing process, air from the environment is drawn into the__________.
9. The pharynx is a muscular first major section of the air passages to the__________.
10. The pharynx is about 5 inches long and consists of how many sections?
11. The nasopharynx, posterior to the__________.
12. The oropharynx, posterior to the__________.
13. The laryngopharynx, above the__________.
14. Within the nasopharynx is a collection of lymphatic tissue known as __________.
15. Palatine tonsils, or more commonly, tonsils, is located in the__________.
16. What is beneath the laryngopharynx is the__________.
17. What is responsible for sound production, or phonation?
18. A leaf-shaped flap on top of the larynx is called the__________.
19. Epiglottis, seals off the air passage to the lungs during__________.
20. Epiglottis ensures that food or liquids do not obstruct the flow of air to the__________.
21. The extension of the air passage tube beneath the larynx is the __________.
22. The trachea is composed of smooth muscle embedded with C-shaped __________.
23. An alveolus expands and contracts with the inflow and outflow of__________.
24. The exchange of gases O_2 from the blood for tissue CO_2 gas is called__________.
25. The space between the right and left lungs is called the__________.

26. Mediastinum contains the heart, aorta, esophagus, and the________.
27. A double fold of serous membrane, eh pleura, surrounds the________.
28. A double fold of serous membrane, the pleura, surrounds the________.
29. A large muscular partition, the diaphragm lies between the chest cavity and________.
30. When the diaphragm relaxes, it slowly re-enters the________.
31. The intercostal muscles assist the diaphragm in changing the volume of the ________.
32. As the diaphragm contacts, the intercostal muscles elevate the _______.

Exercise 2: Complete the Following

1. The organs of the respiratory system are ___________, ___________, ___________, ___________ and ___________.
2. The process of respiration generally involves ___________ and ___________.
3. The pharynx is divided into ___________ parts.
4. The trachea is also known as the ___________.
5. The diaphragm separates the ___________ and ___________ cavities.
6. The diaphragm descends during the ___________ phase of respiration.
7. The ___________ side of the lung is composed of three lobes.
8. The main function of trachea is to ___________.
9. The volume of inhaled air during ordinary respiration is called ___________.
10. The respiratory center is in the ___________.

Exercise 3: Match the Following

1. Air sac of the lung	A. Diaphragm
2. Branch of trachea going to each lobe of the lung	B. Oxygen
3. Warms and moistens entering air	C. Carbon dioxide
4. Odorless, colorless gas formed in tissues and excreted by the lungs	D. Mucous membrane
5. Has a role in respiration, digestion and speech	E. Bronchiole
6. Potential space between the parietal and visceral pleural membranes	F. Pleural cavity
7. Muscular and membranous partition that separates the thoracic cavity from the abdominal cavity	G. Bronchus

8. Epithelial lining of the nose	H. Alveoli
9. Small branch of bronchial tree extending from secondary bronchi	I. Nose
10. Gas present in air, necessary for survival	J. Pharynx

Answers

Exercise 1

1. Carbon dioxide
2. O_2 and CO_2
3. Inspiration
4. Expiration
5. Cellular level
6. In tissues
7. Metabolic process
8. Nose
9. Lungs
10. Three sections
11. Nose
12. Mouth
13. Larynx
14. Adenoids
15. Oropharynx
16. Larynx (voice box)
17. Larynx (voice box)
18. Epiglottis
19. Swallowing
20. Lungs
21. Trachea
22. Cartilage rings
23. Air
24. Internal respiration
25. Mediastinum
26. Bronchi
27. Lungs
28. Lungs
29. Abdominal cavity
30. Thoracic cavity
31. Thoracic cavity
32. Cage

Exercise 2

1. Nose, pharynx, larynx, trachea, bronchi, lungs
2. Inspiration, expiration
3. Three
4. Windpipe
5. Thoracic, abdominal
6. Inspiration
7. Right
8. Maintain its part of airway
9. Tidal
10. Brain

Exercise 3

1. H
2. G
3. I
4. C
5. J
6. F
7. A
8. D
9. E
10. B

9

CHAPTER

Sense Organs

On completion of this chapter, the student will be able to:

- List the special senses of the body
- List the part and functions of the eye
- Explain the physiology of the eye (vision)
- List the parts of ear
- Explain the functioning of the ear
- Describe the structure and function of the ear
- Explain the functions of the nose and tongue
- List the glands present in the skin and their functions

INTRODUCTION

The special senses of the body include the sense of sight, taste, hearing, smell and equilibrium. These senses allow us to detect changes in our environment, and each of them has structurally complex receptors organs. The sense organs are eye, ear, tongue, nose and skin.

EYE

Eye is one of the sense organs. We see the world around us through the eyes by sensing the light that gives off or reflects. Eyes look similar to two balls of jelly each about 2.5 cm apart, set in socket in the skull, on each side of the nose. There are six muscles to each eye, four straight and two sloping muscles. These muscles can move the eyes freely in all directions. The optic nerve joins the eyeball through the back of the eye, which transmits the reflexes to the brain.

The eye's functions are similar to that of a camera. Light rays pass through a small opening and are focused by a lens upon a photoreceptive surface, retina. Then the image is transmitted from retina to the brain through the optic nerves.

The eye is a globe shaped organ that is composed of three distinct layers. They are:

1. *Sclera:* Outer most layer, which is a tough fibrous tissue, acting as a protective shield for the eye and maintains the shape of the eyeball. It also contains the cornea which is transparent.
2. *Choroid:* The middle layer that provides the blood supply for the entire eye. It also contains ciliary body and iris.
3. *Retina:* The innermost layer composed of nerve endings that are responsible for the reception and transmission of light impulses.

Anatomy of Eye

Iris

Iris is a colored, contractile membrane, which functions as a sphincter.

Cornea

Cornea is the transparent layer situated in the external surface of the eyeball. It allows the light to enter into the eye. It is also called as the window of the eye.

Pupil

Pupil is the perforated center for the iris, which regulates the entering of light by varying its size. As the environmental light increases, (bright) the pupil constricts, and as the light decreases (dark), pupil dilates, which can be compared with the aperture of the camera.

Lens

The lens is a biconvex transparent body attached to the ciliary body by the suspensory ligament. When the ligament is taut the lens is flattened and when it slackens the lens becomes thicker.

Ciliary Muscles

Muscle in which the lenses are attached, used to alter the shape of the lens by relaxation and contraction depending upon the distance of the object and environmental light so as to get a clear view. This is like adjusting the camera lens. This process is called accommodation.

Aqueous Humor

Aqueous humor is one of the two major humors (fluids) of the eye. The fluid is filled in between the cornea and lens. The iris divides the aqueous humor into two small chambers, the anterior chamber and posterior chamber.

Vitreous Humor

Vitreous humor is a clear, jelly-like fluid occupying the entire orbit of the eye behind the lens. The vitreous humor, lens and the aqueous humor are the refractive structures of the eye, which are responsible for the focusing of the rays sharply on the retina by bending the rays.

Retina

Retina is the delicate eye membrane, which is attached to the optic nerve. Retina has two types of light receptors on its surface, namely rods and cones. Rods function in dim light and provide black and white vision, whereas the cones functions in bright light and provide color vision.

Optic Nerve

The second cranial nerve is responsible for the sight and transmitting the nerve impulses caused by the chemical changes as the light strikes the retina (on rods and cones).

Accessory Organs of the Eye (Fig. 9.1)

Eyelids

Eyelid is in the anterior portion of the eye, which are movable folds, upper and lower. The upper part is large and more mobile than the lower. It protects the eyes from dust and injuries.

Eyelashes

Eyelashes are short thick hairs projecting from both the eyelids.

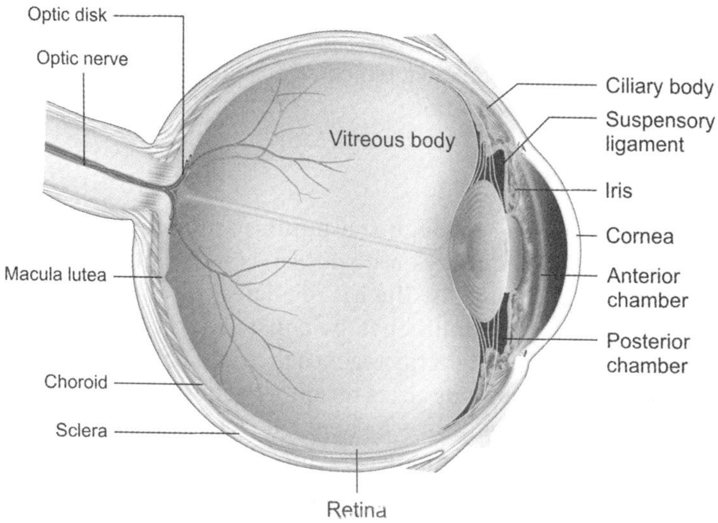

FIG. 9.1 Parts of the eye

Lacrimal Glands

Lacrimal glands situated immediately above the lateral angle of the eye. A number of small canals connect it to the conjunctival sac in the opposite side. It produces tears during the emotional situations and when any foreign body enters. The tears produced by the lacrimal glands keep the eye moist, remove the dust and foreign bodies, and acts as an antiseptic agent.

Lacrimal Duct

The lacrimal duct is a small tubule-like structure, which connects the orbit and lacrimal sac. The lacrimal glands produce tears, these tears when excess, passes down the lacrimal ducts and finally reaches nasal cavity.

Lacrimal Sac

The lacrimal sac is the continuation of the lacrimal duct, which collects the tears produced by the lacrimal glands.

Nasolacrimal Duct

Nasolacrimal duct is the duct, which drains the lacrimal fluid from the lacrimal duct into the nose.

Physiology of Eye

Light enters the eye through the pupil, conjunctiva, lens and cornea where the light rays are bent so as to focus properly on the sensitive receptor cells. The iris regulates the amount of light passing through the conjunctiva by constricting or relaxing the iris muscles. Then the light ray reaches the retina, where 6 million cones and 120 million rods act as receptors of the light. Light when focused on the retina, causes a chemical change in the rods and cones, initiating nerve impulses, which travel from the eye to the brain through optic nerves. The rods and cones in the retina communicate with neurons, connecting to the optic nerve fibers. The optic chiasma is the point where the nerve fibers of the right and left eye meet. Nerve fibers from the right half of each retina now form an optic tract meeting in the thalamus of the brain and ending in the right visual region of the cerebral cortex. Similarly, nerve fibers from the left half of each retina merge to form the optic tract and pass from the thalamus to the left region of the cerebral cortex. The images are fused by a single visual sensation with a three-dimensional effect in the visual area of the cerebral cortex. This is called binocular vision.

EAR

Ear is the sense organ for hearing and for maintaining equilibrium of the body. It is divided into three sections namely, external ear, middle ear, and inner ear (Fig. 9.2).

Parts of External Ear

- Pinna
- External auditory meatus
- Tympanic membrane or eardrum.

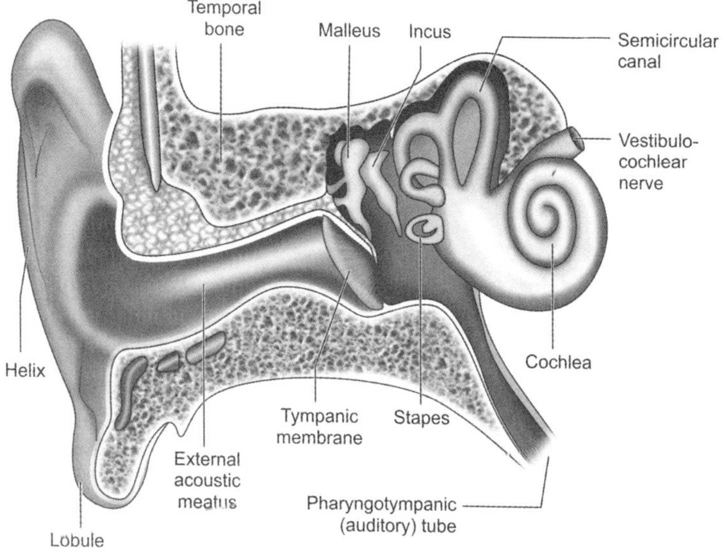

FIG. 9.2 Parts of the ear

Pinna

Pinna is the external structure attached to the side of the head. It has a deep shell-like cavity to collect the sound waves travelling through air.

External Auditory Meatus

External auditory meatus is like a tubule (canal) 2.5 cm long. It leads from the pinna to the tympanic membrane or ear drum (middle ear). The canal is lined with glands that produce a waxy secretion called cerumen. These waxy substances prevent dust and foreign particles from entering into the ear.

Tympanic Membrane

Tympanic membrane is a thin membrane covering the end of the external auditory canal. Sound waves that enter the ear canal, strike against the tympanum.

Eustachian Tube

Eustachian tube is the canal, which connects the middle ear to the nasopharynx. Its functions are to regulate the pressure in the middle ear to that of environment and clear the fluid secretion from the middle ear to the nasopharynx.

Parts of Middle Ear

The middle ear or tympanic cavity is a small chamber containing air to equalize the pressure on both sides of the tympanic membrane. It has a narrow and bony membranous wall, which communicates with the nasopharynx through the eustachian tube. The tympanic cavity contains three small bones or ossicles namely malleus, incus and stapes that are responsible for transmission of sound waves from the external ear (tympanic membrane) to the inner ear cochlea by conduction. Malleus the external bone, which is shaped similar to a hammer with its handle attached to the tympanic membrane and its head in the tympanic cavity, articulating with the incus and the inner most bone the stapes, which is attached to the oval base of the fenestra vestibuli, transmit the sound vibration to the inner ear.

Parts of Inner Ear

- Cochlea
- Semicircular canals
- Vestibule.

Cochlea

Cochlea is similar to a snail, which contains cochlear fluid and its inner surface is lined with nerve endings called corti. Disturbance of the fluid stimulates the hairs of corti, causing them to generate a series of nerve impulses. These impulses are transmitted to the brain by the auditory nerves that are interpreted as sound.

Semicircular Canals

Semicircular canal is situated to the posterior of the vestibule. Its main function is to maintain the balance and equilibrium.

Vestibule

It lies in the central part of the bony labyrinth. It is in the shape of oval. It connects the cochlea and semicircular canals.

Functioning of Ear

Sound is produced due to the vibrations of atmosphere. Sound waves vary by the rate and volume. The units to measure the sound waves frequency and intensity are hertz (speed) and decibels (dB), respectively. The human ear is able to hear the frequency of 20 to 20,000 hertz and is sensitive to the intensity of 10 to 140 dB.

A sound waves passes along the external auditory canal and makes the eardrum vibrate. This causes the malleus to pass vibrations to the incus and stapes. The three bones moving against one another cause the vibrations to be magnified and thus they are passed through the vestibular membrane to the perilymph. Vibrations in the perilymph are transmitted to the endolymph in the canal of the cochlea and the stimuli reach the nerve endings to be passed to the brain by the auditory nerve.

SKIN

The outer surface of the body is covered by the skin. The skin and its accessory organs (hairs, nails and glands) are known as the integumentary system of the body. The skin consists of two layers, epidermis and dermis (corium). Integument means covering, and the skin is the outer covering of the body, hence, it is called integumentary system. The skin has specialized tissues, contains glands, which secrete several types of fluids, nerves that carry impulses and regulates the body temperature.

Functions of Skin

The important functions of the skin are:

- Provides protection against injuries and invasion of the bacteria
- Regulates the body temperature and the prevention of dehydration

- Works as a sensory receptor and is responsible for synthesis of vitamin D.

Structure of Skin

The structure of the skin consists of two layers (Fig. 9.3) embedding one above the other. The two layers are as follows:

Epidermis

Epidermis is the outermost cellular membrane layer of the skin. It has no blood supply. The cells of the epidermis will shed continuously. The mature cells of the dermis are pushed above which are finally sloughed off and replaced by new cells. The deepest layer of the epidermis is called basal layer. The cells in the basal layer are constantly growing and multiplying and give rise to all the other cells in the epidermis. As the basal layer cells divide, they are pushed upward and away from the blood supply of the corium layer by a

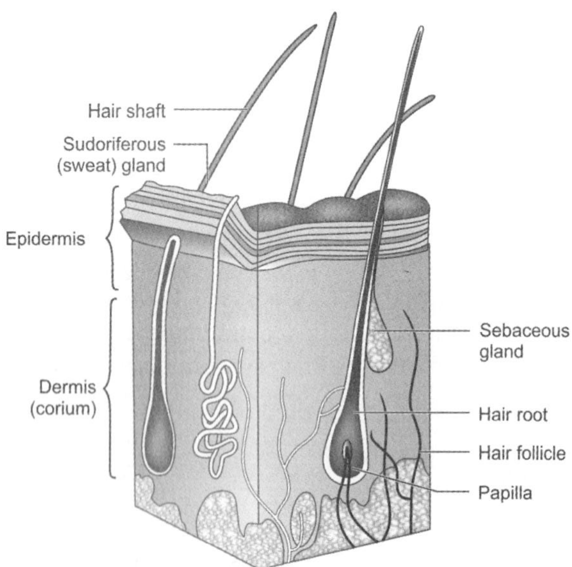

FIG. 9.3 Cross-section of structure of the skin

steady stream of younger cells and finally these cells shed from our body. This process of dividing, pushing upward and shedding of these cells takes 3–4 weeks. Thus, it is constantly renewing itself, cells dying at the same rate at which they are born. The basal layer of the epidermis contains special cells called melanocytes. Melanocytes form and contain a black pigment called melanin. The amount of black pigments accounts for the color variations. The presence of melanin in the epidermis protects against the harmful effects of ultraviolet radiation, which can cause skin cancer.

Dermis

Dermis is the layer of skin lies under the epidermis. It is a dense, fibrous, connective tissue layer. It has nerve endings and numerous capillaries for blood supply. Apart from these, hair follicles, sebaceous glands and sweat glands are also present in the dermis. This layer is also called as corium.

Subcutaneous

The subcutaneous layer of the skin is another connective tissue layer where the formation of fat is more. Lipocytes (fat cells) are predominant in the subcutaneous layer and they manufacture and store large quantities of fat. Functionally, this layer of the skin protects the deeper tissues of the body and serves as a heat insulator.

Hair

The hair has three parts namely, hair shaft, hair root and hair follicle. The hair shaft is visible in the epidermis; the hair root and hair follicle are lying under the dermis. The hair follicle is a collection of capillaries enclosed in a covering called the papilla. Deep-lying cells in the hair root produce horny cells, which move upward through the follicles for the formation of the hair shaft. As long as these cells remain alive, hair will regenerate even though it is cut or plucked or otherwise removed. Baldness (alopecia) is evident when the hairs of the scalp are not replaced. Men rather than women are more susceptible to this condition, which is because of hereditary factors. Presence of the melanin pigment makes the hair look black and the pigment is supported by the melanocytes, which are located at the root of the hair follicle. Hair turns gray when the melanocytes stop producing melanin.

Glands

There are two types of glands present under the skin, they are sebaceous and sweat glands. The sebaceous gland produces an oily secretion called sebum, while the sweat glands produce a watery secretion called sweat.

Sebaceous Glands

Sebaceous glands are filled with fatty substances, when these cells disintegrate; they yield an oily secretion called sebum. The acidic nature of sebum helps to destroy harmful organisms on the surface of the skin, and thus, prevents infections. Sebaceous glands are present over the entire body except the soles of the feet and palms of the hands.

Sweat Glands

Sweat glands are small structures that open as pores on the surface of the skin. They are found on the palms, soles, forehead and armpits. On the palms of the hands, there are approximately 3,000 sweat glands per square inch of skin. Sweat is a clear watery fluid containing 0.5% of solids such as sodium chloride, small amount of other mineral salts and urea. Sweating is one of the mechanisms by which the human body regulates its body temperature. Secretion of sweat is controlled by hypothalamus through the sympathetic nervous system. Sweating may also be induced by the emotional stress, anxiety and fear. The main functions of the sudoriferous glands are to cool the body by evaporation, to excrete waste products through the pores of the skin and to moisturize surface cells. The ceruminous glands are modified sweat glands located in the skin that lines the external auditory canal. Instead of sweat, they secrete wax (cerumen). These secretions are carried out to the outer edges of the skin by ducts and excreted from the skin through opening or pores.

Nails

Nails are solid plates present at dorsal end of fingers, which protect fingers and toes. The nail plate or body is firmly attached to the underlying nail bed, which consists of modified epidermal cells. The nail body is pink because of the underlying vascular tissue. The half-moon shaped white area near the root of the nail bed is the lunula. The lunula is the area where the new growth occurs. The average growth rate is approximately 1 mm per week for finger nails and slower for the toenails. The main function of the nails is to protect the tips of the fingers and toes from bruises and other kinds of injuries.

TONGUE

The tongue is a highly mobile organ composed of voluntary muscles. It is essential for speech, taste (bitter, sweet, sour and salt), mastication and swallowing. The root of the tongue is attached to the hyoid bone in the neck. On the dorsum of the tongue are numerous minute elevations of the mucous membrane called papillae (Fig. 9.4).

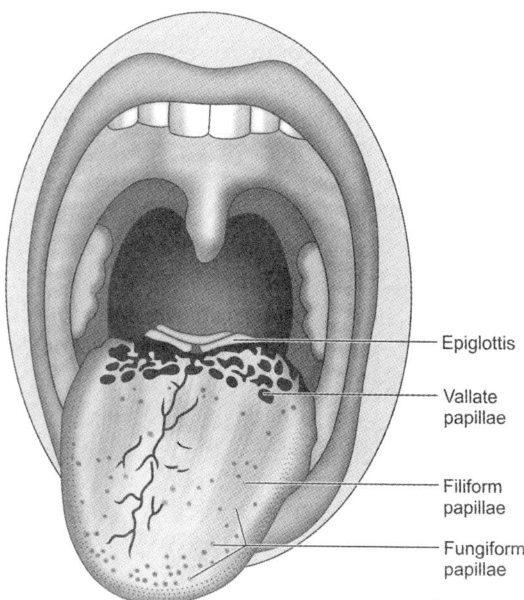

FIG. 9.4 Parts of the tongue

Embedded in the papillae are the taste buds, which are situated more densely at the tip, sides and base of the tongue (up to 9,000 tiny papillae). There are three types of papillae, namely fungiform, filiform and circumvallate papillae. The tongue is governed by facial and glossopharyngeal nerves (Fig. 9.4).

NOSE

Nose is the organ for smell. Sensory nerve ends of the olfactory nerves are situated (Fig. 9.5) in the olfactory mucosa which forms the upper one-third of the nasal mucosa. Olfactory nerves transmit these signals to olfactory bulbs then through olfactory tracts to the smell center in the temporal lobes of the cerebral cortex. Nose smell the substances whose molecules are breathed into the roof of each nasal cavity and dissolved on a patch of olfactory membrane along with 100 million smell receptor cells equipped with tiny sensitive hairs. Smell molecules react with these to stimulate nerve impulses in the receptor cells. Some people can identify 10,000 odors all evidently based on combinations of just seven (Fig. 9.6).

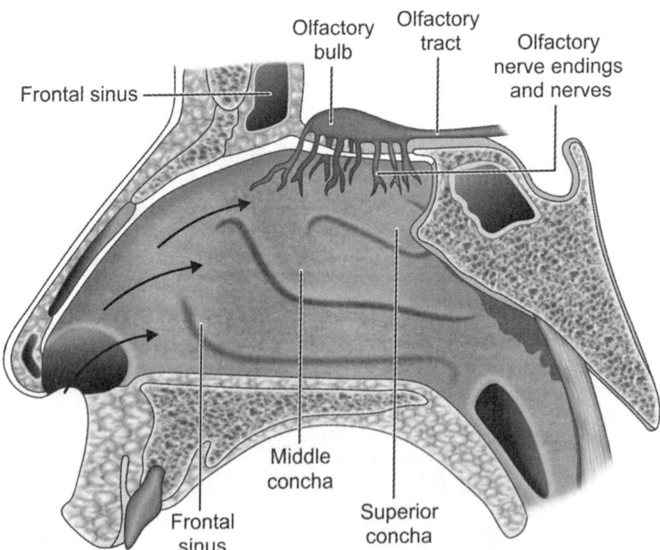

Fig. 9.5 Cross-section of the structures of olfactory mucosa with different parts names

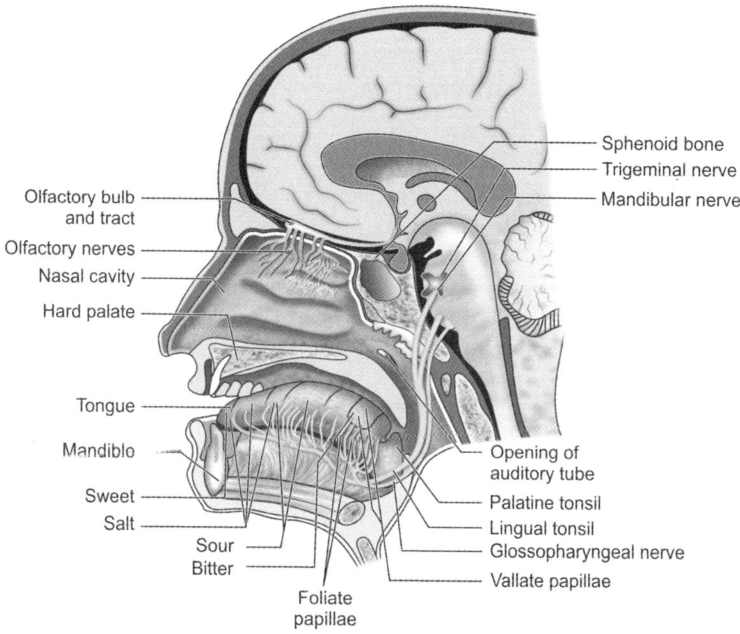

FIG. 9.6 Centers of smell and taste

Chapter Summary

All outer surfaces of the body are covered by the (1)..................... The word integument (L) means covering. The integument system consists of skin and its appendages such as hair, nails, sebaceous glands, sweat glands and breasts.

The skin performs many vital functions that include protection against injuries and invasion of bacteria and acids in the regulation of body temperature and the prevention of dehydration. It also functions as a reservoir for food and water, works as a sensory receptor and is responsible for synthesis of vitamin D.

The skin contains two layers, e.g. (2)..................... The epidermis, which is a layer of tissue with no blood or nerve supply, is the outermost layer of skin. It is in a state of continuous shedding. Cells that are formed in the innermost part of epidermis mature and are pushed to the outermost layer. These cells are finally sloughed off and replaced with new cells. The dermis or corium is a layer, lying immediately under epidermis. It is composed of living tissue that consists of numerous capillaries, lymphatics and nerve endings. Hair follicles, sebaceous glands and sweat glands are also located in the (3)....................

Hair

The visible part of the hair is referred to as the hair shaft and which is embedded in the dermis is called (4)..................... The root, together with its coverings forms the hair follicle. At the bottom of the follicle is a loop of capillaries enclosed in a covering called papilla. The cluster of epithelial cells lying over the papilla reproduced and is responsible for the eventual formation of the hair shaft. As long as these cells remain alive, hair will regenerate despite it is plucked or cut or otherwise removed. When the hair is not replaced, the result is (5)..................... men are more vulnerable and this could be due to hereditary.

Nails

The nail bed covers the dorsal surface of the terminal phalanges, the most distant bones of each finger and toe. Due to underlying vascular tissue, the most nail body is pink. The crescent-shaped white area near the root of the nail bed is the lunula. It has a whitish appearance because the vascular tissue underneath does not show through. The lunula is the area in which new growth occurs. The average growth rate is approximately 1 mm per week for fingernails, and somewhat slower for toenails. The major function of the nails is to protect the (6) .... from bruises and other kinds of injuries.

Glands

There are three kinds of microscopic glands within the skin that are (7).....................

Sweat Glands or Sudoriferous Glands

Sweat glands or sudoriferous glands are small structures that open as pores on the surface of skin. They are found in the palms, soles, forehead and armpits (axillae). There are about 3,000 sweat glands per square inch of skin on the palms of the hand. The functions of the sweat glands are to cool the body by evaporation, to excrete waste products through the pores of the skin and to moisturize surface cells.

Sebaceous Glands

Sebaceous glands are the oil-secreting glands of the skin. These glands are filled with cells, the centers of which are saturated with fatty droplets. As these cells disintegrate, they yield an oily secretion called sebum. The acidic nature of sebum helps to destroy harmful organisms on the surface of the skin end, thus prevent infections. Sebaceous glands are present over the entire body except the palms of the hand and soles of the feet. They are prevalent on face and scalp, and around opening such as the nose, mouth, external ear and anus, as well as the upper back and scrotum.

Ceruminous Glands

Ceruminous glands are modified sweat glands located in the skin that lines external auditory canal. They secret wax (cerumen) instead of sweat.

Breasts

The breasts or (8)..................... are located in the upper anterior aspect of the chest. During puberty, girl's breasts begin to develop because they are exposed to periodic stimulation of two ovarian hormones, estrogen and progesterone. Estrogen is responsible for the fatty growth (adipose tissue) and increased size of the breasts as they reach full maturity. The size of the breast is basically determined by the amount of fat around the glandular tissue and is not indicative of functional ability. The outer ovarian hormone, progesterone, forms the lobules that are present in the breast. Each breast has approximately twenty lobes of glandular tissue. These lobes are drained by a lactiferous duct that carries milk that opens on the tip of the raised (9).................... Circling the nipple, there is a border of slightly darker skin referred to as the areola.

In females, full development of the breasts is achieved by the age of 16. The main purpose of the breasts is secretion of milk for the nourishment of newborn infants. Thus, pregnancy causes the breasts to enlarge for this function. At menopause, breast tissue begins to atrophy.

Special Senses

The special senses of the body include the senses of taste, smell, equilibrium, sight, and hearing. Theses senses allow us to detect changes in the environment, and each of them has a structurally complex receptor organs.

Taste

The ability to taste is accomplished by numerous structures located on the tongue, the (10).................... In order for taste buds to be stimulated, substances must be dissolved in saliva. When this occurs, the solution containing the dissolved substance enters the taste bud and stimulates the particular receptor, producing taste. Despite the fact that one tastes many flavors, the taste buds of the tongue respond to only four sensations, i.e. sour, salty, bitter and sweet. All other 'tastes' are actually odors that are stimulating the olfactory bulb in the nose.

Smell

Olfactory sensation or the sensation of smell, is accomplished by a highly specialized collection of nervous tissue, the olfactory bulb. Odors emitted from substances enter the nasal passageways and stimulate the olfactory bulb, producing the sensation of (11).................... The taste of burger and tea is actually the sensation of smell, not taste.

Equilibrium

The ability to maintain equilibrium is attained, to a large extent by complex structure located in the inner portion of the ear, the semicircular canals. The posture and orientation of the body is sensed by this structure, which transmits impulses to the brain. As the brain integrates these impulses, it makes the necessary physiological adjustments that are required to maintain equilibrium.

Eye

The eye functions in a manner similar to that of a (12)..................... Light rays pass through a small opening and are focused by a lens upon a photoreceptive surface. In a camera, this surface is photographic film; in the eye, it is the retina. The eye is globe-shaped organ that is composed of three distinct layers. Its outermost layer is the sclera. As the name suggests, it is a tough fibrous tissue that serves as a protective shield for the more sensitive beneath. The sclera is also known as white of the eye. A highly vascular middle layer, the choroid, provides the blood supply for the entire eye. The innermost layer of the eye, (13)..................... is composed of nerve endings that are responsible for the reception and transmission of light impulses.

A specialized portion of the sclera, cornea, passes in front of the lens. Rather than being opaque, it is transparent and thus permits the entrance of light into the interior of the eye. One of the two major humors or fluids, of the eye is the aqueous humor. The iris divides the aqueous humor into two small chambers, the (14)..................... A colored, contractile membrane, iris, functions as a sphincter. Its perforated center is the pupil. The amount of light entering the eye is regulated by the size of pupil. As the environmental light increases, the pupil constricts; as the light decreases, the pupil dilates. Located behind the posterior chamber is the lens. This crystalline structure is suspended between the ciliary muscles. As these muscles relax or contract, they alter the shape of the lens, making it thicker or thinner, respectively, thus enabling the light rays to focus upon the retina. This process is called accommodation.

The second major humor of the eye is the (15)..................... This clear, jelly-like fluid occupies the entire orbit of the eye behind the lens. The vitreous humor, lens and aqueous humor are the refractive structures of the eye. They are responsible for the bending of light rays, so that they focus sharply on the retina. If any one of these structures does not function properly, vision is impaired. The retina is an extremely delicate eye membrane. It is continuous with the optic nerve and has two types of light receptor upon its surface or rods and cones. Rods, function in dim light and provide black and white vision. Cones function in bright light and provide color vision. Rods and cones contain chemicals called photopigments. As light strikes the pigments, a chemical change occurs that produces a nerve impulse. These impulses are then transmitted to the brain through the optic nerve. The brain interprets them as vision. Both optic nerve and blood vessels of the eye enter the eyeball at the optic disk. Its center is referred to as the blind spot because the area has neither rods nor cones. Such muscles control the movement of the eye; the superior, inferior, lateral and medial rectus muscles and superior and inferior oblique muscles. These muscles are coordinated to move both eyes in a synchronized manner.

The font of the eye is protected by two movable folds of skin, the eyelids. Their edges are lined with two or three rows of eyelashes, which protect the surface of the eye. A thin mucous membrane called conjunctiva lines the inner surface of the eyelids and passes over the cornea. Lying superior and to the outer edges of each eye are the inner edges of the eyes, the canthi (singular, canthus), and pass though pinpoint openings, the lacrimal canaliculi to the nose.

Ear

The ear is the sense organ of (16)..................... It consists of three major sections, i.e. the external or outer ear, the middle ear or tympanic cavity and the inner ear or labyrinth. Although, each of these sections transmits sound waves, each accomplishes the task in a different way. The external ear conducts sound waves through air; the middle ear, through bone; and the inner ear, through fluid. It is subsequently explained, this series of transmissions plays an integral part in hearing.

The external ear is designed to channel sound waves from the environment to the middle and inner ears. An (17)..................... is the external structure designed to collect waves travelling through air. The auricle channels the waves through the ear canal, which is a slender tube that leads to the middle ear. The canal is lined with glands that produce a waxy secretion called (18).....................

(19)..................... prevents foreign particles from entering the ear. A flat membranous structure, the (tympani membrane, or ear-drum) is drawn over the end of the canal. Sound waves that enter the ear canal strike against the tympanum.

In the middle ear, vibrations of the tympanum are picked up by three tiny articulating bones called ossicles. These bones are responsible for the transmission of sound waves through the middle ear. The three bones are the (20).....................

These bones form a chain that stretches from the inner surface of the tympanum to an inner ear structure called cochlea.

A tube called (21)..................... connects the nose and throat with cavity of the middle ear. Its purpose is to equalize pressure on the outer and inner surfaces of the eardrum. In situations in which sudden pressure change occurs, equalization of pressure is achieved by deliberate swallowing. The inner ear, sometimes referred to as the labyrinth because of its complicated maze-like design, is composed of three structures; a snail-shaped cochlea, semicircular canals and vestibule, which is a chamber that joins the cochlea and semicircular canals.

The cochlea is filled with fluid. Lining is inner surface are tiny nerve endings called hairs of corti. There is a membrane-covered opening on the external surface of the cochlea, called oval window. It is on this membrane that the stapes is attached to the cochlea. Transmission of sound along ossicles in the middle ear causes the stapes to exert a gentle pumping action against the oval window. The pumping action forces the cochlear fluid to move. Disturbance of the fluid stimulates the hair of Corti, causing them to generate a series of nerve impulses. The impulses are transmitted to the brain by way of the auditory nerve, where they are interpreted sound.

Answers

1. Skin
2. Epidermis and dermis or corium
3. Corium
4. Hair root
5. Alopecia (baldness)
6. Tip of the fingers and toes
7. i Sweat glands or sudoriferous glands
   ii. Sebaceous glands and
   iii. Ceruminous glands
8. Mammary glands
9. Nipple
10. Taste buds
11. Smell
12. Camera
13. Retina
14. Anterior chamber and the posterior chamber
15. Vitreous humor
16. Hearing
17. Auricle or pinna
18. Cerumen
19. Cerumen
20. Malleus (hammer), the incus (anvil) and the stapes (stirrups)
21. Eustachian tube

Review Questions

Exercise 1: Answer in One Word

1. The special senses include the senses of taste, smell, equilibrium, sight, and __________.
2. Taste is accomplished by numerous structures located on the tongue, the __________.
3. The feeling of the smell is felt by the collection of nervous tissue, the __________.
4. The ability to maintain equilibrium is by the inner portion of the __________.
5. The eye functions in a manner similar to that of a __________.
6. The eye is a globe-shaped organ that is composed of three distinct __________.
7. The outermost layer of eye is the __________.
8. The sclera is also known as the white of the __________.
9. One of the two major humors, or fluids, of the eye is the __________.
10. The second major humor of the eye is the __________.
11. What is an extremely delicate eye membrane?
12. Both the optic nerve and the blood vessels of the eye enter the eyeball at the __________.
13. How many muscles control the movement of the eye?
14. The front of the eye is protected by two moveable folds of skin, the __________.
15. A thin mucous membrane called the __________.
16. Conjunctive lines the inner surface of the __________.
17. The ear is the sense organ of __________.
18. The ear consists of the external ear; the middle ear, and the __________.
19. The external ear conducts sound waves through __________.
20. The middle ear conducts sound waves through __________.
21. The inner ear conducts sound waves through __________.
22. An auricle, or pinna, is designed to collect waves travelling through __________.
23. Sound waves that enter the ear canal strike against the __________.
24. The tympanum vibrations are picked up by 3 tiny articulating bones called __________.
25. Ossicles are responsible for the transmission of sound waves through the __________.

26. Ossicles three bones are the malleus (hammer), the incus anvil), and the ___________.
27. The Eustachian tube connects the nose and the throat with the cavity of the ___________.
28. The inner ear, is sometimes referred to as the ___________.
29. The cochlea fluid-lining its inner surface are tiny nerve endings called the ___________.
30. Disturbance of the fluid stimulates the ___________.
31. Hairs of Corti, causing them to generate a series of ___________.
32. The impulses are conveyed to the brain by the auditory nerve, where they ___________.

Exercise 2: Complete the Following

1. The transparent portion of the fibrous coat of the eyeball is ___________.
2. The innermost of the three coats of the eyeball is ___________.
3. Tears are secreted by ___________.
4. The receptors of light stimuli are the ___________ and ___________.
5. The 'white of the eye' is called the ___________.
6. The divisions of the ear are the ___________, ___________ and ___________.
7. The ear has two functions ___________ and ___________.
8. The three ossicles are the ___________, ___________ and ___________.
9. The tympanic membrane is also known as the ___________.
10. Hair cells transmit sound stimulation to the brain by way of the ___________ nerve.
11. The ___________ is the organ for smell.
12. The organs of taste are located mainly on the ___________.
13. Skin is composed of two principal layers ___________ and ___________.
14. The skin is the receptor for ___________, ___________, ___________ and ___________.
15. Sebaceous glands secrete ___________.

Exercise 3: Match the Following

1. Special cylindrical neuroepithelial cells in the retina, highly sensitive to low light	A. Dense, gibbous connective tissue
2. The partition separating the external nares	B. Secretions of sebaceous glands

3. The projecting posterior part of the ear that lies outside the head	C. Rods
4. Structure leading from the ear to the throat	D. Pinna
5. Structure that separates the middle ear from the external ear	E. Septum
6. Sebaceous glands	F. Tympanic membrane
7. Dermis	G. Area around the nipple
8. Areola	H. Glands with ducts opening around hair follicles
9. Melanin pigment	I. Eustachian tube
10. Sebum	J. Pigment of skin or hair

Answers

Exercise 1

1. Hearing
2. Taste buds
3. Olfactory bulb
4. Ear
5. Camera
6. Layers
7. Sclera
8. Eye
9. Aqueous humor
10. Vitreous humor
11. The retina
12. Optic disc
13. Six
14. Eyeballs
15. Conjunctive
16. Eye-lids
17. Hearing
18. Inner ear
19. Air
20. Bone
21. Fluid
22. Air
23. Tympanum
24. Ossicles
25. Middle ear
26. Stapes (stirrups)
27. Middle ear
28. Labyrinth
29. Hairs of Corti
30. Hairs of Corti
31. Nerve impulses
32. Interpreted a sound

Exercise 2

1. Cornea
2. Retina
3. Lacrimal
4. Rods, cones
5. Sclera
6. External, middle, inner
7. Hearing and equilibrium
8. Malleus, incus, stapes

9. Eardrum
10. Auditory
11. Nose
12. Tongue
13. Epidermis, dermis
14. Touch, heat, cold and pain
15. Sebum

Exercise 3

1. C
2. E
3. D
4. I
5. F
6. H
7. A
8. G
9. J
10. B

10

CHAPTER

Excretory System

On completion of this chapter, the student will be able to:

- List the organs of the excretory system
- Explain the structure and functions of nephron
- Describe the excretion process of urine
- Explain the peripheral nervous system and their divisions

INTRODUCTION

The urinary system is one of the important systems, which excretes the waste (end) products of metabolism that tend to change the normal internal and external environment of the cell. This is also called excretory system (Fig. 10.1). The wastes produced by the body such as carbon dioxide and water in the form of vapor are removed from the body by the exhalation through the lungs. Whereas the nitrous waste, produced when proteins combine with oxygen is

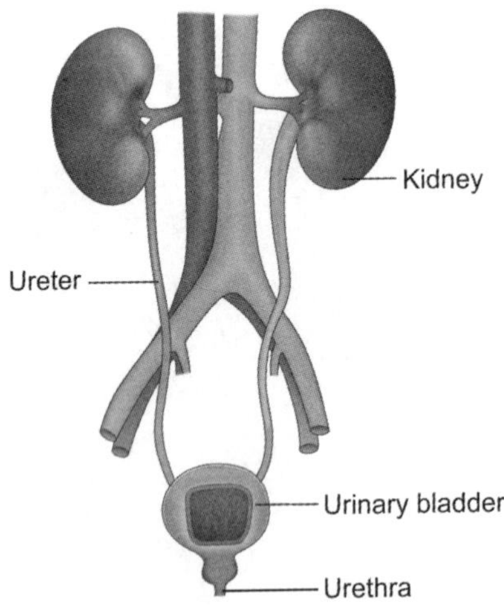

FIG. 10.1 Excretory system

more difficult to excrete from the body by exhalation. Hence, the body excretes it in the form of a water-soluble substance called urea. The major function of the urinary system is to remove urea from the bloodstream, so that it does not accumulate in the body and become toxic. Besides removing the urea, the urinary system maintains the proper balance of water, salts and acids in the body fluids, salts such as sodium, potassium and some acids known as electrolytes. Nephrology is the study of the urinary system or kidney and a specialist in this field is called nephrologist.

PARTS OF URINARY SYSTEM

The urinary system is composed of:

- Two kidneys
- Two ureters
- Urinary bladder
- Urethra.

Kidneys

There are two kidneys, which are bean-shaped organs situated behind the abdominal cavity on either side of the vertebral column in the lumbar region of the spine. They lie behind the peritoneum and are embedded in renal fat for protection. They are dark reddish brown in color, measuring the size of a fist and about half a pound each. The left kidney is situated at higher level on the posterior abdominal wall than the right kidney (Figs. 10.2 and 10.3).

The kidney can be divided into three parts namely:

1. The cortex or outer part
2. The medulla or inner part
3. The hilum depression at the medial part of the kidney.

The cortex (outer) part of the kidney contains tiny glomeruli, together with the renal tubules, which lie partly in the medulla also. These two are commonly called nephron (Fig. 10.4), the functional units of the kidney. There are about 1 million nephron.

Each nephron has a renal corpuscle and a renal tubule. The renal corpuscle is composed of a tuft of capillaries, the glomerulus and a modified funnel-shaped end of the renal tubule called Bowman's capsule, which encases the glomerulus. An afferent

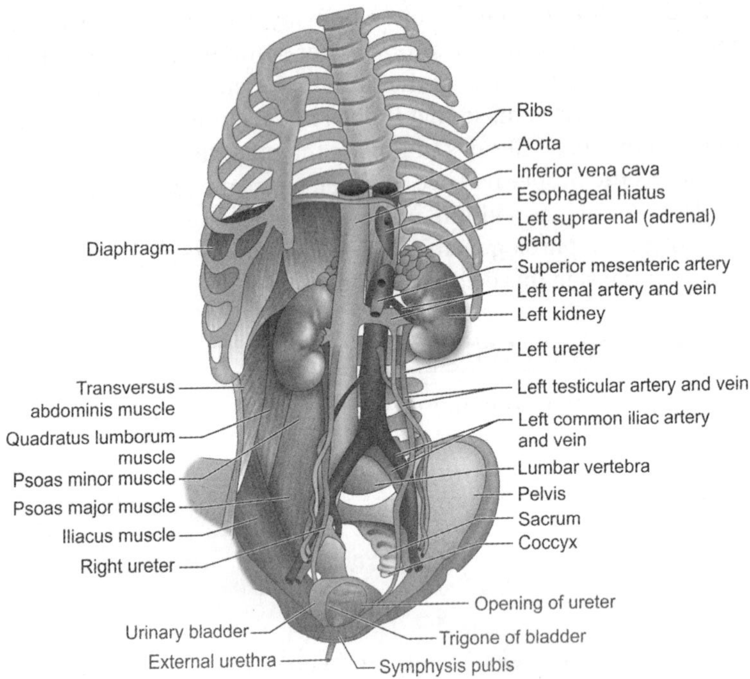

FIG. 10.2 Urinary system comprising names of different parts including kidneys

arteriole conveys blood to the glomerulus and an efferent arteriole carries the blood away from the glomerulus. The renal tubule has four sections, the proximal convoluted tubule, Henle's loop, distal convoluted tubule, and collecting tubule, where the excretion process for removing the waste products from the blood takes place. After this process, blood leaves the kidney by way of the renal vein. The waste material is carried out to the hollow chamber, the renal pelvis that is situated in the hilus. The adrenal gland lies on top of each kidney.

The concave central part of the kidney is called hilum, where the renal artery enters the kidney and renal vein leaves the kidney. The inner area is called medulla. Calices are the ducts, which join the renal pelvis. Pelvis is the collection point of urine as it is formed. The main function of the urinary system is to filter and remove waste products from the blood.

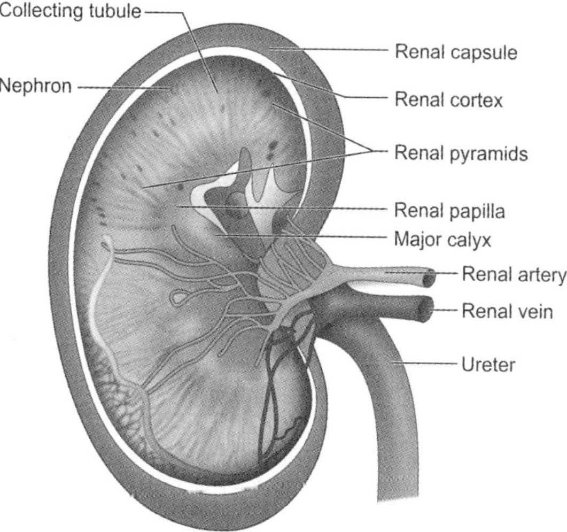

FIG. 10.3 Longitudinal section of right kidney with names of different parts

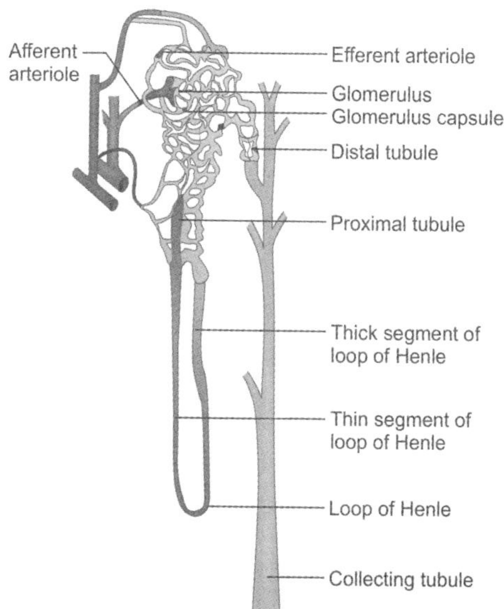

FIG. 10.4 Nephron with the names of different parts

Ureters

There are two ureters, which start from the pelvis of each kidney and opens into the urinary bladder. Each ureter is 25 cm long and they are fine, muscular tubes lined with mucous membrane. They convey urine in peristaltic waves from the kidney to the urinary bladder.

Urinary Bladder

The urinary bladder is a triangle-shaped muscular bag, situated in the pelvic cavity. It acts as a temporary reservoir for the urine. The neck of the bladder has a sphincter muscle to stop the backflow of the urine from the bladder. The voluntary action controls the external muscle sphincter, which opens only when the desire to void arises. The trigone is a triangular space at the base of the bladder where the ureters enter and the urethra leads out.

Urethra

Urethra is a canal leading from the bladder to discharge urine from the urinary bladder. The external opening of the urethra is called urethral or urinary meatus. Urethra is a common passage for urine and seminal fluid in the male, while in the female it is the passage for urine only. The length of the male urethra is longer than the female. It measures about 20 cm in male and 8 cm in female. The male urethra has three parts, prostatic part is surrounded by the prostate gland; the ejaculatory ducts and the ducts of the prostate gland open into it, the membranous part and penile part is surrounded by the corpus spongiosum of the penis.

Adrenal Glands (Suprarenal Glands)

There are two glands, which are endocrine glands located above each kidney. The functioning of the adrenal glands are explained in the endocrine system.

EXCRETION PROCESS OF URINE (FLOWCHART 10.1)

Blood enters each kidney through the renal artery. These arteries, divides into small arteries called arterioles and these are located

FLOWCHART 10.1 Excretion process of urine

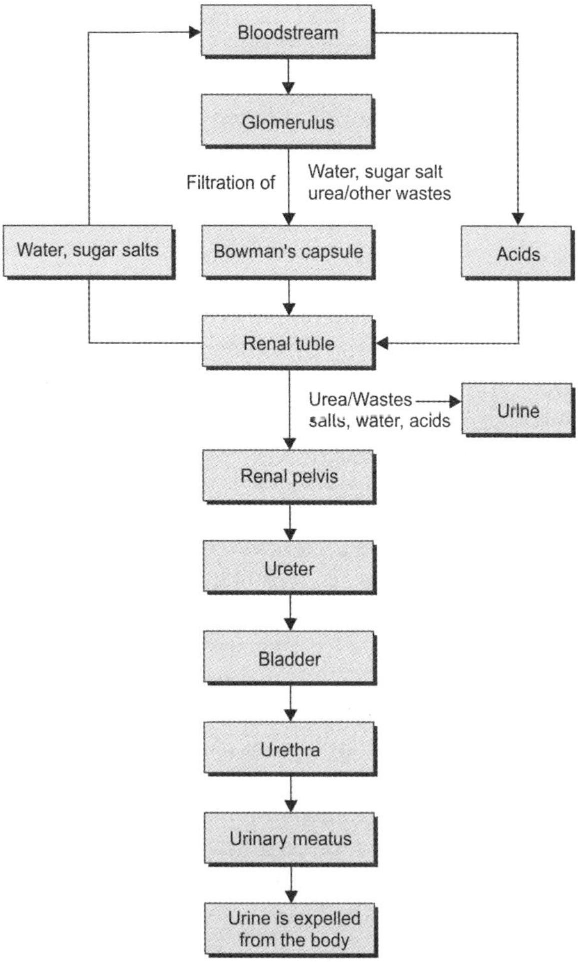

throughout the cortex of the kidney. The blood from the arteriole leads to the tiny smaller blood vessels called capillaries, which are collectively called glomeruli, and here the process of formation of urine begins. The three steps involved in this process are filtration, reabsorption and secretion.

The filtration process starts at the glomeruli, where the water, salts, sugar and nitrogenous waste such as urea, creatinine, and uric acid are filtered out through the thin walls of the glomeruli. These filtered products are collected by the Bowman's capsule, a cup-like structure holding the glomeruli and the fluid formed is called filtrate. During filtration, some of the essential chemicals for healthy living such as water, sugar, salts are also filtered out with the wastes.

When this filtrate passes through the four sections of the renal tubule, certain amount of these filtered products such as water, some of the electrolytes and amino acids are absorbed by the peritubular capillaries, thus re-entering the circulating blood. In the convoluted tubules much of the water, salts, etc. are returned to the blood supply while the remainder is passed into the collecting tubules, and then into the kidney pelvis via the pyramids and calyces as urine. The final stage of urine production occurs when specialized cells of the collecting tubules secrete ammonia, uric acid and other substances directly into the lumen of the tubule. Here thousands of renal tubule deposit urine into the central renal pelvis, a space that fills most of the medulla of the kidney. Blood leaves the kidney via the renal vein. The urine is then passed via the ureters into the urinary bladder, where it is temporarily stored. The exit area of the bladder to the urethra is closed by sphincters, which do not permit urine to leave the bladder. As the bladder fills up, however, there is a point at which muscular contractions of the walls of the bladder begin and pressure is placed on the base of the urethra, which causes the desire to urinate. This process of muscular contractions, so as to pass urine is called *micturition.*

Blood flow should be maintained constantly through the kidneys. When the flow of blood is reduced, a substance called renin is released by the kidney, which ultimately increases the blood pressure and blood flow in the kidneys is restored to normal.

Chapter Summary

The male and female urinary systems consist of four major structures they are (1) ....

Urinary System

The urinary system act as the regulator of extracellular products of the body by determining the harmful products in the blood plasma and selectively filtering them from the blood. Included in the products that must be removed from the body are nitrogen wastes and excess fluid electrolytes (sodium, potassium and calcium). One of the nitrogenous products is urea. This substance is produced when body tissues metabolize protein. High concentration of urea in the blood causes a toxic condition known (2) ....

The blood collects urea and other waste materials from body tissues and conveys these materials to the kidneys. In the kidneys, microscopic structures called nephrons filter these substances from the blood as they form a complex fluid called urine. It eventually expelled from the body.

Answers

1. A pair of kidneys, two ureters, a bladder and a urethra
2. Uremia

Review Questions

Exercise 1: Answer in One Word

1. The male and female urinary systems consist of ___________ major structures.
2. One of the nitrogenous products is ___________.
3. Urea is produced when body tissues metabolize ___________.
4. High concentrations of urea in the blood cause a toxic condition known as ___________.
5. The blood collects urea and other waste materials from ___________.
6. The urea and other waste materials collected convey these materials to the ___________.
7. In the kidneys, microscopic structures called ___________.
8. Nephrons filter waste materials from the blood, fluid called ___________.
9. Two kidneys are located in the retroperitoneal area of the ___________.
10. Near the medial border is a slit like aperture, the hilus or ___________.
11. The hilum as an opening for a renal vein and a renal artery to enter the ___________.
12. Each ureter that conveys urine, in peristaltic waves, to the ___________.
13. The bladder is an expandable hollow organ, acts as a temporary reservoir for ___________.
14. During micturition (voiding), urine is expelled from the bladder through the ___________.
15. Kidney tissue comprises 1 million tiny functional structures called ___________.
16. The end products of urea, uric acid, and creatinine are removed by ___________.
17. Each nephron includes a renal corpuscle and a renal ___________.
18. What capsule encases the glomerulus?
19. How may sections each renal tubule consists of?
20. The phase of urine production, filtration, takes place in the ___________.

Exercise 2: Complete the Following

1. The organs of the urinary system are the ___________, ___________, ___________ and ___________.
2. The concave depression on the medial margin of the kidney is called ___________.
3. The ___________ is the functional unit of the kidney.

4. The main function of the kidney is to ___________ in the blood.
5. The wrinkles on the mucous membrane lining the bladder are called ___________.
6. The twisted cluster of capillary channels called ___________ is contained in the ___________ capsule.
7. Sectioning of kidney shows it to have an internal ___________.
8. Sectioning of kidney shows it to have an external ___________.
9. The process of muscular contractions so as to pass urine is called ___________.
10. ___________ endocrine glands are located above each kidney.

Answers

Exercise 1

1. Four
2. Urea
3. Protein
4. Uraemia
5. Body tissues
6. Kidney
7. Nephrons
8. Urine
9. Abdominal cavity
10. Hilum
11. Kidney
12. Bladder
13. Urine
14. Urethra
15. Urethra
16. Nephrons
17. Tubule
18. Bowman's capsule
19. Four sections
20. Renal corpuscle

Exercise 2

1. Kidneys (two), ureters (two), bladder, urethra
2. Hilum
3. Nephrons
4. Filter the waste and toxins
5. Rugae
6. Glomerulus, Bowman's
7. Medulla
8. Cortex
9. Micturition
10. Adrenal

11

CHAPTER

Reproductive System

On completion of this chapter, the student will be able to:

- List the organs of male and female reproductive system
- Know the process of reproduction (birth)
- Explain the series of events associated with maturation of the ovum (menstrual cycle)
- Describe the condition and stages of pregnancy

INTRODUCTION

The reproductive system plays a vital role in the reproduction of an individual. The organs and functions of the reproductive system differ in male and female. Reproduction is the union of the female sex cell (ovum) and male sex cell (sperm), which contains the genetic material called chromosomes. Each sex cell (male and female) has exactly 23 chromosomes. Male has 21 chromosomes and 2 autosomes (X and Y), which decides the sex of the newborn, whereas female has 23 chromosomes, when the ovum and sperm cell unite, the cell produced receives half of its genetic material complement of hereditary material. These sex cells are produced in special organs called gonads in the male and female. The female gonads are the ovaries and male gonads are the testes.

MALE REPRODUCTIVE SYSTEM

The male reproductive system performs two important functions, viz. production of the male sex cells (sperm), storage and transportation of the sperm. The parts of the male reproductive system (Fig. 11.1) are:

- Testes (singular: testis)
- Scrotum
- Seminiferous tubules
- Epididymis

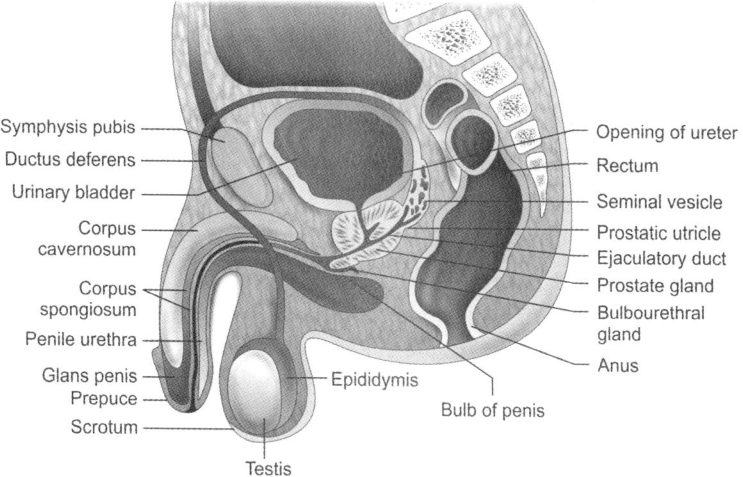

FIG. 11.1 Parts of the male reproductive system

- Vas deferens
- Seminal vesicles
- Ejaculatory duct
- Prostate gland
- Penis
- Urethra

Testes

The primary organ of male reproductive system is testis. The male gonad consists of pair of testes. The testes develop in the kidney region of the body and descends into the scrotum during embryonic development. They produce an important male hormone called testosterone, which is responsible for the secondary sexual character such as beard, pubic hair, voice deepening, proper development of male gonads and accessory organs, which secretes fluid to insure the lubrication and viability of the sperm.

Scrotum

The scrotum is a muscular sac enclosing the testes on the outside of the body. It lies between the thighs, and maintains the testes at lower temperature than that of the body, facilitating adequate maturation and development of sperm, which requires quite low temperature.

Seminiferous Tubules

Seminiferous tubules are small-coiled tubules in the testis and they produce sperm.

Epididymis

Epididymis is the tightly coiled tubule lying over the surface of the testis. The seminiferous tubule collectively meets at the epididymis. The spermatozoa become motile and are temporarily stored in epididymis.

Vas Deferens

The vas deferens is a narrow tubule, which starts from the epididymis runs down through the length of testes then turns upward again to reach the seminal vesicle. The vas deferens is about 2 feet long and carries the sperm up into the pelvic region, around the urinary bladder and down toward the urethra.

Seminal Vesicle

The seminal vesicles are glands located at the base of the urinary bladder and open into the vas deferens as it joins the urethra. It secretes a thick yellowish substance that nourishes the sperm cells and forms much of the volume of ejaculated semen.

Ejaculatory Duct

The ejaculatory duct is a tubule like structure where the vas deferens and seminal vesicle meet together.

Prostate Gland

The prostate gland is triple lobed cone-shaped organ, situated below the urinary bladder and surrounding the upper part of the urethra near the bladder neck. The prostate gland secretes a thin, alkaline substance that accounts for about 30% of seminal fluid and helps to protect the sperms from the acidic environment, and aids the motility of the sperms.

Two pea-shaped glands Cowper's gland or bulbourethral glands are located below the prostate and they also secrete fluid into the urethra.

Penis

The penis is the organ for copulation. It is cylindrical in shape composed of erectile tissue made up of three cylindrical bodies, viz. a pair of corpus cavernosum and one corpus spongiosum. It is enclosed by the urethra. The tip of the penis is soft and sensitive region called glans penis. A fold of skin known as the prepuce, which is freely movable, protects the glans penis.

Urethra

The urethra expels both semen and urine from the body. During ejaculation, the sphincter at the base of the bladder is closed. This not only stops the urine from being expelled with the semen but also prevents the sperm from entering the bladder.

Semen

Semen is a combination of fluid and spermatozoa, which is ejected from the body through the urethra. In the male, as opposed to the female, the genital orifice combines with the urinary opening.

The male sex cell, the spermatozoon (sperm) is microscopic-in volume, only one-third of the size of an erythrocyte and less than 1/100,000 th size of female ovum. It is relatively uncomplicated cell, composed of a head region, which contains nuclear hereditary material and a tail region, consisting of flagellum (hair like process), which makes the sperm motile, somewhat resembling a tadpole.

Only one spermatozoon of approximately 100 million sperm cells, which may be released during a single ejaculation can penetrate a single ovum and produce fertilization of the ovum. If more than one egg is passing down the fallopian tube when sperms are present, multiple fertilization are possible and twins, triplets, quadruplets and so fifth one may occur. Twins resulting from the fertilization of separate ova by a separate sperm called fraternal twins. These twins develop in separate placentae. Identical twins are formed from the fertilization of a single egg cell by a single sperm, where both the embryos share the same placenta.

FEMALE REPRODUCTIVE SYSTEM

The female reproductive system consists of organs, which produce ova and provide space for the growth of embryo. The female reproductive organs (Figs. 11.2 and 11.3) also secrete hormones such as estrogen and progesterone that contribute the secondary female sexual characteristics such as body hair, breast development, structural changes in bones and fat. The period when the secondary female sexual characteristics develop is called puberty. Ova are produced during the onset of the puberty period. When the ova is not fertilized the hormonal changes result in the shedding of the uterine lining and bleeding. This is called menstruation. When ova is fertilized in uterus that condition is called pregnancy, the normal gestation period is approximately 9 calendar months. The cessation of the fertility and diminishing of the hormone production is called menopause. The

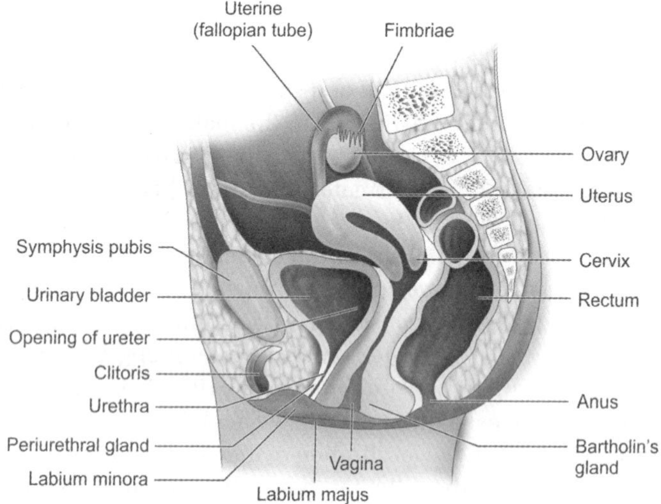

FIG. 11.2 Parts of the female reproductive system (lateral view)

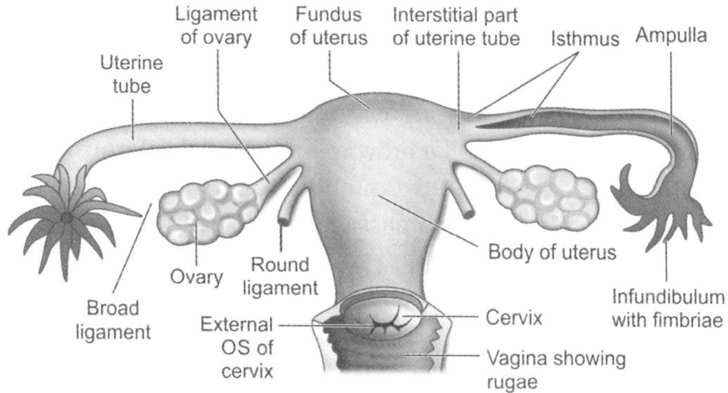

FIG. 11.3 Parts of the female reproductive system (anterior view)

TABLE 11.1 Organs of the internal and external genitalia

Internal genitalia	External genitalia
Ovaries	Vulva
Fallopian tubes	Labia majora
Uterus	Labia minora
Vagina	Hymen

period between the puberty and menopause is called reproductive period or childbearing age, it is normally between age of 15–44 years of a woman's age.

The major organs of female reproductive system can be divided into two, they are internal genitalia and external genitalia. The organs of the internal and external genitalia are detailed in Table 11.1.

The accessory organ of the female reproductive system is breasts.

Ovaries

Ovaries are the bean-shaped glands located in the pelvic cavity on either side of the uterus to which they are attached by the ovarian ligament. They produce ovum, which is the female reproductive cell and hormones such as progesterone and estrogen. These hormones are responsible for the menstrual cycle and prepare the uterus for pregnancy when the fertilization takes place and also plays a vital role in development of secondary sexual characteristics.

Fallopian Tubes

The fallopian tubes are the muscular tube like structure measuring 5½ inches which extends from ovaries to either side of the uterus. It transport ovum by a wavelike movement (peristalsis) from the ovary to the uterus. It takes for an ovum about 5 days to pass through the fallopian tube. It also acts as a passage for the ovum to pass from the uterus towards the ovaries.

Uterus

Uterus is a muscular pear-shaped organ. It lies in the pelvic cavity behind the urinary bladder and in front of the rectum. It is supported in position by ligaments and covered by three layers of tissue:

1. *Endometrium:* Inner lining of the uterus.
2. *Myometrium:* Middle muscular lining of the uterus.
3. *Perimetrium:* Outer covering of the uterus.

It is the organ, which stores and nourishes the embryo from the time of fertilization until the fetus is born. It has three parts namely, the fundus, which is the upper round part; the corpus, which is the central part and the cervix the external part, which extends to vagina.

Vagina

The vagina is a muscular tube of 7.5 cm long, extending from the uterus to the exterior of the body. It is lined by mucous membranous fold, which provides elastic quality. It serves as an organ for sexual intercourse and receptor of semen and passageway for the delivery of the fetus. Besides these, it discharges the menstrual flow.

There are two glands situated on either side of the vaginal orifice, they are called Bartholin's gland. The clitoris is an organ of sensitive erectile tissue located anterior to the vaginal orifice and in front of the urethral meatus. The clitoris is similar in structure to the penis in the male.

External Genitalia

The organs of the external genitalia are collectively called vulva. The vulva consists of labia majora the outer lips of the vagina and labia minora are the small and inner lips. The hymen is a mucous membrane, partially covering the entrance to the vagina. It is normally perforated, which permits the exit of menstrual discharge. The clitoris and Bartholin's gland are also parts of the vulva.

Breast

The breasts (Fig. 11.4) are two mammary (milk producing) organs, located in the upper anterior region of the chest. The breasts also contain fatty tissue, special lactiferous ducts and sinuses, which carry milk to the opening of nipple. The breast nipple is called mammary papilla and the dark-pigmented area around the mammary papilla is called areola. They are in rudimentary stage during the birth and they develop during the puberty period and the size of the breast increases during the pregnancy and when lactation takes place.

Menstrual Cycle

The menstrual cycle, which last long for 28 days is divided into four phases:

1. *Menstrual phase (1–5 days):* These are the days during which bloody fluid containing disintegrated endometrial cells, glandular secretion and blood cells passing from the uterus are discharged through vagina.
2. *Preovulatory phase (6–13 days):* Estrogen is released by the ovarian follicles to repair the endometrium (uterus lining). During this phase, one of the secondary follicles matures into a Graafian follicle, which is ready for ovulation.

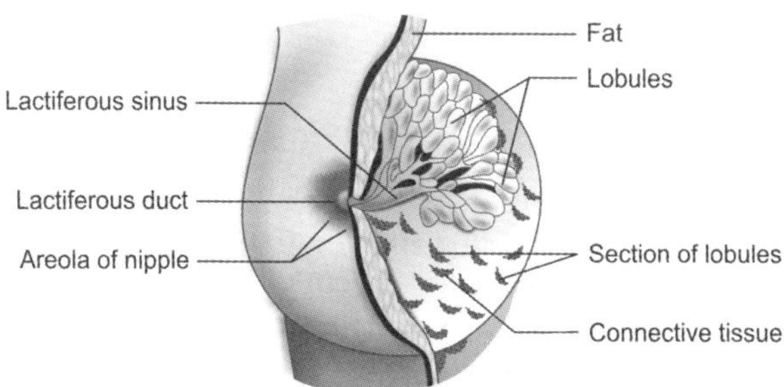

FIG. 11.4 Cross section of the breast and its parts

3. *Ovulatory phase (13–14 days):* On about the 14th day of the cycle, the Graafian follicle ruptures (ovulation) and the egg leaves the ovary to travel slowly down to the fallopian tube. This phase (14th day) is said to be the best period of copulation for the fertilization of ovum.
4. *Menstrual phase (15–28 days):* This represents the time between ovulation and the onset of next menses.

Following ovulation, the Graafian follicle collapses and forms a clot which is absorbed by the remaining follicular cells. These follicular cells enlarge, change character and form the corpus luteum or yellow body. The corpus luteum then secretes increasing quantities of estrogen and progesterone.

If fertilization and implantation do not occur, the decreased secretion of progesterone and estrogen then initiates the next menstrual cycle.

PREGNANCY

Pregnancy is the condition in which a zygote (the union of male gonad and female ovum) develops in the uterus. The placenta, which is the organ of communication between the mother and embryo, now forms within the uterine wall. The placenta is filled with a fluid called amniotic fluid, which breaks during the onset of labor. The hormone oxytocin instigate the vigorous contraction of the uterus to effect the delivery of the fetus. The normal gestation period is about 40 weeks. Immediately after delivery, a hormone called prolactin promotes the milk secretion to feed the newborn.

The product of conception up to the 3rd month is called embryo and later it is referred as fetus. During pregnancy, there will be a change in uterus, vagina and breasts.

Labor and Birth

The labor and birth can be classified into three stages:

1. *Dilation stage:* During this stage, the uterus contracts and the complete dilation of the cervix occurs.
2. *Expulsion stage:* This stage starts from complete dilation of the cervix to the birth of baby.
3. *Placental stage:* After the childbirth, when the uterine contractions discharge the placenta from the uterus.

Chapter Summary

Male Reproductive System

The male reproductive system serves two important functions. First it produces sperm, the male sex cell, which consists on half of the genetic material necessary to produce a living being. Second, it provides the structure necessary to transport and maintain viable sperm. The primary male reproductive organ consists of a pair of testes (singular testis), which are located in the external sac, the scrotum. Within the testes are numerous small tubes that twist and coil to form the (1)..................... These structures produce sperm, which is the male sex cell. The testes also secret testosterone, an androgenic hormone that develops and maintains secondary sex characteristics and influences adult male sexual behavior. Lying over the superior surface of each testis is a single, tightly coiled tube, the (2)..................... This structure stores sperm after it leaves the seminiferous tubules. The epididymis is the first duct through which firm passes after its production in the testes. Tracing the duct upward, the epididymis forms the vas deferens (seminal duct or ductus deferens), which is narrow tube that passes through the inguinal canal into the abdominal cavity. The vas extends over the top and down the posterior surface of the bladder, where it joins a duct leading from an accessory sex gland, the seminal vesicle. The union of the vas and the duct from the seminal vesicle forms the ejaculatory duct.

The seminal vesicle secrets approximately 60% of the fluid that is usually ejaculated during (3)..................... Thus, fluid contains nutrients that support sperm viability. The ejaculatory duct passes at an angle the rough the prostate gland, which is a triple-lobed organ fused to the base of the bladder where it joins the urethra. The prostate secretes a thin, alkaline substance that accounts for about 30% of the seminal fluid. Its alkalinity helps protect the sperm from the acidic environments of both male urethra and female vagina. Two pea-shaped glands, Cowper's glands or bulbourethral glands, are located below the (4).....................

They are connected by small duct to the urethra. Cowper's glands also provide an alkaline fluid that is necessary for the viability of the sperm. The penis is the male organ of copulation. It is a cylindrical organ composed of erectile tissue and it encloses the urethra. The urethra expels both (5)..................... from the body. During ejaculation, the sphincter at the base of the bladder is closed. This not only stops the urine from being expelled with the semen but also prevents the sperm from entering the bladder. The enlarged tip of the penis is the glans penis. It contains the urethral orifice (meatus). A movable hood of skin, called prepuce or foreskin, covers the glans penis.

Female Reproductive System

The female reproductive system consists of internal and external organs. The internal or essential organs of reproduction are the (6)....................

The external genitalia include the labia majora, labia minora, clitoris, vestibule of the vagina and the greater vestibular glands or Bartholin's glands. The combined structures of the external genitalia are known as vulva. Both the cervix and vagina are lubricated by the mucus secretions of the Bartholin's glands. These glands provide lubrication during sexual intercourse by secreting a mucoid acid substance.

Ovaries

The ovaries are almond-shaped glands located in the pelvic cavity, one on each side of the uterus. They produce both the ovum and egg, which is the female reproductive cell and various hormones. Two of the hormones secreted by the ovaries are estrogen and progesterone. These hormones are responsible for the menstrual cycle and menopause. In addition, both hormones prepare the uterus for implantation of the fertilized egg, help maintain pregnancy and promote growth of the placenta. Estrogen and progesterone also play an important role in the development of secondary sex characteristics.

Fallopian Tubes or Oviducts

Two fallopian tubes or oviducts extend laterally from superior angles of the (7).................... They transport ovum by a wave-like current (peristalsis) from the ovary to the uterus. In addition to conveying the ovum, an oviduct provides a passageway through which sperm travel from the uterus toward the ovary. Union of the ovum and sperm results in fertilization. Thus 9-month period of development (gestation, pregnancy within the uterus) begins with the fertilization of the egg.

Uterus and Vagina

The uterus is an organ that contains and nourishes the embryo from the time the fertilized eggs is implanted until the fetus is born. It is a muscular hollow, pear-shaped structure and is located in the pelvic area between the bladder and rectum. The uterus is normally in a position of antiflexion (bent forward), and it consists of three parts—the fundus, which is the upper-rounded part; the corpus or body, which is the central part and the cervix, which is sometime referred to as the (8)..................... and it extends into the top portion of the vagina. The vagina is a muscular tube ranges from 6.5 to 12.5 centimeters in length, and its lining consists of a mucous membrane fold that gives the organ an elastic quality. The vagina extends from the receptor of semen, the vagina discharges the menstrual flow. The vagina also acts as a passageway for the delivery of the fetus.

Menstrual Cycle

The menstrual cycle consists of approximately 28 days and can be grouped into four phases, which are used in describing the events of the cycle. The initial menstrual period (menarche) occurs between the ages of 9 and 18, the average being 12–13 years of age.

Menstrual cycle with four phases		
Phase I	Menstrual phase (first 5 day)	A discharge that is mixture of endometrium, blood, mucus and vaginal cells passes from the uterine cavity to the cervix, through the vagina and ultimately to the exterior
Phase II	Preovulatory phase (day 6-13)	Ovarian follicles produce more estrogen, which stimulates the repair of the endometrium. During this phase, one of the secondary follicles matures into a graafian follicle, which is ready for ovulation
Phase III	Ovulation (day 14)	About the 14th day, the graafian follicle ruptures (ovulation), and the egg cell leaves the ovary and enters the peritoneal cavity. The egg cell then drawn into the uterine tubes
Phase IV	Postovulatory phase (day 15–28)	This represents the time between ovulation and onset of the next menses
Following ovulation, the graafian follicle collapses and forms a clot, which is absorbed by the remaining follicular cells. These follicular cells enlarge, change character and form the corpus luteum or yellow body. The corpus luteum then secrets the increasing quantities of estrogens and progesterone.		

Menopause Manifestations

Menopause is the cessation of the (9) .... for the remainder of women's life time. It is usually diagnosed, if menorrhea (absence of menses) has persisted for 1 year and there are no other complications. The period of time in which symptoms of approaching menopause occur is known as climacteric period. Some common manifestations during the climacteric are shown in table given below.

Menopausal manifestations during the climacteric period	
Premenopausal	• Nervous • Irregular menses • Vasomotor symptoms (due to an effect on the diameter of blood vessels) • Instability (hot flashes)
Menopausal	• Frequent vasomotor symptoms • Cessation of menses • Atrophy of genitourinary tissue (wasting; a decrease in size of an organ or tissue
Postmenopausal	• Occasional vasomotor symptoms • Atrophic vaginitis • Atrophy of genitourinary tissue with decreased support • Osteoporosis

Pregnancy

Pregnancy is the condition in which a zygote (fertilized ovum) develops in the uterus. The normal gestation period is approximately 9 calendar months. The product of conception up to the 3rd month of pregnancy is referred to as the embryo. From the 3rd month to the time of birth, the unborn offspring is referred to as the fetus.

During pregnancy, the uterus changes its shape, size and consistency. The peritoneal covering becomes enlarged and there is an enormous increase in the muscle mass. The vaginal canal becomes elongated by the rise of the uterus in the pelvis. The mucosa thickens and secretions increases and there is a rise in the vascularity and elasticity of both the cervix and vagina. Pregnancy also causes enlargement of the (10) .... sometimes to the point of painfulness. On the whole, many changes are evident in all of body symptoms in order to accommodate the development and birth of the fetus.

Labor and Birth

Labor is the physiological process by which the fetus is expelled from the uterus. Labor occurs in three stages; the first stage of dilation, which begins with uterine contractions and terminates when there is complete dilation (10 cm) of the cervix. The second is the stage of expulsion. This is the time from complete cervical dilation to the birth of the baby. The last is the placental stage, or after birth. It begins shortly after childbirth when the uterine contractions discharge the placental from the uterus. The actual birth usually occurs in a short period of time provided there are no complications.

Answers

1. Seminiferous tubules
2. Epididymis
3. Sexual climax
4. Prostate
5. Semen and urine
6. Ovaries, fallopian tubes, uterus and vagina
7. Uterus
8. Neck of the uterus
9. Menses
10. Breasts

Review Questions

Exercise 1: Answer in One Word

1. What do male sex cell produce?
2. What do male sex cells contain to produce a living being?
3. The male reproductive organ consists of pair of ___________.
4. Testes are located in an external sac called the ___________.
5. Within the testes are numerous small tubes that twist and coil to form the ___________.
6. Lying over the superior surface of each testis is a single, tightly coiled tube, ___________.
7. The union of the vas and the duct from the seminal vesicle forms the ___________.
8. What percentage of fluid does the seminal vesicle secrete?
9. The seminal vesicle secretes fluid which contains nutrients that support ___________.
10. What is ejaculated during sexual climax is secreted by the seminal vesicle?
11. The prostate secretes a thin, alkaline substance about 30% of the ___________.
12. Two Cowper's glands, or bulbourethral glands, are located below the ___________.
13. What expels both semen and urine from the body?
14. During ejaculation, the sphincter at the base of the bladder is ___________.
15. The enlarged tip of the penis is called ___________.
16. A movable hood of skin, called the prepuce of foreskin that, covers the ___________.
17. The female reproduction system consists of internal and ___________.
18. The organs of the reproduction are the ovaries, fallopian tubes, uterus, and ___________.
19. Two fallopian tubes or oviducts extend laterally from superior angles of the ___________.
20. Both the cervix and vagina are lubricated by the mucus secretions of the ___________.
21. The ovaries are almond-shaped glands located in the ___________.
22. Two of the hormones secreted by the ovaries are estrogen and ___________.
23. The union of the ovum and sperm results in ___________.

24. The cervix is the neck of the uterus, and it extends into the top portion of the ___________.
25. The vagina also as a passageway for the delivery of the ___________.
26. How many days does the menstrual cycle consist of?
27. The corpus luteum secretes increasing quantities of estrogenic and ___________.
28. Menopause is the cessation of ___________.
29. How many days does the first phase of menstrual cycle consist of?
30. The menstrual preovulatory phase consists of how many days?
31. How many days does the menstrual ovulation phase consist of and when?
32. How many days does menstrual postovulatory phase consist of?
33. Pregnancy is the state in which a zygote (fertilized ovum) develops in the ___________.
34. How many months is the normal gestation period?
35. The product of conception up to the month of pregnancy is stated as the ___________.
36. The vaginal canal extended during pregnancy by rise of the uterus in the ___________.
37. Pregnancy also causes enlargement of the ___________.
38. Labor is the physiological process by which the fetus is expelled from the ___________.
39. The first stage of labor is called ___________.
40. The second stage of labor is called ___________.

Exercise 2: Complete the Following

1. The male reproductive cell is called ___________.
2. The chief male sex hormone is ___________.
3. The vase deferens are encased by the ___________.
4. The female reproductive cells are called ___________.
5. The functions of the ovaries are ___________.
6. The onset of menstruation is called ___________.
7. The cessation of the menstrual cycle is called ___________.
8. The smooth muscle, elastic tube extending from the uterine is called ___________.
9. The ___________ stage last from the second through the 8 week of pregnancy.
10. The only connection between the mother and fetus is the ___________.

Exercise 3: Match the Following

1. Pair of tubes encased by spermatic cords
2. Secretion discharged by male reproductive organ
3. Foreskin of penis
4. Male gland producing spermatozoa
5. Reproductive cells of the female
6. External female genitalia
7. Mucous membrane lining of the uterus
8. Interior of cervix
9. Saclike male structure
10. Neck of uterus
11. Elastic muscular tube below cervix, extending to body exterior
12. Developing human beginning with ninth week
13. Pad of fat in front of symphysis pubis
14. Pigmented portion of nipple
15. Reproductive cells of the male

A. Testis
B. Endocervix
C. Vagina
D. Mons pubis
E. Vas deferens
F. Prepuce
G. Areola
H. Vulva
I. Ova
J. Spermatozoa
K. Fetus
L. Cervix
M. Endometrium
N. Semen
O. Scrotum

Answers

Exercise 1

1. Sperm
2. Genetic material
3. Testes
4. Scrotum
5. Seminiferous tubule
6. The epididymis
7. Ejaculatory duct
8. 60
9. Sperm viability
10. Fluid
11. Seminal fluid
12. Prostate
13. Urethra
14. Closed
15. Glans penis
16. Glans penis
17. External organs
18. Vagina
19. Uterus
20. Bartholdi's glands
21. Pelvic cavity
22. Progesterone
23. Fertilization
24. Vagina
25. Fetus
26. 28 days
27. Progesterone
28. Menses
29. 5 days
30. 6–13 days
31. Day 14
32. Days 15–28

33. Uterus
34. 9
35. Fetus
36. Pelvis
37. Breasts
38. Uterus
39. Dilation
40. Expulsion

Exercise 2

1. Sperm cell
2. Testosterone
3. Spermatic cord
4. Ova
5. Ovulation, hormonal secretion
6. Menarche
7. Menopause
8. Vagina
9. Embryonic
10. Placenta

Exercise 3

1. E
2. N
3. F
4. A
5. I
6. H
7. M
8. B
9. O
10. L
11. C
12. K
13. D
14. G
15. J

12

CHAPTER

Oncology

> **On completion of this chapter, the student will be able to:**
>
> - Explain briefly about oncology
> - Differentiate between the malignant and benign tumors
> - List various types of malignant tumors
> - Describe the staging and grading of the cancer
> - List various types of cancer treatment

INTRODUCTION

Oncology is the study of tumors. Unrestrained and excessive multiplication of body cells producing lump or swelling, known as tumor or neoplasm. The neoplasm may be either benign or malignant. Malignant tumors or neoplasm accumulate as growth, which penetrate, compress and ultimately destroy the surrounding normal tissue. The malignant cells from the primary tumor site find their way into lymph channels or blood vessels and are carried to remote body structures by which secondary malignant neoplasms develop. This is called metastasis. Benign neoplasms are new growths that develop in body tissues. They are composed of the same type of cells as the tissue in which they are growing. When they grow bigger in size, then they harm the place by exerting pressure on surrounding structures. In general, benign tumors are not life-threatening; once they are removed, they usually do not reoccur.

DIFFERENCES BETWEEN MALIGNANT AND BENIGN NEOPLASMS

See Table 12.1.

DIFFERENT TYPES OF TUMORS

Carcinomas

Carcinomas, the largest group, are solid tumors, which are derived from epithelial tissue. Epithelial tissue is found on external and

TABLE 12.1 Differences between malignant and benign neoplasm

Malignant	Benign
Rapid growth could be seen	Grows slowly
Invasive and infiltrative	Encapsulated
Composed of tissue that does not resemble the tissue in which the neoplasm arises	Composed of highly organized and specialized tissue, that closely resembles the tissue in which the neoplasm arises
If left untreated, establish a new tumor site by infiltrating through blood and lymphatic vessels in the remote regions of the body	Does not spread to remote areas to form a secondary tumor
If left untreated, poses a risk to the patient	Generally, poses little risk, if any, to the patient

internal body surfaces, including skin, glands, digestive, urinary and reproductive organs. Almost all malignant neoplasms are carcinomas.

Sarcomas

Sarcomas are a rare type of cancer when compared to carcinomas and are derived from supportive and connective tissue, such as bone, fat, muscle, cartilage, bone marrow and lymphatic tissue or from blood cells. Sarcomas account approximately 10% of all malignant neoplasm.

Mixed Tissue Tumors

Mixed tissue tumors are derived from tissue which is capable of differentiating into epithelial as well as connective tissue. The tumors are thus composed of several different types of cells. Examples are mixed tissue tumors can be found in kidney, ovaries and testes.

STAGING

Staging is an attempt to define the extent of cancer by classifying it into three categories—T, N, and M. T represents the primary tumor site or place of origin; N represents local or regional node involvement; and M indicates whether metastasis is there or not. When the primary site

TABLE 12.2 Staging

T N M	Primary tumor Regional lymph nodes Distant metastasis
Tumor	
T_0 T_{IS} T_1, T_2, T_3, T_4 T_X	No evidence of primary tumor Carcinoma in situ Progressive increase in tumor size and involvement Tumor cannot be assessed
Nodes	
N_0 N_1, N_2, N_3, etc. N_X	Regional lymph nodes not demonstrably abnormal Increasing degrees of demonstrable abnormality of regional lymph nodes Regional lymph nodes cannot be assessed clinically
Metastasis	
M_0 M_1, M_2, M_3	No evidence of distant metastasis Ascending degrees of distant metastasis, including metastasis to distant lymph nodes TNM assignments may be grouped into small number of stages

contains classifications of T_1, T_2, T_3 or T_4, the higher number indicates progressive increases in tumor size and involvement. Similarly N_0, N_1, N_2 or N_3, represent progressively advancing nodular involvement. Finally, M_0, or M+ defines absence or presence of metastasis, respectively (Table 12.2).

GRADING

Grading is concerned with the microscopic appearance of the tumor cells, in other words, the degree of anaplasia. Generally, four grades are employed, which are numbered from 1 through 4. Neoplasms that are composed of cells that closely resemble the tissue from which they arise are given a grade 1 rating. The tissue demonstrates a minimum amount of anaplasia. Patients with grade 1 tumors have high survival rate, while patients with grades 2, 3, and 4 tumors, have a poorer survival rate. At the other extreme is grade 4, in which there is a great deal of anaplasia within the tumor. Such tumors are more serious and the prognosis is very poor. Grades 2 and 3 are intermediate grades between these two extremes.

CANCER TREATMENT

Cancer is treated by three major approaches, namely, surgery, radiation therapy and chemotherapy.

Surgery

The surgery is performed when the tumor is localized and gets the effective means of cure. Some common cancers in which surgery may be curative are those of the stomach, large bowel, breasts and endometrium, especially the accessory organs of the system.

Radiation Therapy

The goal of the radiation therapy is to deliver a maximal dose of ionizing radiation to the tumor tissue and a minimal dose to the surrounding normal tissue. In reality, this goal is difficult to obtain and usually one accepts a degree of residual normal cell damage as a sequel to the destruction of the tumor. The effect of high-dose radiation to cells is to produce damage to deoxyribonucleic acid (DNA) and thus inhibit cell replication and growth.

Chemotherapy

Chemotherapy is the treatment of cancer using drugs. It is probably the most important factor responsible for long-term survival in several types of cancer. Chemotherapy may be used alone or in combination with surgery and radiation.

Review Questions

Exercise 1: Answer in One Word

1. The newly formed cells increase at an uncontrolled rate, producing a ____________.
2. Lump or swelling is known as a tumor or ____________.
3. These neoplasms may be either benign or malignant ____________.
4. Benign neoplasms are new growths that develop in the body ____________.
5. Benign neoplasms are within a capsule-don't invade the surrounding ____________.
6. When benign tumor is there is no pressure on other organs excision is ____________.
7. As a general rule, however, benign tumors are not life-____________.
8. Once benign tumors are removed, they usually do not ____________.
9. The malignant neoplasm cells do not resemble tissue in which they are ____________.
10. Malignant tumor cells lack specialization in both structure and ____________.
11. Malignant neoplasms spread to normal tissues due to non-____________.
12. The malignant is invasive growth develops by either direct extensions or ____________.
13. In direct extension, the malignant tumor grows directly into normal ____________.
14. Which tumors encapsulated the tissues—Malignant or Benign?
15. Which tumor non-encapsulated the tissues—Malignant or Benign?
16. Which tumor does not spread to remote areas of the body? Malignant or ____________.
17. Which cells of the neoplasm metastasise to remote regions of the body?
18. Which neoplasms generally poses little risk, if any, to the patient?
19. Which neoplasm if left untreated poses a risk to the patient?
20. Oncology is the study of ____________.

Answers

Exercise 1

1. Lump
2. Neoplasm
3. Malignant
4. Tissues
5. Tissues
6. Necessary
7. Threatening
8. Re-grow
9. Growing
10. Function
11. Encapsulated
12. Metastasis
13. Tissue
14. Benign
15. Malignant
16. Benign
17. Malignant
18. Benign
19. Malignant
20. Tumor

13

CHAPTER

Psychiatry

On completion of this chapter, the student will be able to:

- Understand briefly about psychiatry, and psychotherapy
- Know different techniques involved in psychotherapy
- Define terms, which describe psychiatric symptoms

INTRODUCTION

The branch of medicine, which deals with study, treatment and prevention of mental illness. Madness is different from psychiatry. A psychiatric condition, if untreated, may develop into insane condition, which may become madness.

Psychotherapy is the treatment of emotional problems by psychological techniques (Table 13.1). There are different techniques involved in psychotherapy.

PSYCHIATRY DISORDERS

Affective Disorders

Disorder of mood, e.g., manic-depressive illness, major depressions, etc. Manic depressive illness is characterized by alternating moods of mania such as excitement, activity, exalted feelings and decreased in need for sleep. Major depression, involves, severe, dysphoric mood, such as sadness, hopelessness, irritability and worry, etc.

Anxiety Disorders

Anxiety disorders are characterized by the experience of unpleasant tension, distress and troubled feelings, such as phobias and anxiety states.

TABLE 13.1 Description of different types of psychotherapy

Types	Explanation
Behavior therapy	Conditioning the primary feelings of the patients
Group therapy	Patients are educated through group discussions in front of invited audience
Sex therapy	Mainly deals with solving psychosexual disorders such as frigidity, impotence and premature ejaculation
Family therapy	This deals with the common problems of a family
Psychoanalysis	This is a long-term form of psychotherapy, to resolve internal conflicts, by allowing the patients to bring their unconscious emotions, such as free association and transference (recollecting the early past incidence)
Hypnosis	Therapy by recovery of deeply repressed memories
Play therapy	Therapy given to children through toys and plays to express conflicts, and feelings, which he/she is unable to communicate directly
Electroshock therapy	Treatment applied to the brain by producing convulsions, through electric current, chiefly for severe depressions
Drug therapy	Treatment by drugs such as antianxiety agents (diazepam), antipsychotic tranquilizers (chlorpromazine), lithium, anti-depressants, etc.

Somatoform Disorders

Somatoform disorders in which the patient's mental conflicts, are expressed as physical symptoms, such as abdominal pain, nausea, vomiting, chest pain, loss of functions in parts of body (difficulty in swallowing), loss of voice, deafness, etc. In conversion disorders (hysterical neurosis), the patient usually has a feared, but unconscious conflict, which threatens to escape from repression. Hypochondriasis is a somatoform disorders, in which the patient has preoccupation, with body pains, and discomforts.

Disassociate Disorders (Hysterical Neurosis)

The symptoms of this disorder are psychogenic amnesia and multiple personality. This disorder is characterized by inability to remember important personal information, unexpected travel away from home or work (with amnesia).

Psychosexual Disorders

Psychosexual disorders include sexual perversion, in which the patient's psychological sexual identity from his/her gender identity.

Transvestism

Dressing in the clothes of opposite sex.

Exhibitionism

Compulsive need to expose one's genitals.

Sexual Masochism

Achievement of sexual pleasure from suffering.

Transsexualism

Desire to change anatomic sexual characteristics, stemming from the fixed conviction that one is a member of the opposite sex. Such a person often seeks medical and surgical treatment to bring their anatomy into conformity with their belief.

Fetishism

Achieving sexual gratification by substituting an inanimate object for a human love object.

Voyeurism

An abnormal desire, to look at sexual organs or acts.

Sexual Sadism

Achievement of sexual pleasure, by inflicting physical or psychological pain.

Personality Disorders

Personality disorders are behavioral disorders acceptable to the individuals, but produce, conflict with others who interact with the same individuals.

Antisocial

No loyalty or concern for others and without moral standards.

Passive Aggression

Individual shows aggressive feelings in passive ways, such as stubbornness, helplessness, etc.

Histrionic

Emotional immaturity, and dependent having general dissatisfaction with themselves and angry feelings about the world.

Narcissistic

Pompous sense of self-importance and preoccupation, with the fantasy of success, and power.

Paranoid

Pervasive, suspiciousness and mistrust of people, jealous and quick to take offence.

Delirium

Mental disturbances associated with illness characterized by mental cloudiness and visual hallucinations.

Dementia

Characterized by loss of memory and intelligence. The most common is senile dementia.

Schizophrenic Disorders

Schizophrenic disorders is a major psychotic disorder characterized by withdrawal from reality into inner world of disorganized thinking and feeling. Symptoms are bizarre delusions, auditory hallucinations, hearing imaginary voices, and incoherent speech.

Paranoic Disorders

In this disorder, patient will have persistent delusions or persecution and jealousy.

Chronic Alcoholism

Addition to alcohol consumption, may present psychological symptoms such as hallucinations, amnesia, with physical ailments, such as cirrhosis of liver and brain damage. Patient will be unable to remember and resorts to confabulation (lying).

Drug Dependence (Substance Induced Disorders)

Diseases due to addiction to drugs such as opioids (heroin, morphine, etc.), sedatives (barbiturates, diazepam, etc.), cocaine and hallucinogen-type drugs.

14

CHAPTER

Medical Psychology

On completion of this chapter, the student will be able to:

- Understand briefly about psychology and psychologists
- Describe abnormal, clinical, cognitive psychology
- Explain community, comparative and counseling psychology
- Know health, industrial, organizational and occupational health psychology
- Illustrate personality, social and qualitative and quantitative psychology

DEFINITION

Psychology (literally means 'study of the soul' or 'study of the mind') is an academic and applied discipline, which involves the scientific study of human or animal mental functions and behaviors. In the field of psychology, a professional researcher or practitioner is called psychologist. In addition or opposition to employing scientific methods, psychologists often rely upon symbolic interpretation and critical analysis, although less frequently than other social sciences such as sociology.

Psychologists generally study such observable fact such as perception, cognition, attention, emotion, motivation, personality, behavior and interpersonal relationships and also consider the mind. A neuropsychologist attempts to understand the role of mental functions in individual and social behavior, in order to explore the underlying physiological and neurological processes.

Psychological knowledge is applied to various areas of human activity including the family, education, employment and the treatment of mental health problems. Psychology includes many subfields as diverse as human development, sports, health, industry, media and law, and integrate research from the social sciences, natural sciences and humanities.

Psychology encompasses a vast domain and includes many different approaches to the study of mental processes and behavior.

Below are the major areas of inquiry that comprise psychology. A comprehensive list of the subfields and areas within psychology can be found at the list of psychology topics and list of psychology disciplines.

ABNORMAL PSYCHOLOGY

Abnormal psychology is the study of abnormal behavior in order to describe, predict, explain and change abnormal patterns of functioning. Abnormal psychology studies the nature of psychopathology and its causes, and this knowledge is applied in clinical psychology to treat patients with psychological disorders.

It is normally difficult to draw the line between normal and abnormal behaviors. In general, abnormal behaviors must be maladaptive and cause an individual significant discomfort in order to be of clinical and research importance. According to the DSM-IV-TR, behaviors may be considered abnormal if they are associated with disability, personal distress, the violation of social norms or dysfunction (Fig. 14.1).

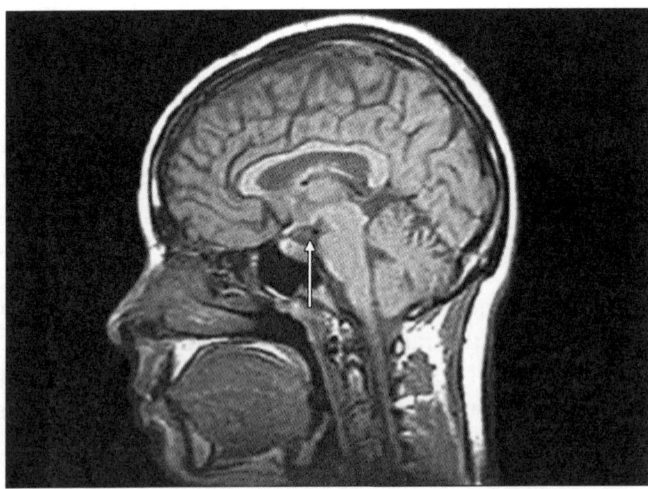

FIG. 14.1 Magnetic resonance imaging (MRI) depicting the human brain. The arrow indicates the position of the hypothalamus

BIOLOGICAL PSYCHOLOGY

Biological psychology is the scientific study of the biological, status of behavior and mental states. Bearing in mind all behavior as entangled with the nervous system, biological psychologists feel it is sensible to study how the brain functions in order to understand behavior. This is the approach taken in behavioral neuroscience, cognitive neuroscience and neuropsychology. Neuropsychology is the branch of psychology that aims to understand how the structure and function of the brain relate to specific behavioral, and psychological processes. Neuropsychology is particularly concerned with the understanding of brain injury in an attempt to work out normal psychological function. Cognitive neuroscientists often use neuroimaging tools, which can help them to observe, which areas of the brain are active during a particular task.

CLINICAL PSYCHOLOGY

Clinical psychology includes the study and application of psychology for the purpose of understanding, preventing and relieving psychologically-related distress or dysfunction and to promote subjective well-being, and personal development. The psychological assessment and psychotherapy are part of general study, and clinical psychologists may also engage in research, teaching, consultation, and program development and administration. Some clinical psychologists may focus on the clinical management of patients with brain injury, which is known as clinical neuropsychology. In many countries, clinical psychology is a profession that deals with mental health.

The clinical psychologist perform the work that likely to be influenced by various therapeutic approaches, all of which involve a formal relationship between professional and client that could be an individual, couple, family or small group of community. The various therapeutic approaches and practices are associated with different theoretical perspectives, and employ different procedures anticipated to form a therapeutic alliance, explore the nature of psychological problems, and persuade new ways of thinking, feeling or behaving. There are four major theoretical perspectives that are psychodynamic, cognitive behavioral, existential-humanistic and systems or family therapy. There has been a growing movement to integrate the various therapeutic approaches, especially with an increased understanding of issues regarding culture, gender, spirituality and sexual orientation. With the advent of more vigorous research findings regarding psychotherapy, there is evidence that most of the major therapies are about of equal effectiveness, with the key common element being a strong therapeutic association. In view of new findings and conducting various training programs, psychologists are now adopting an eclectic therapeutic orientation that has been found very useful and significant outcome.

COGNITIVE PSYCHOLOGY

Cognitive psychology studies cognition, the mental processes underlying mental activity. The research that made interesting to explore more on learning, perception, problem solving, reasoning, thinking, memory, attention, language and emotion, and other related areas. Classical cognitive psychology is associated with a school of thought known as cognitivism, whose adherents argue for an information processing model of mental function that consist of functionalism and experimental psychology.

As far as the cognitive science is concerned is an interdisciplinary enterprise of cognitive psychologists, cognitive neuroscientists, researchers in artificial intelligence, linguists, human-computer interaction, computational neuroscience, logicians and social scientists. In order to stimulate phenomena of interest computational models are occasionally used. Computational models provide a tool for studying the functional organization of the mind and neuroscience provides measures of brain activity. To understand the activities of both models play an important role.

COMMUNITY PSYCHOLOGY

In a social welfare state, community is one of fundamental ingredient in the society and in that community psychology plays a vital role and deals with the relationships of the individual to communities and the wider humanity. Community psychologists seek to understand the quality of life of individuals, families, communities and society.

Their aim is to enhance improve quality of life through collaborative research and efficient practice.

Community psychology as a routine makes use of various perspectives within and outside of psychology to address issues of communities, the relationships within them and people's attitudes, and behaviors about them. Through collaborative research and practice, community psychologists hunt for to understand, and enhance to improve quality of life for individuals, families, communities, and society as whole. Community psychology besides curative, takes a public health approach and focuses on prevention and early intervention as a means to solve problems in addition to treatment. The psychologist had in-depth deliberations and discussions found that the perspective of community psychology as an ecological perspective with the person-environment fit being the focus of study and action instead of attempting to change the person or the environment when an individual or family is seen as having a problem. Timely understand the problem and providing appropriate solution would improve greatly.

COMPARATIVE PSYCHOLOGY

Comparative psychology refers to the study of the behavior and mental life of human being as well as animals. It is extended disciplines outside of psychology that study animal behavior such as etiology. Although the field of psychology is primarily concerned with humans, their behavior and mental processes of animals is also an important part of psychological research. This being either as a subject in with strong emphasis about evolutionary links and somewhat more controversially, as a way of gaining an insight into human psychology.

COUNSELING PSYCHOLOGY

Counseling psychology seeks to facilitate personal and interpersonal functioning across the life span with a focus on emotional, social, vocational, educational, health related, developmental, and organizational concerns. Counselors are primarily clinicians, using psychotherapy and other interventions in order to treat patients and potential patients. As conventionally, counseling psychology has been focusing more on normal developmental issues and on a daily basis stress rather than psychopathology, but this distinction has softened over time. Counseling psychologists are employed in a variety of settings, including hospitals, schools, universities, governmental organizations, businesses, private practice and community mental health centers, and also nonprofit religious healthcare organizations.

CRITICAL PSYCHOLOGY

Critical psychology its name indicates the seriousness that applies the methodology of critical theory to psychology. Accordingly, it seeks the supportive roles that psychology and psychologists play, often inadvertently, in oppressive ideologies, and it tries to replace these roles with ones that can transform oppressive social structures. Critical psychology operates on the belief "that mainstream psychology has institutionalized a narrow view of the field's ethical mandate to promote human welfare", and critical psychology endeavors to broaden the view of that mandate. The critical psychology is under transformation to find new ways and methods to deal cases in an effective ways.

A critical psychologist might ask whether a case with work stress necessitate efforts to change the macrolevel systems that control the work, rather than to treat in isolation those individuals who experience the anxiety and pressure. One might also ask why peoples efforts fail to incorporate a focus on human rights and social justice in complex societies. In short, critical psychology seeks, where it considers appropriate, to raise psychology's level of analysis from the individual to family and society, and to render psychology more transformative than superficially ameliorative. Critical psychology has been applied to a wide range of psychologies other subfields and many of its practitioners are employed in conventional psychological professions. As the lifestyle of people all over the globe is changing in a rapid manner, the critical psychology's role would become inevitable.

DEVELOPMENTAL PSYCHOLOGY

The growth of the human mind through the course of lifetime, the developmental psychology seeks to understand how people come to understand, perceive and act within their life span, and how these processes transform as the child grow older. This change focuses mainly on intellectual, cognitive, neural, social or moral development. Researchers who study children use a number of different types of research methods and techniques to make observations in natural settings or to employ them in experimental situation to find the results. Such methods and techniques often applied in specially designed games and activities that are both enjoyable for the child and scientifically useful to the executors and researchers to study the mental processes of small infants and children of less IQ. In addition to studying children, developmental psychologists also study aging and processes throughout the life span, from the infant stage to child growth, youth, adolescent and old age. Developmental psychologists has become a regular and continuous field to conduct research to evolve news techniques and methods to deal with newly emanating problems in the individual, families and community as a whole.

EDUCATIONAL PSYCHOLOGY

The work of child psychologists such as Lev Vygotsky, Jean Piaget and Jerome Bruner has been influential in creating teaching methods and educational practices. Educational psychology is often included in the syllabus of teacher education programs, at least in North America, Australia and New Zealand. Educational psychology is the study of how humans learn in educational settings, the effectiveness of educational interference within the set educational program, add value to the effective teaching psychology and the social psychology. The institutions where the child psychology and social psychology are imparted have to bear the practical needs of modern medicine, and psychological issues that are in vogue.

EVOLUTIONARY PSYCHOLOGY

Evolutionary psychology explores the genetic roots of mental and behavioral patterns, and that common patterns may have emerged because they were highly adaptive for humans in the environments of their evolutionary past. Fields closely related to evolutionary psychology are animal behavioral ecology, human behavioral ecology, dual inheritance theory and sociobiology. Memetics, founded by Richard Dawkins, is a related, but competing field that proposes cultural evolution can occur in a Darwinian sense, but independently of Mendelian mechanisms; it is therefore, examines the ways in which thoughts or memes, may evolve independently of genes in an evolutionary span of period.

FORENSIC PSYCHOLOGY

The legal, especially medical legal, are closely related with forensic psychology. The subject encompasses a broad range of practices including the clinical evaluations of defendants, reports to judges and attorneys, and courtroom testimony on given issues. Forensic psychologists are appointed by the court or hired by attorneys to evaluate defendants' competency to stand trial, competency to be executed, sanity and need for involuntary commitment. Forensic psychologists are involved in variety of psychological cases related to evaluate sex offenders and treatments and provide recommendations to the court through written reports, and testimony. Many of the questions, the court asks the forensic psychologist are generally concerned to legal issues. As a psychologist in some instance cannot answer all legal questions. For example, there is no definition of sanity in psychology. Rather, sanity is a legal definition that varies from place to place throughout the world. Therefore, a prime qualification of a forensic psychologist is an intimate understanding of the law, especially criminal law and now this has become a practicing profession, many lawyers have adopted as their specialized profession.

GLOBAL PSYCHOLOGY

The global psychology expands the aim of psychology to macrolevel trends; it examines the overwhelming consequences of global warming, economic destabilization and other large-scale phenomena, while recognizing that global sustainability can best be achieved by psychologically marinating sound individuals and cultures that could be useful to society. Global psychologists advocate a comprehensive, psychology, whose strength is its focus on the long-term well-being of all of humanity. Global psychology is matter of fact is a subfield of psychology that addresses the issues raised in the global sustainability debate for solutions to various psychological issues that emanate time-to-time.

HEALTH PSYCHOLOGY

Health psychology is mainly related to health illness and health care of needy clients. As we have seen the clinical psychology focuses on mental health and neurological illness. The health psychology is mainly concerned with the psychology of a much wider range of health-related behavior including healthy eating and living. The health psychology closely create working link between the doctor-patient relationship, a patient's understanding of health information and viewpoint about illness. Health psychologists generally involved in public health campaigns, examining the impact of illness or health policy on quality of life as a preventive promotive of psychological impact of health and social care that would build-up healthy society.

INDUSTRIAL/ORGANIZATIONAL PSYCHOLOGY

Industrial and organizational psychology (I/O) applies psychological concepts and methods to optimize human potential in the industrial and organizational workplaces. Personnel psychology, a subfield of industrial and organizational psychology that applies the principles and methods of psychology in selecting, and evaluating workers. The I/O psychology's and organizational psychology, surveys the effects of work environments, and its conditions, management involvement on worker motivation, job satisfaction, and welfare of workers in addition to maximize the productivity.

LEGAL PSYCHOLOGY

In the modern days with competitive society, along with the advancements in all the fields, there also parallel growing of criminality, unethical methods and sexual abuses and accidental, suicidal and homogenous issues are creeping heavily all over the globe. The need for legal settlements has become part of judiciary and prevent the growth, need for legal psychologist is inevitable. Legal psychology is a specialized field to study various issues prevalent in the society, public areas to explore the possibility of assisting the judiciary and society in minimizing the crime and other prevailing legal issues related to human elements that could be addressed. This profession has been engaged as an advisory body in policy makers for the security and well-being of people.

OCCUPATIONAL HEALTH PSYCHOLOGY

Occupational health psychology (OHP) is a discipline that emerged out of health psychology, industrial/organizational psychology, and occupational health. The OHP is concerned with identifying psycho-social characteristics of workplaces that give rise to problems in physical and mental health, e.g. depression. The OHP is concerned with psychosocial characteristics of workplaces as workers' way of working and employers decision, and attitudes of supervisors in getting the work done. The OHP also concerns itself with interference that can prevent or improve work-related health problems. Such interventions have definite beneficial implications for the employees and employers, and economic success of organizations. The OHP spends more on research areas of concern include workplace violence, unemployment and workplace safety.

PERSONALITY PSYCHOLOGY

Personality psychology studies enduring patterns of behavior, thought, and emotion in individuals, commonly referred to as personality. Theories of personality vary across different psychological schools of thought. According to Freud, personality is based on the dynamic interactions of the ego, superego. Trait theorists, in contrast, attempt to analyze personality in terms of a discrete number of key traits by the statistical method of factor analysis. The number of proposed traits has varied widely. An early model proposed by Hans Eysenck suggested that there are three traits that comprise human personality—extraversion-introversion, neuroticism, and psychoticism. Raymond Cattell proposed a theory of 16 personality factors. The 'Big Five', or Five-factor Model, proposed by Lewis Goldberg, currently has strong support among trait theorists. The personality theory carry different assumptions about such issues as the role of the childhood experience, behavior, forgets, strong and weak personality.

QUANTITATIVE PSYCHOLOGY

The term 'quantitative psychology' is relatively new and gradually gaining the ground as specialize branch of psychology. This covers the longer standing subfields psychometrics and mathematical psychology. Quantitative psychology involves the application of mathematical and statistical modeling in psychological research, and the development of statistical methods for analyzing and explaining behavioral data. Psychometrics is the field of psychology concerned with the theory and technique of psychological measurement, which includes the measurement of knowledge, abilities, attitudes and personality traits. Measurement of these phenomena is difficult and much research has been developed to define, and analyze such phenomena. Psychometric research typically involves two major research tasks, namely:

1. The construction of instruments and procedures for measurement.
2. The development and refinement of theoretical approaches to measurement.

MATHEMATICAL PSYCHOLOGY

Mathematical psychology is the subdiscipline that is concerned with the development of psychological theory in relation with mathematics and statistics. Basic topics in mathematical psychology include measurement theory and mathematical learning theory as well as the modeling and analysis of mental, and motor processes. Psychometrics is more associated with educational psychology, personality and clinical psychology. Mathematical psychology is more closely related to psychonomics/experimental and cognitive and physiological psychology, and (cognitive) neuroscience.

SOCIAL PSYCHOLOGY (FIG. 14.2)

The social psychology is playing very important role in hospital and patient care environment. These professionals have become indispensable in the care of patients. Social psychology is the study of social behavior and mental processes, with an emphasis on how humans think about each other and how they relate to each other. Social psychologists are especially interested in how people react to

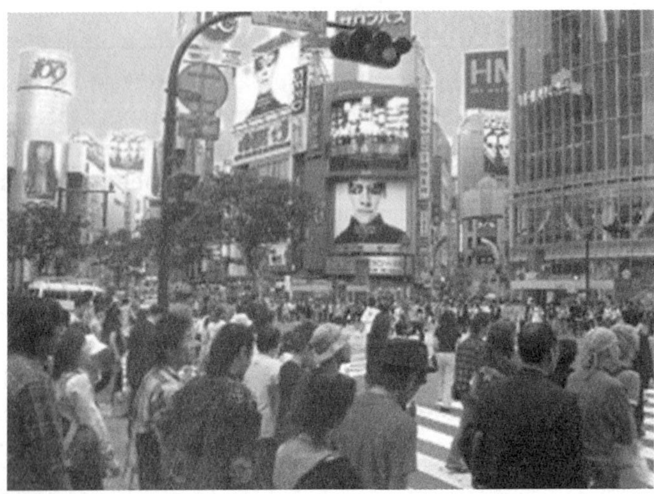

FIG. 14.2 Social psychology studies the nature and causes of social behavior

social situations. They study such topics as the influence of others on an individual's behavior and the formation of beliefs, attitudes, and stereotypes about other people. Social cognition fuses elements of social and cognitive psychology. In order to understand how people process, remember, and distort social information. The study of group dynamics reveals information about the nature and potential optimization of leadership, communication, and other phenomena that emerge at least at the microsocial level. In recent years, many social psychologists have become increasingly interested in implicit measures, mediational models and the interaction of both person, and social variables in accounting for behavior.

SCHOOL PSYCHOLOGY

School psychology is also an integral part of educational psychology and clinical psychology to understand and treat students with learning disabilities, to promote the intellectual growth of students in general and weak, and below average students in particular. The main object is also promoting safe, supportive and effective learning environments. School psychologists are trained in educational and behavioral assessment, intervention and prevention, and these psychologist are called professional 'psychologist'.

RESEARCH METHODS (FIG. 14.3)

Psychology leans to be drawing on knowledge from other fields to help explain and understand psychological phenomena. Additionally, psychologists make extensive use of the three modes of inference that were identified by CS Peirce—deduction, induction and abduction (hypothesis generation). While often employing deductive-nomological reasoning, they also rely on inductive reasoning to generate explanations. For example, evolutionary psychologists propose explanations of human behavior in terms of such behaviors' advantages for hunter-gatherers.

Academic psychologists may focus purely on research and psychological theory, aiming to further psychological understanding in a specific area, while other psychologists may work in applied psychology to deploy such knowledge for immediate and practical benefit. These approaches are not mutually exclusive and many psychologists will be involved in both researching, and applying psychology at some point during their career. Many clinical psychology programs aim to develop in practicing psychologists both knowledge of and experience with research and experimental

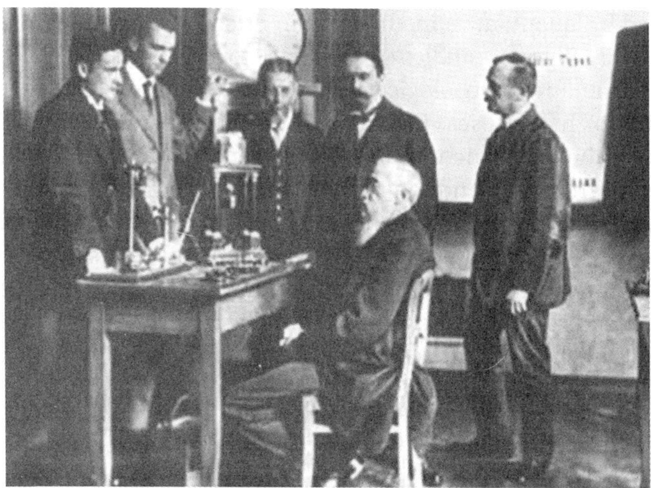

FIG. 14.3 Wilhelm Maximilian Wundt (seated) was a German psychologist, generally acknowledged as a founder of experimental psychology

methods, which they may interpret and employ as they treat individuals with psychological issues.

When an area of interest requires specific training and specialist knowledge, especially in applied areas, psychological associations are formed, and the association in collaboration with educational institutions establish educational and training requirements. These requirements may be laid down for institutional diplomas or university degrees in psychology, so that students acquire an adequate knowledge in a number of areas in order to provide manpower in this specialty, where psychologists are required to offer treatment.

QUALITATIVE AND QUANTITATIVE RESEARCH

Qualitative psychological research methods include interviews, first-hand observation and participant observation. Qualitative researchers aim to enrich interpretations or critiques of symbols, subjective experiences, or social structures. Research in most areas of psychology is conducted in accordance with the standards of the scientific method. Psychological researchers seek theoretically interesting categories and hypotheses from data, using qualitative or quantitative methods or both to explore the unknown to known knowledge. Similar hermeneutic and critical aims have also been served by 'quantitative methods', as in Erich Fromm's study of Nazi voting or Milgram's studies of obedience to authority.

Quantitative psychological research renders itself to the statistical testing of hypotheses. Quantitatively oriented research designs include the experiment, quasi-experiment, cross-sectional study, case-control study and longitudinal study. The measurement and operationalization of important constructs is an essential part of these research designs. Statistical methods include the Pearson product-moment correlation coefficient, the analysis of variance, multiple linear regression, logistic regression, structural equation modeling and hierarchical linear modeling. The quantitative and qualitative research is gaining foothold in all the fields.

PRACTICE

Some observers distinguish a gap between scientific theory and its application—in particular, the application of unsupported or unsound clinical practices. Critics say there has been an increase in the number of mental health training programs that are mainly remain theoretical knowledge and do not inspire scientific competence that help in practice. One disbeliever asserts that practices, such as 'facilitated communication for infantile autism'; memory-recovery techniques including body work; and other therapies, such as rebirthing and reparenting, may be doubtful or even dangerous, despite their qualification to practice. In 1984, Allen Neuringer had made a similar point regarding the experimental analysis of behavior. The institutions impart more practical knowledge and required skills to practice efficiently.

Chapter Summary

Clinical psychology includes the study and application of psychology for the purpose of understanding, preventing and relieving psychologically-related distress or dysfunction and to promote subjective well-being, and personal development. The psychological assessment and psychotherapy are part of general study, and clinical psychologists may also engage in research, teaching, consultation, and program development and administration. Some clinical psychologists may focus on the clinical management of patients with brain injury, which is known as clinical neuropsychology. In many countries, clinical psychology is a profession that deals with mental health. The clinical psychologist performs the work especially related to children with abnormal behavior and activities either they are too intelligent or too feeble to their age or parents or society is more concern about their future.

There are four major theoretical perspectives that are psychodynamic, cognitive behavioral, existential-humanistic and systems or family therapy. Cognitive psychology studies cognition, the mental processes underlying mental activity. The research that made interesting to explore more on learning, perception, problem solving, reasoning, thinking, memory, attention, language and emotion, and other related areas. Community psychologists seek to understand the quality of life of individuals, families, communities and their aim is to enhance improve quality of life through collaborative research and efficient practice. Counselors are primarily clinicians, using psychotherapy and other interventions in order to treat patients and potential patients. As conventionally, counseling psychology has been focusing more on normal developmental issues and on a daily basis stress rather than psychopathology. The critical psychology is under transformation to find new ways and methods to deal cases within an effective ways to promote human welfare, and critical psychology endeavors to broaden the view of that mandate.

Educational psychology is the effectiveness of educational interference within the set educational program, adds value to the effective teaching psychology and the social psychology. Evolutionary psychology explores the genetic roots of mental and behavioral patterns, and that common patterns may have emerged because they were highly adaptive for humans in the environments of their evolutionary past. The child psychology and social psychology concerned with the practical needs of modern medicine, and psychological issues that are in vogue. The medical legal, with forensic psychology are involved with the practices including the clinical evaluations of defendants, reports to judges, and courtroom testimony on given issues.

Forensic psychologists are involved in variety of psychological cases related to evaluate sex offenders and treatments and provide recommendations to the court through written reports, and testimony.

Health psychology is mainly related to health illness and health care of needy clients and the clinical psychology focuses on mental health and neurological illness. The health psychology is mainly concerned with the wider range of health-related behavior including healthy eating and living. The health psychology closely create working link between the doctor-patient relationship, a patient's understanding of health information and viewpoint about illness and involve in public health campaigns, examining the impact of illness or health policy on quality of life as a preventive promotive of psychological impact of health and social care that would build-up healthy society. The social psychology professionals have become indispensable in the care of patients social psychology is the study of social behavior and mental processes with an emphasis on how humans think about each other and how they relate to each other. Social psychologists are especially interested in how people react to social situations.

Personality psychology studies enduring patterns of behavior, thought, and emotion in individuals, commonly referred to as personality. Abnormal psychology studies the nature of psychopathology and its causes, and this knowledge is applied in clinical psychology to treat patients with psychological disorders. Biological psychology is the scientific study of the biological, status of behavior and mental states. There has been a growing movement to integrate the various therapeutic approaches, especially with an increased understanding of issues regarding culture, gender, spirituality and sexual orientation. With the advent of more vigorous research findings regarding psychotherapy, there is evidence that most of the major therapies are about of equal effectiveness, with the key common element being a strong therapeutic association. In view of new findings and conducting various training programs, psychologists are now adopting an eclectic therapeutic orientation that has been found very useful and significant outcome.

15

CHAPTER

Human Body Part Identification Exercises and Answers

EXERCISES

1. Identify the figure and name each level.

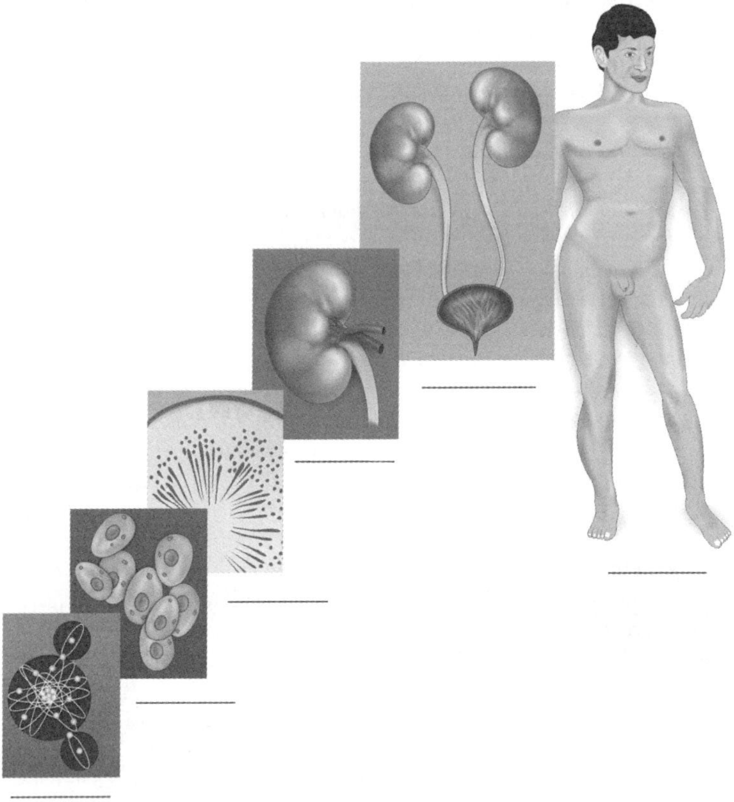

FIG. 1 AP evolution of human body

2. Identify the part name on indicated lines.

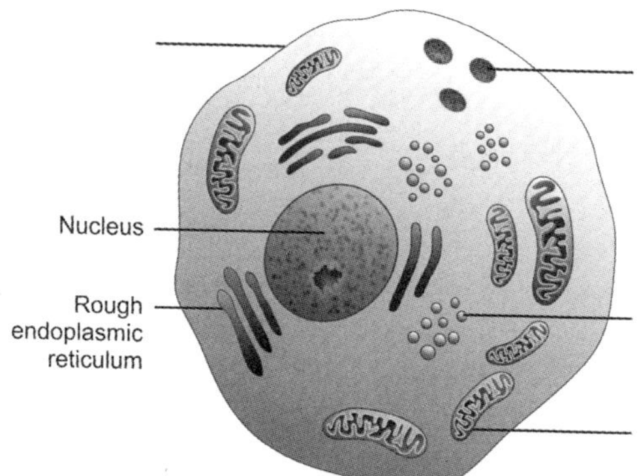

FIG. 1.1 Structure of cell

3. Identify the part name on indicated lines.

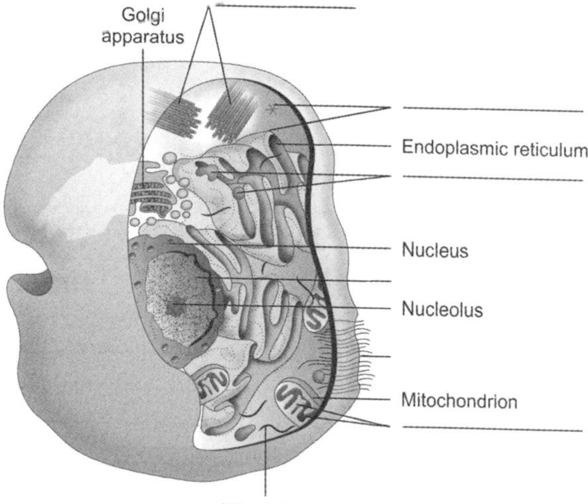

FIG. 1.2 Parts of the cell

4. Identify the part name on indicated lines.

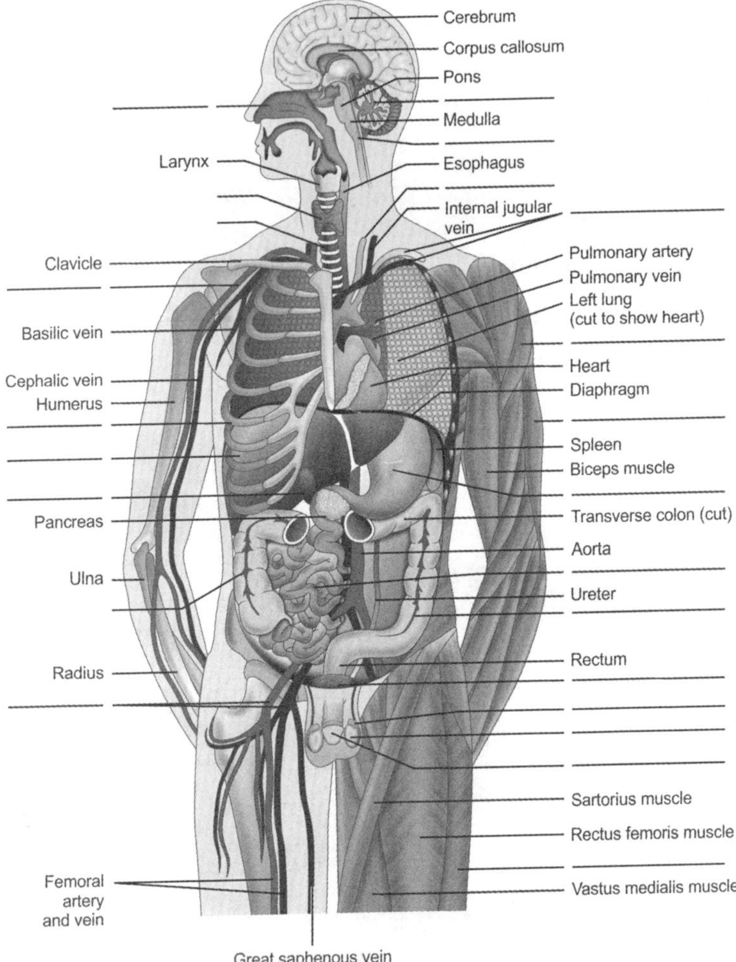

FIG. 1.3 Overview of body structure and organs

5. Identify the part name on indicated lines.

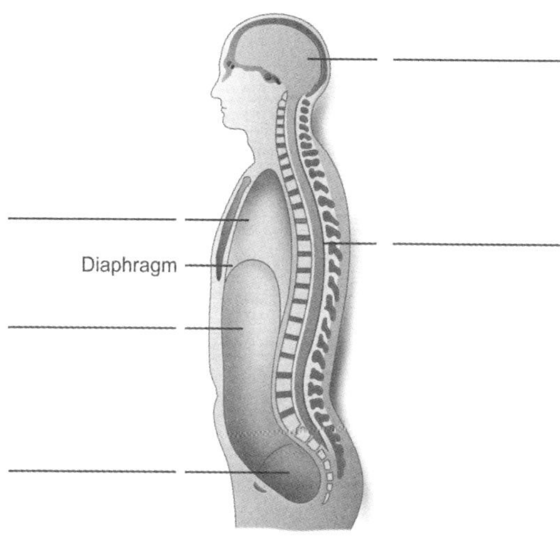

FIG. 1.4 Body cavities

6. Identify the part name on indicated lines.

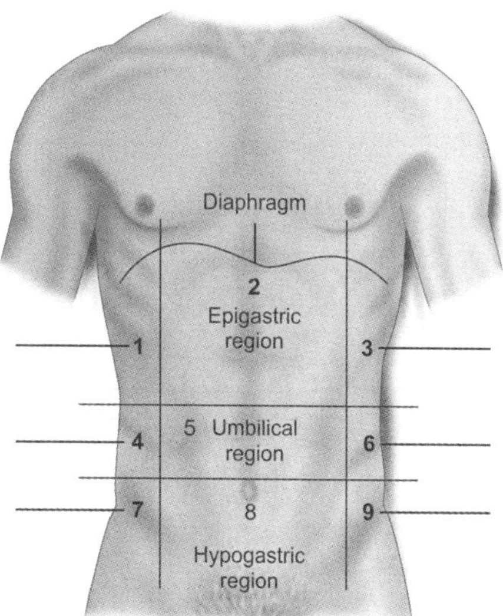

FIG. 1.5 Anatomical divisions of the body

7. Identify the part name on indicated lines.

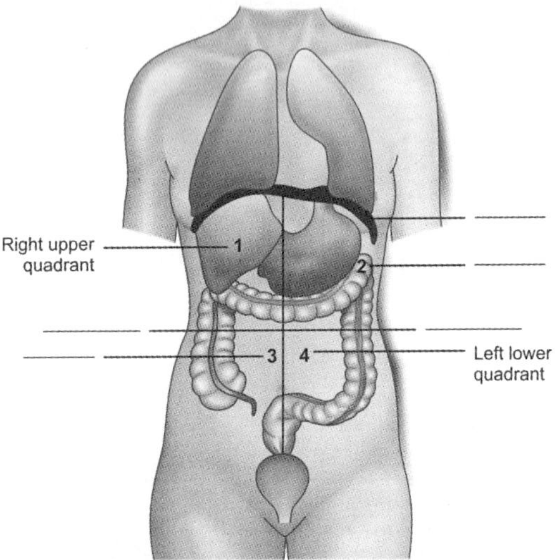

FIG. 1.6 Clinical divisions of the abdomen

8. Identify the part name on indicated lines.

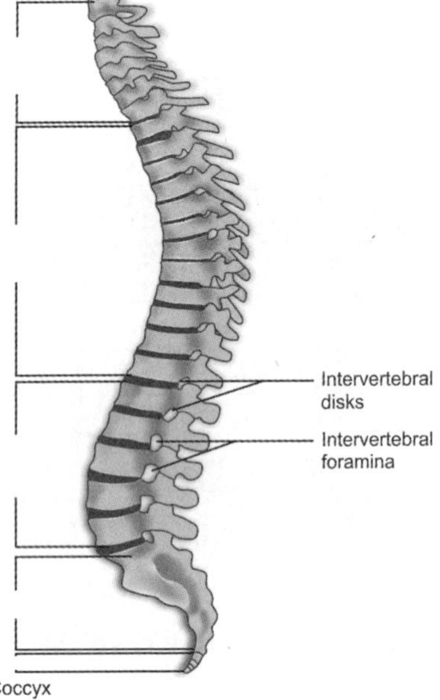

FIG. 1.7 Anatomical divisions of the back (spinal column)

9. Identify the part name on indicated lines.

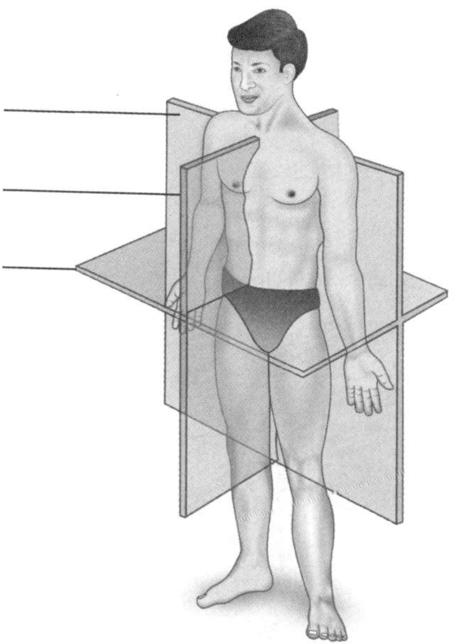

FIG. 1.8 Planes of the body

10. Identify the part name on indicated lines.

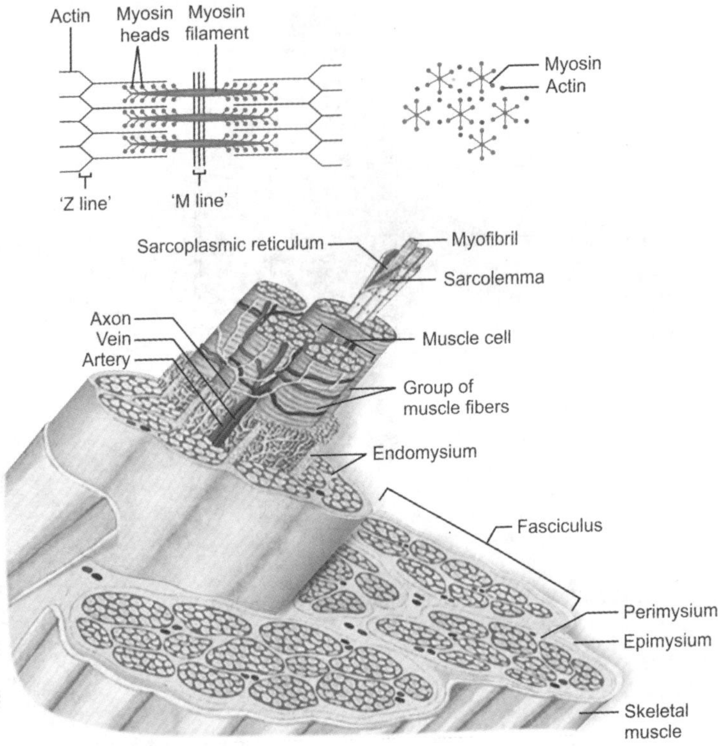

FIG. 2.1 Cross-section of skeletal muscle with names of important points of the muscle

11. Identify the part name on indicated lines.

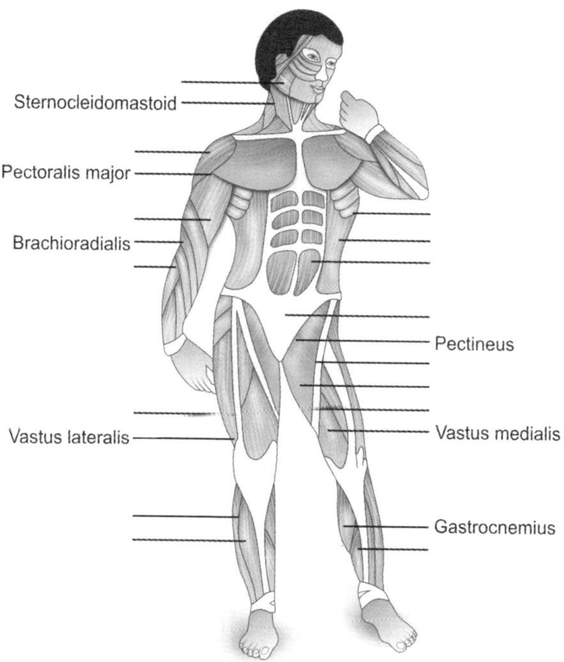

FIG. 2.2 Muscles—(anterior view)

12. Identify the part name on indicated lines.

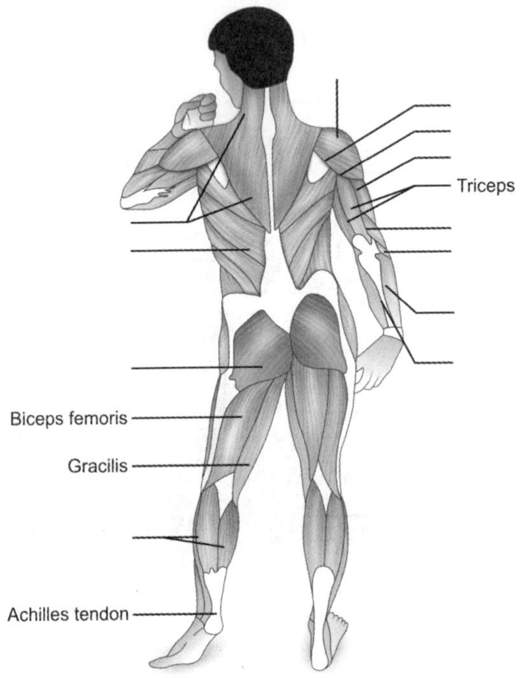

FIG. 2.3 Muscles—(posterior view)

13. Identify the part name on indicated lines.

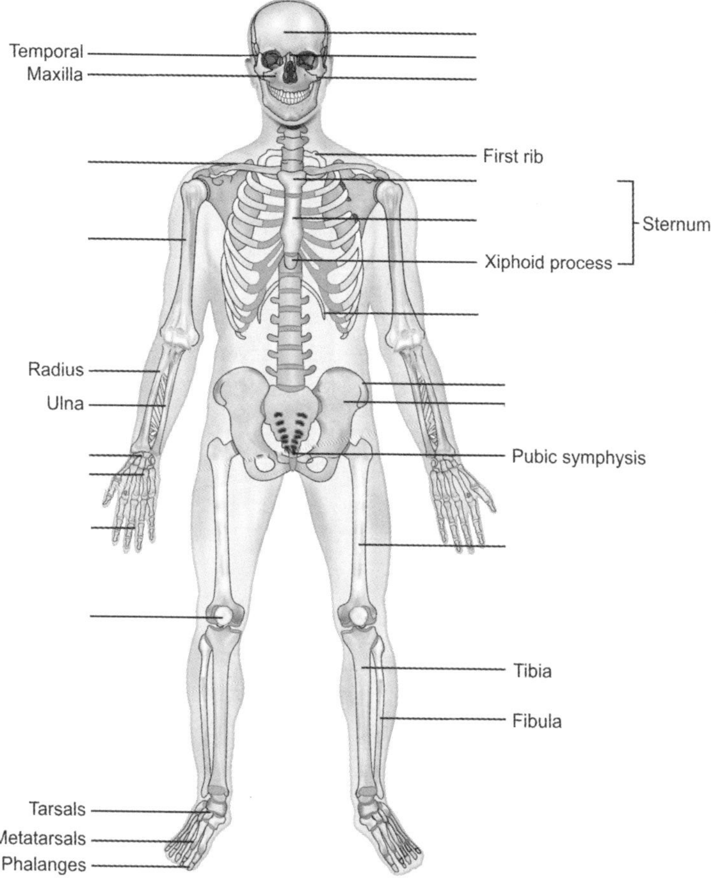

FIG. 2.4 Bones—(anterior view)

14. Identify the part name on indicated lines.

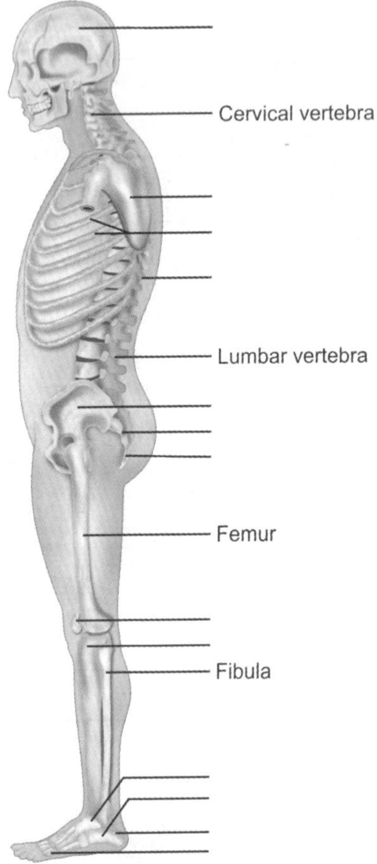

FIG. 2.5 Bones—(lateral view)

15. Identify the part name on indicated lines.

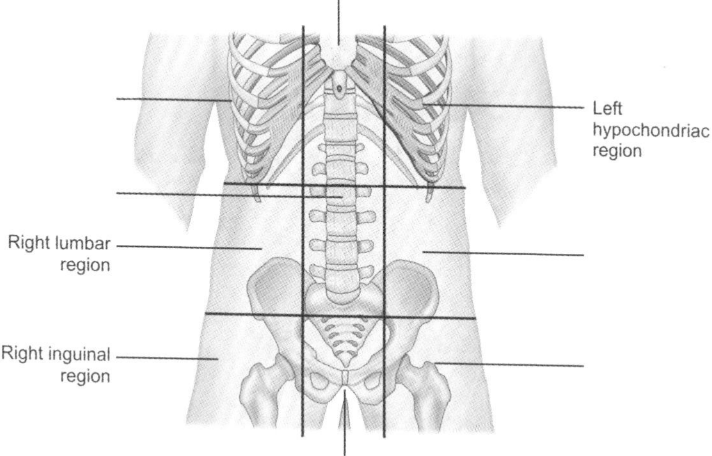

FIG. 2.6 Anatomical division of the abdominopelvic region with locality of hypochondriac, lumbar and inguinal regions.

16. Identify the part name on indicated lines.

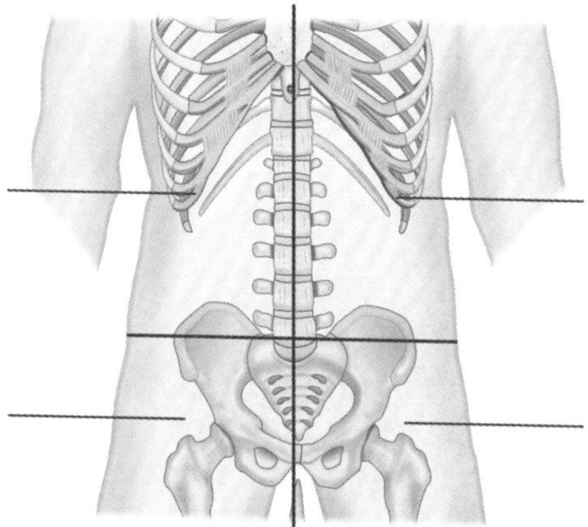

FIG. 2.7 Anatomical division of upper and lower, right and left quadrants

17. Identify the part name on indicated lines.

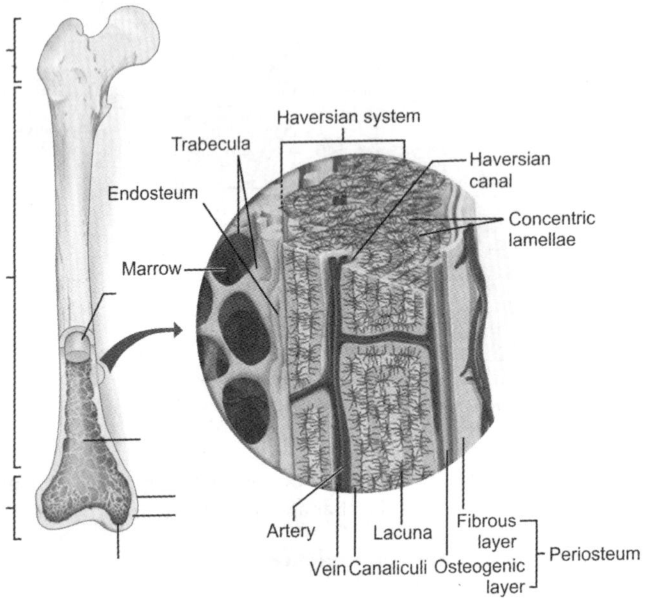

FIG. 2.8 Longitudinal section of a long bone

18. Identify the part name on indicated lines.

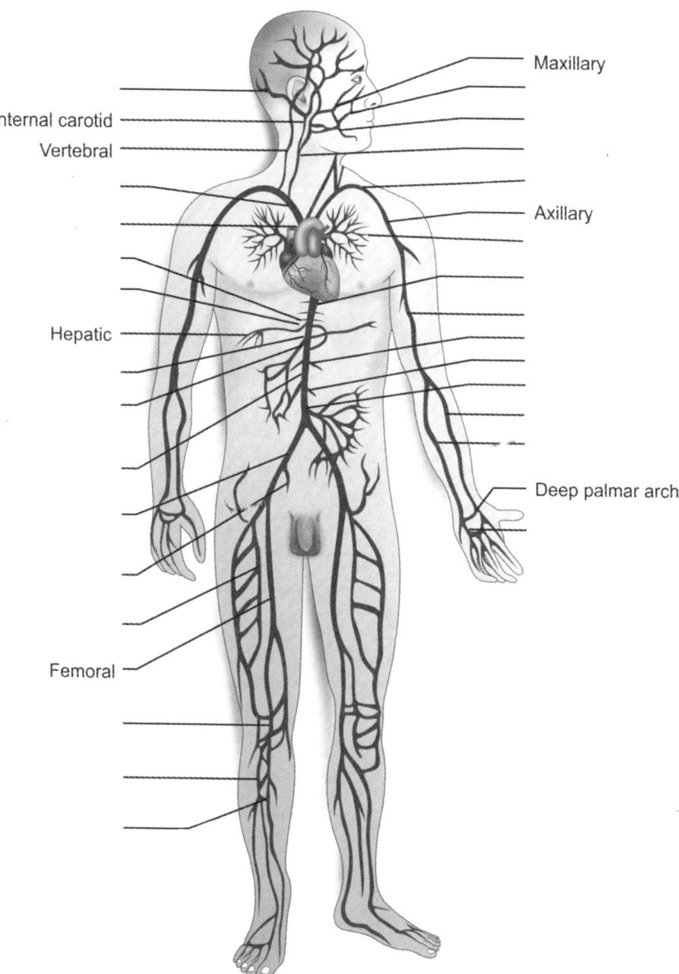

FIG. 3.1 Important arteries

19. Identify the part name on indicated lines.

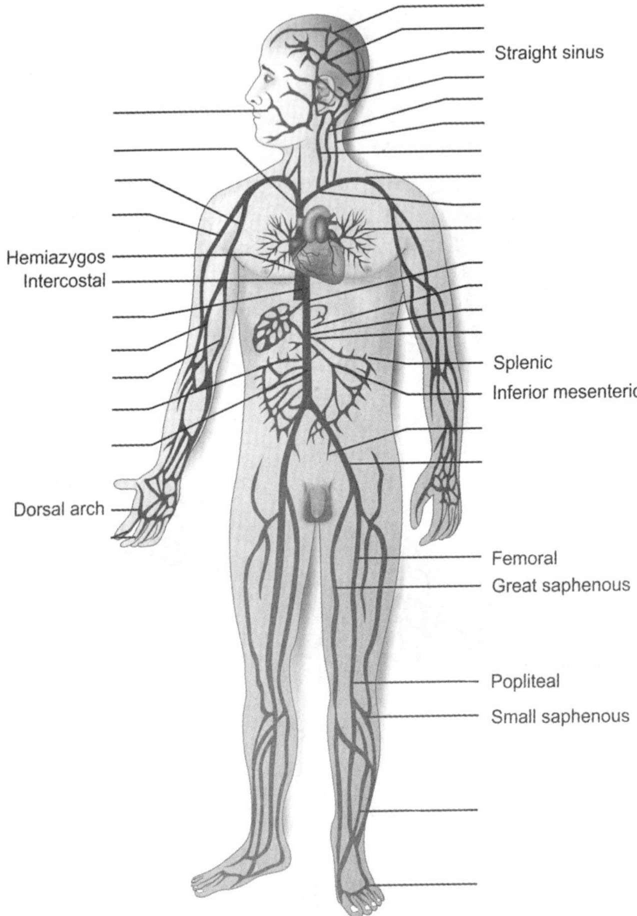

FIG. 3.2 Important veins

20. Identify the part name on indicated lines.

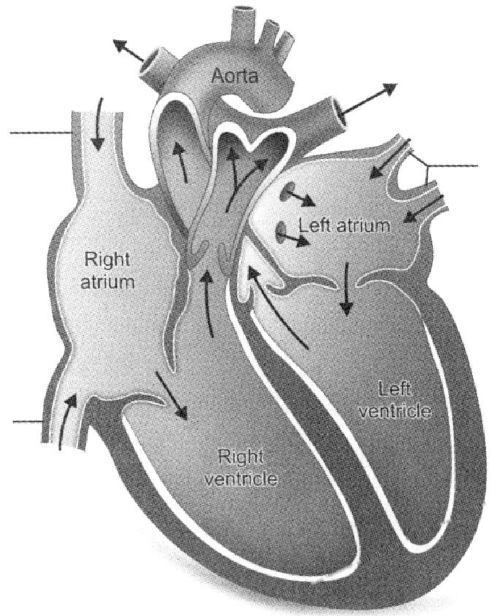

FIG. 3.3 Structure of heart

21. Identify the part name on indicated lines.

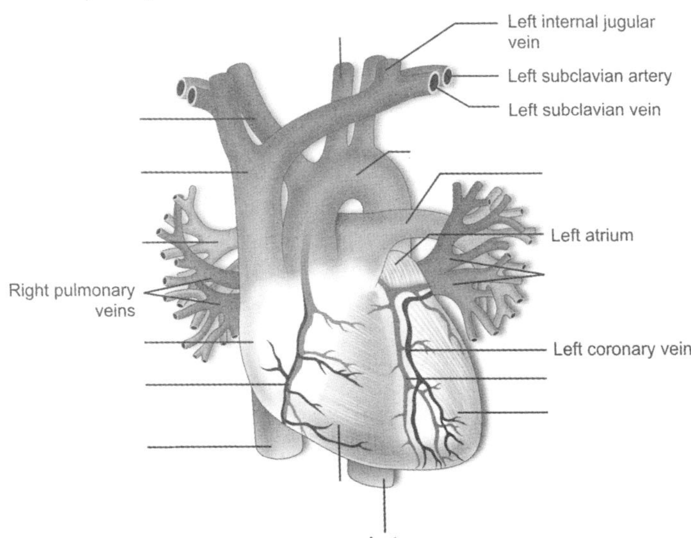

FIG. 3.4 Exterior section of the heart with blood flow

22. Identify the part name on indicated lines.

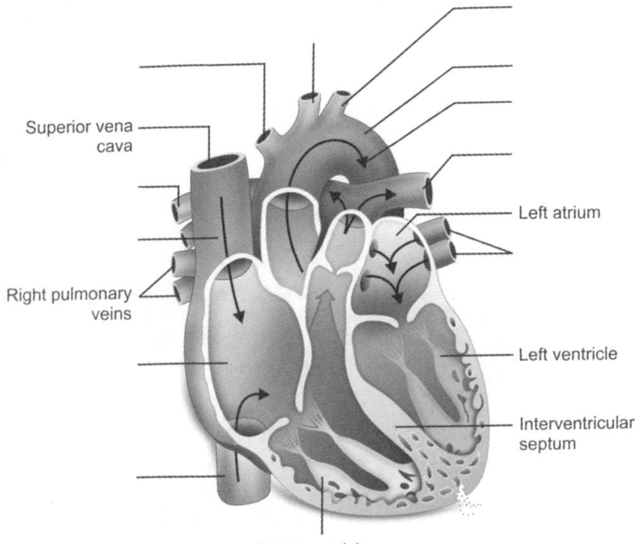

FIG. 3.5 Interior section of the heart with blood flow

23. Identify the part name on indicated lines.

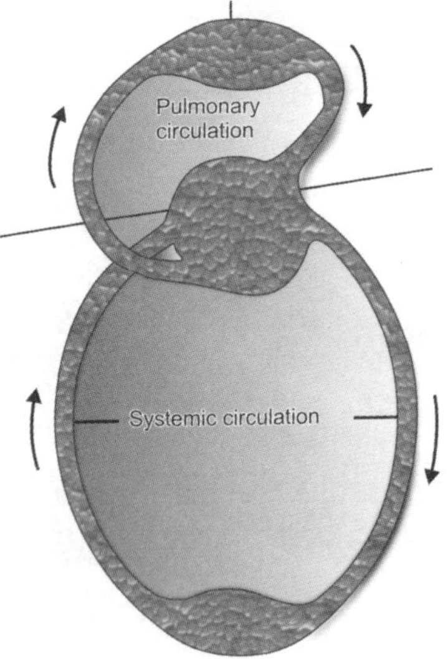

FIG. 3.7 Systemic circulation

24. Identify the part name on indicated lines.

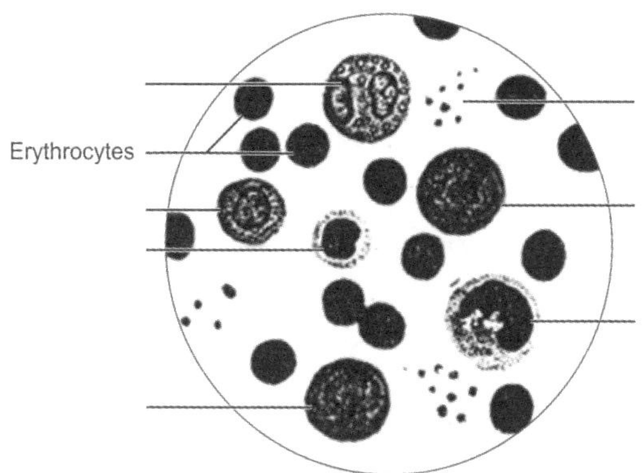

FIG. 4.1 Blood cell

25. Identify the part name on indicated lines.

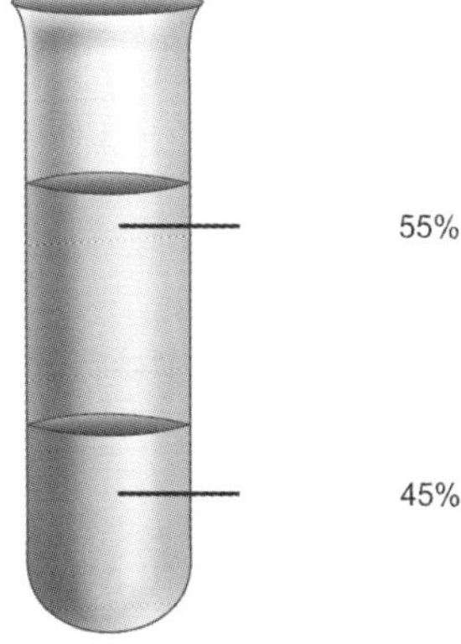

FIG. 4.2 The blood in the test tube shows the percentage composition of plasma and cells

26. Identify the part name on indicated lines.

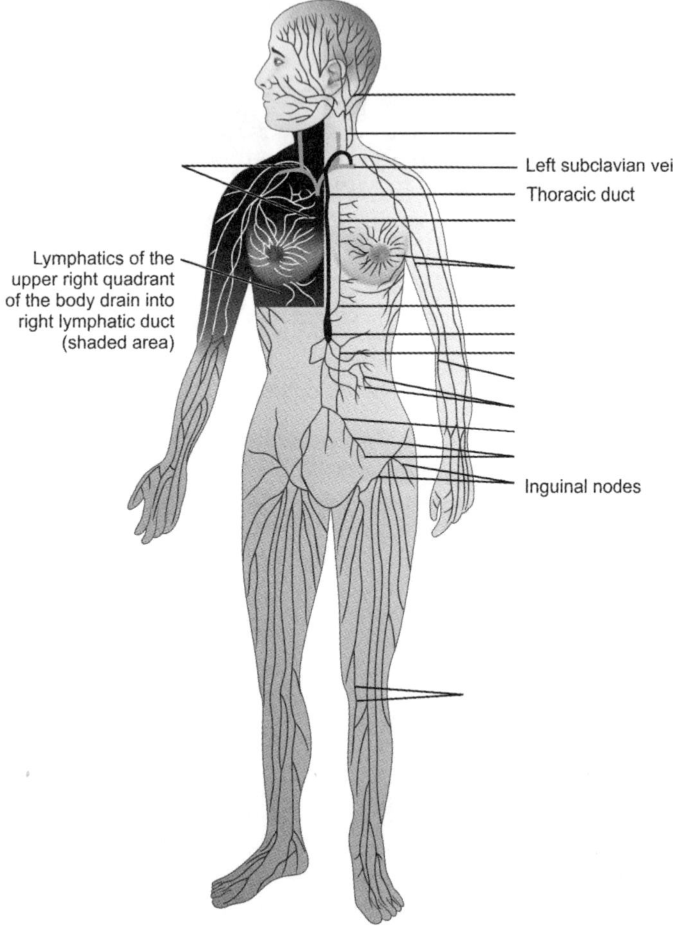

FIG. 4.3 Lymph nodes and their location

27. Identify the part name on indicated lines.

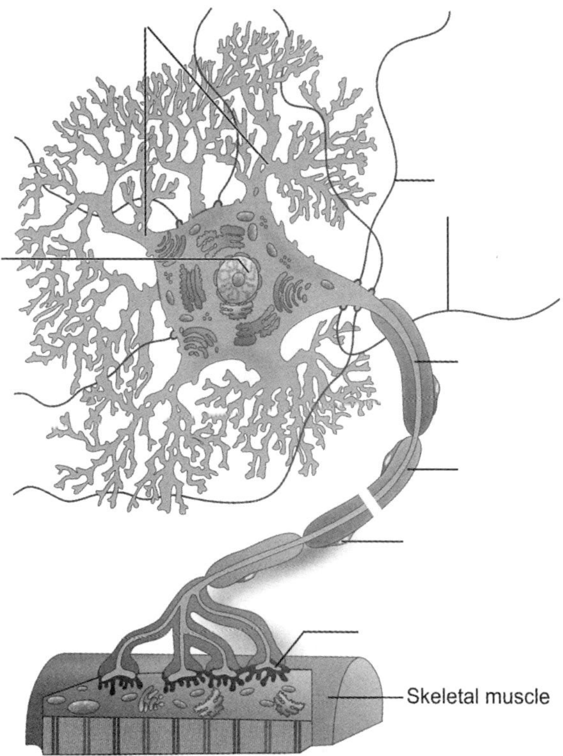

FIG. 5.1 A motor or efferent neuron

28. Identify the part name on indicated lines.

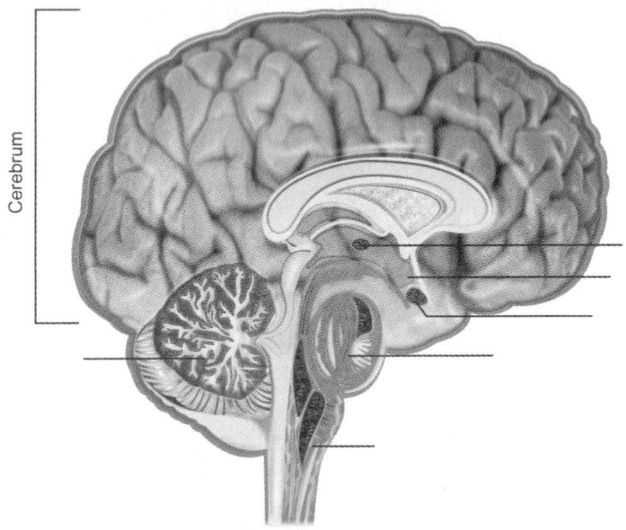

FIG. 5.2 Parts of the brain

29. Identify the part name on indicated lines.

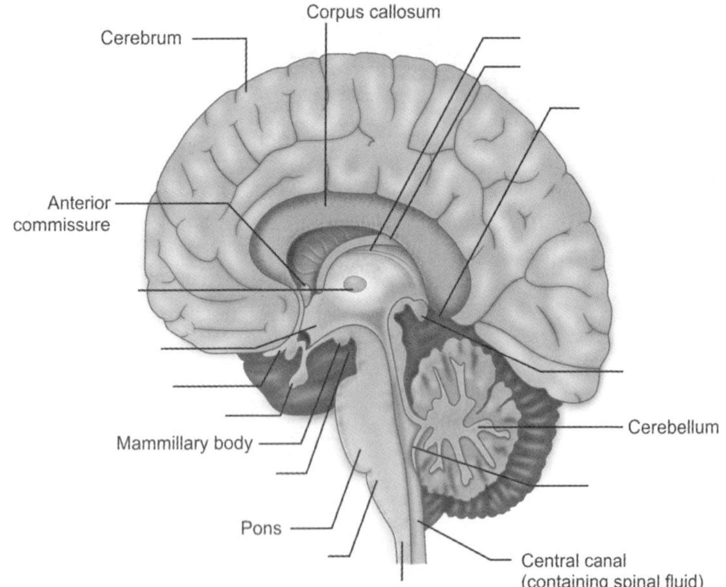

FIG. 5.3 The cross-section of brain

30. Identify the part name on indicated lines.

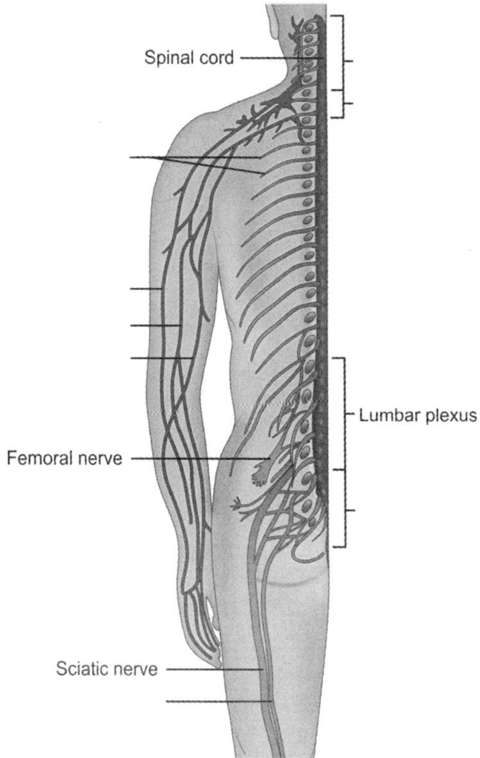

FIG. 5.4 Peripheral parts of nervous system

31. Identify the part name on indicated lines.

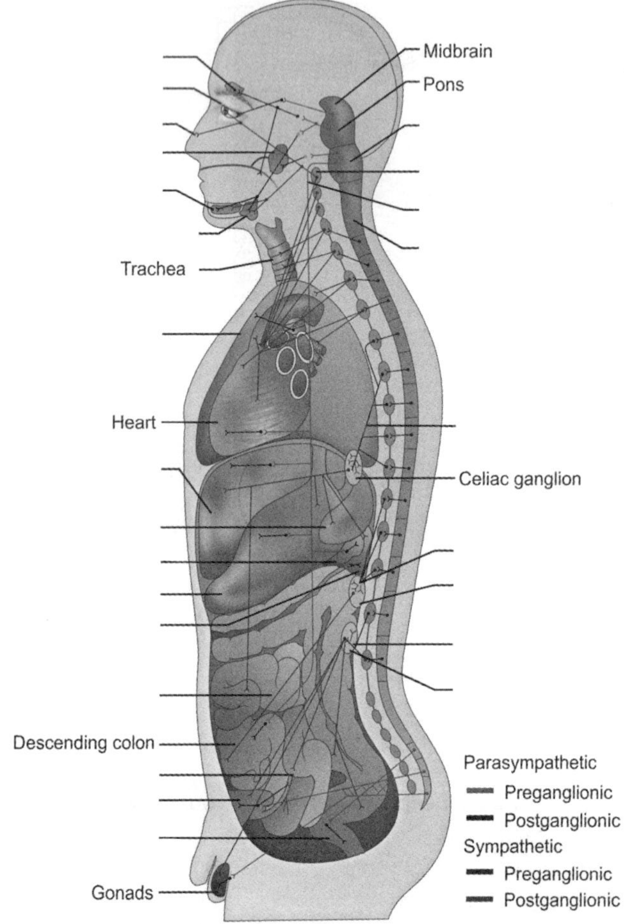

FIG. 5.5 Autonomic nervous system

32. Identify the part name on indicated lines.

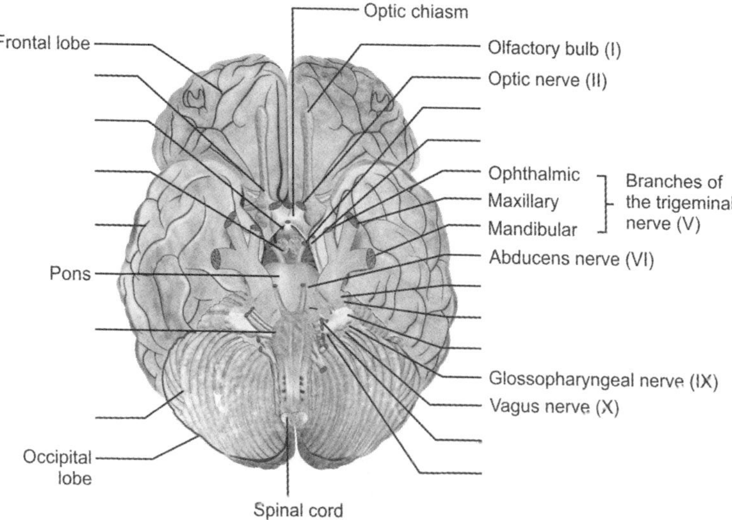

FIG. 5.6 Cross-section of brain with cranial nerves

33. Identify the part name on indicated lines.

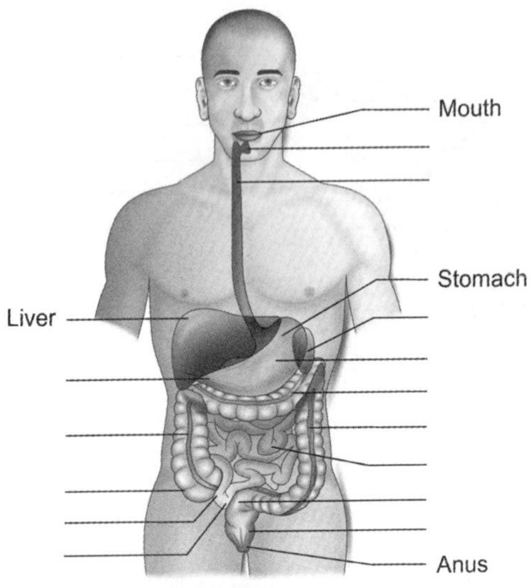

FIG. 6.1 Organs of digestive system

34. Identify the part name on indicated lines.

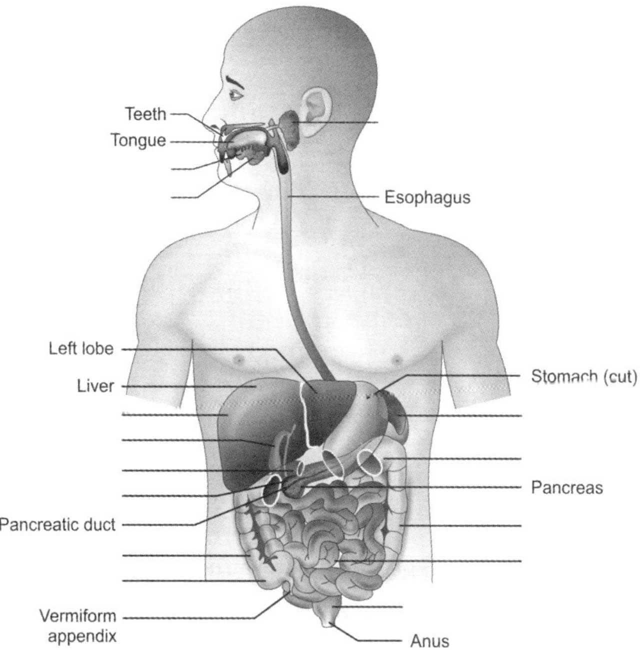

FIG. 6.2 Parts of the digestive system

35. Identify the part name on indicated lines.

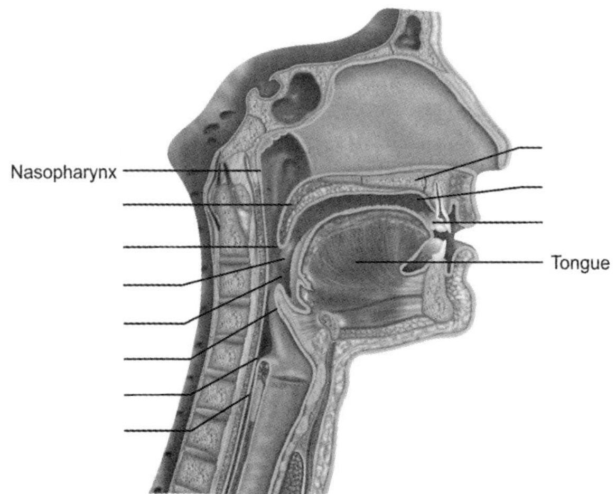

FIG. 6.3 Cross-section of oral cavity

36. Identify the part name on indicated lines.

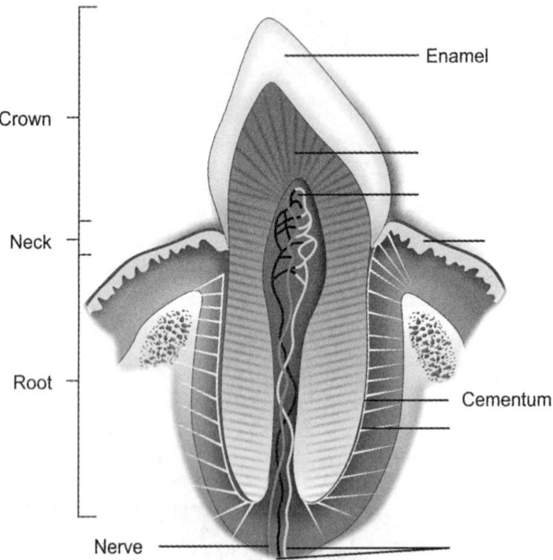

FIG. 6.4 Parts of a tooth—crown, neck and root

37. Identify the part name on indicated lines.

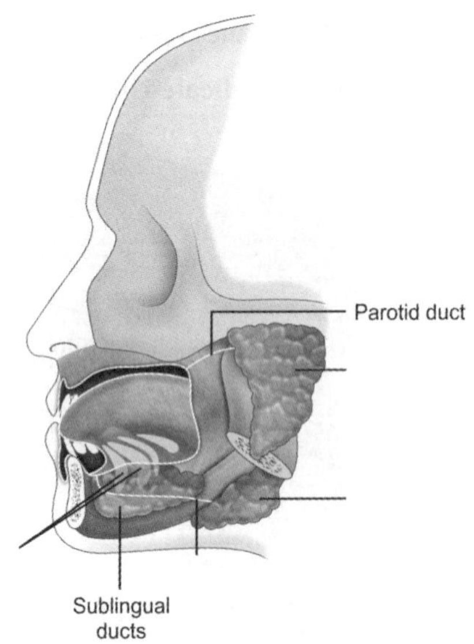

FIG. 6.5 Salivary glands comprising names of diferent ducts and glands

38. Identify the part name on indicated lines.

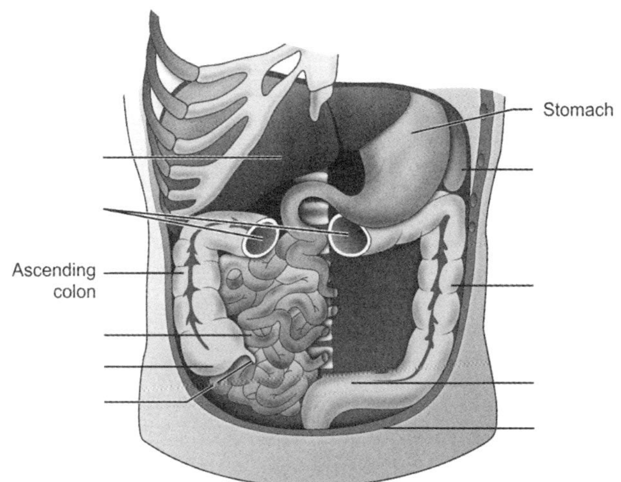

FIG. 6.6 Organs of abdominal region with names of different parts

39. Identify the part name on indicated lines.

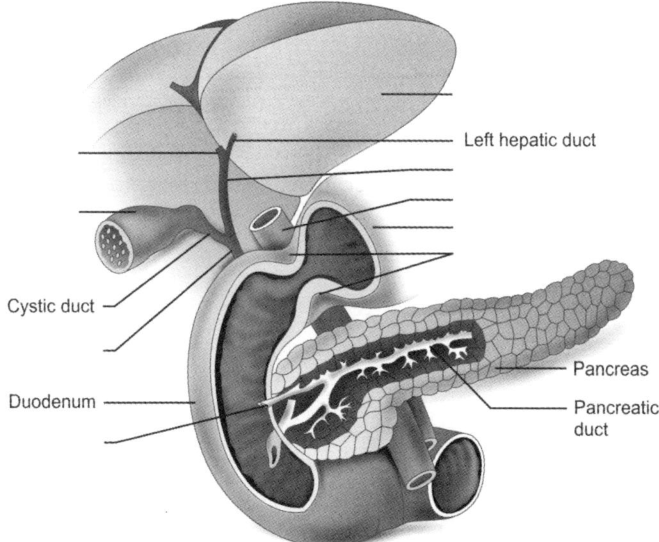

FIG. 6.7 Liver, gallbladder, pancreas, and duodenum with associated names of blood vessels and ducts

40. Identify the part name on indicated lines.

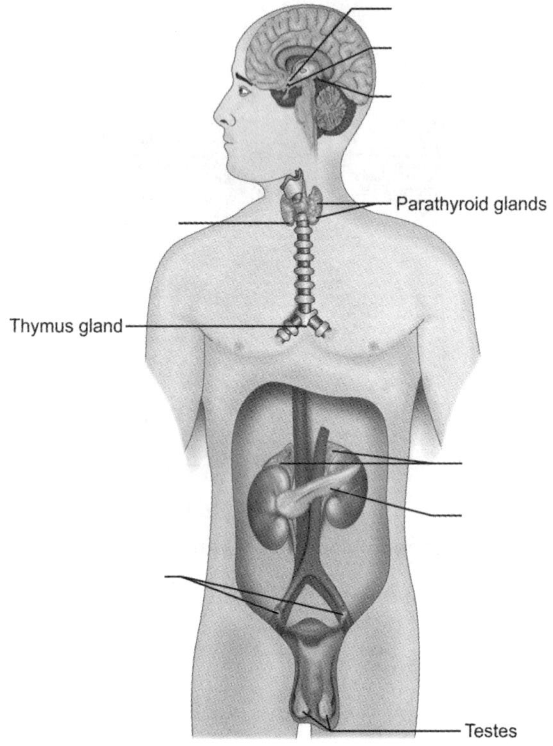

FIG. 7.1 Endocrine system with location of glands that produce hormones

41. Identify the part name on indicated lines.

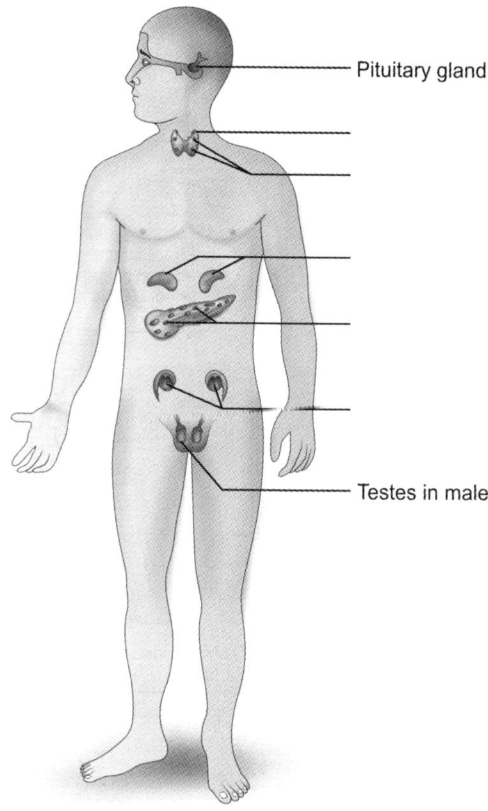

FIG. 7.2 Endocrine glands of human body with their names and location

42. Identify the part name on indicated lines.

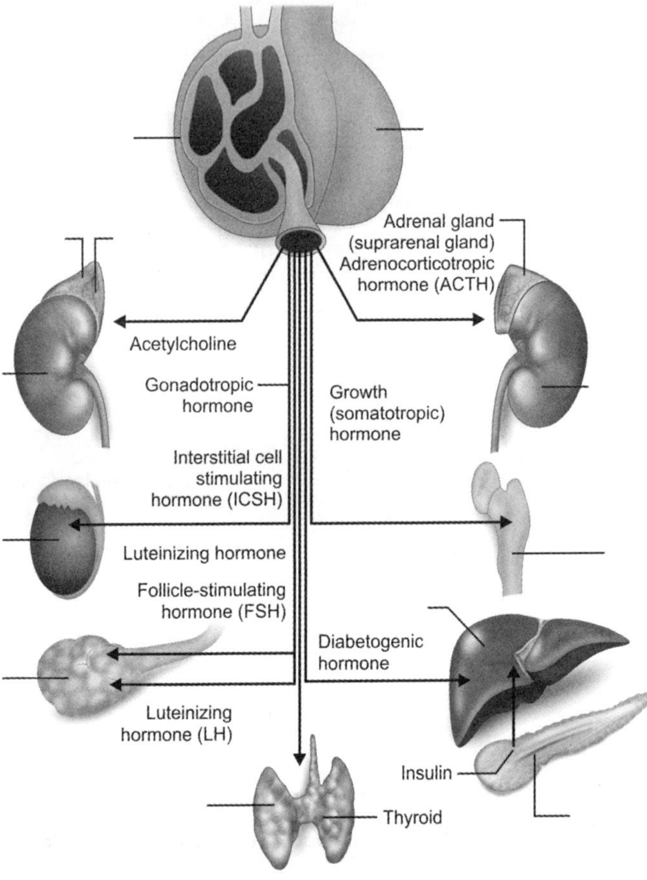

FIG. 7.3 Hormones of pituitary gland—direct and indirect effect on target organs

43. Identify the part name on indicated lines.

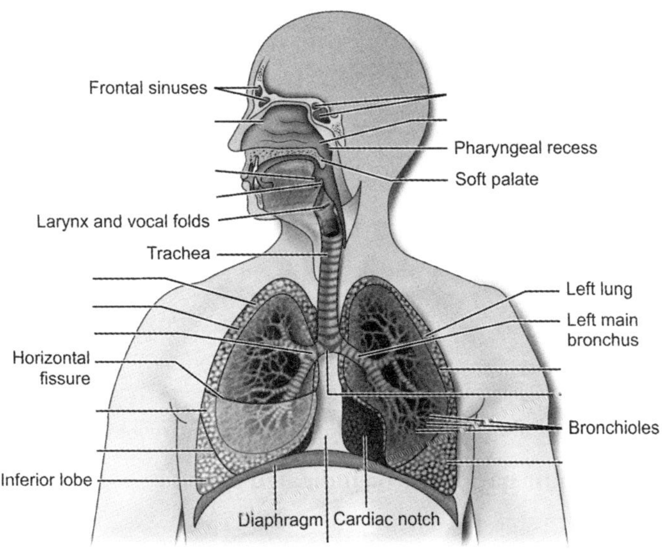

FIG. 8.1 Cross-section with names of different parts of respiratory system

44. Identify the part name on indicated lines.

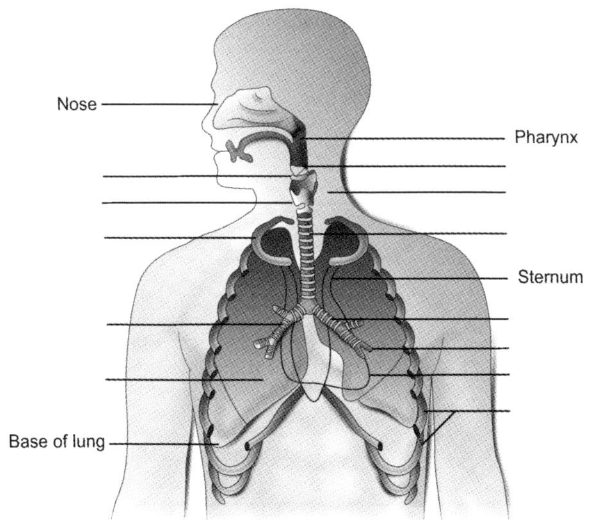

FIG. 8.2 ImPortant parts of the organs of respiratory system

45. Identify the part name on indicated lines.

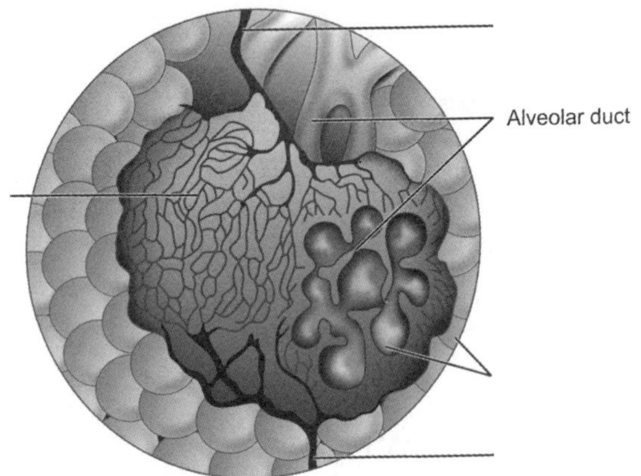

FIG. 8.3 Mechanism of internal or tissue respiration

46. Identify the part name on indicated lines.

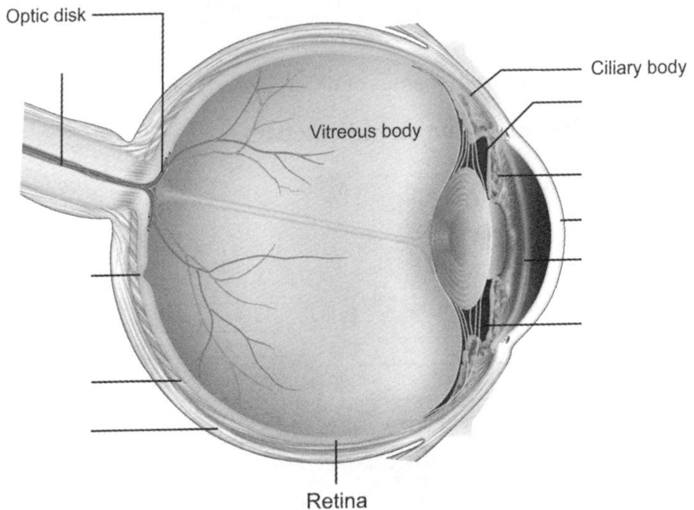

FIG. 9.1 Parts of the eye

47. Identify the part name on indicated lines.

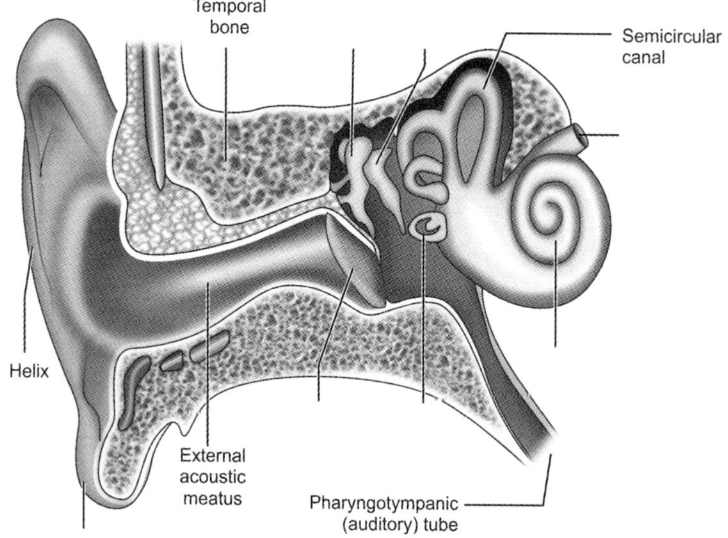

FIG. 9.2 Parts of the ear

48. Identify the part name on indicated lines.

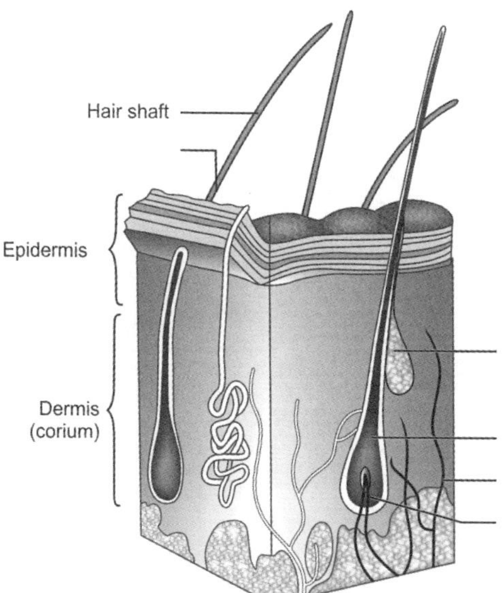

FIG. 9.3 Cross-section of structure of the skin

49. Identify the part name on indicated lines.

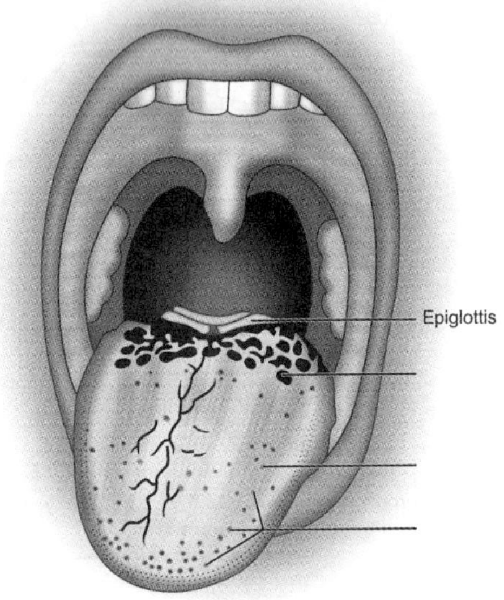

FIG. 9.4 Parts of the tongue

50. Identify the part name on indicated lines.

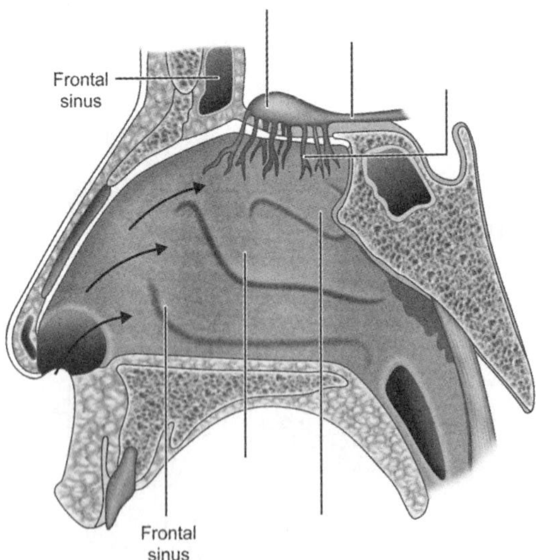

FIG. 9.5 Cross-section of the structures of olfactory mucosa with different parts names

51. Identify the part name on indicated lines.

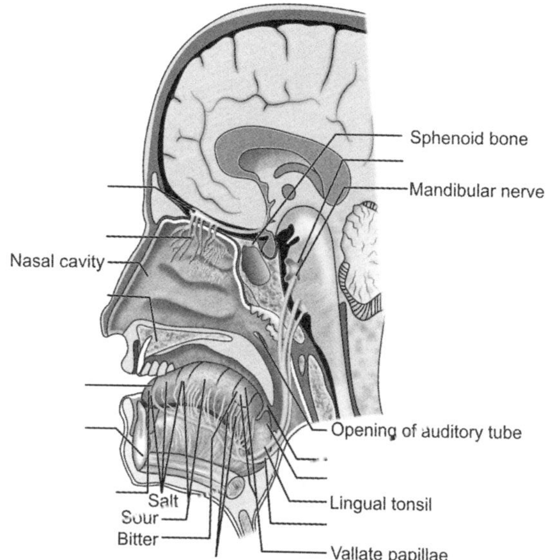

FIG. 9.6 Centers of smell and taste

52. Identify the part name on indicated lines.

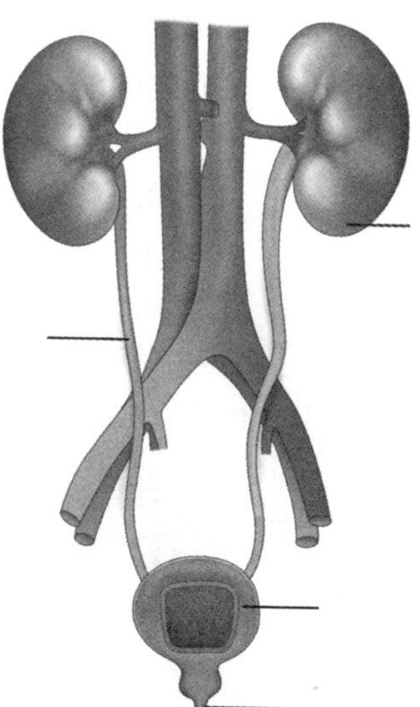

FIG. 10.1 Excretory system

53. Identify the part name on indicated lines.

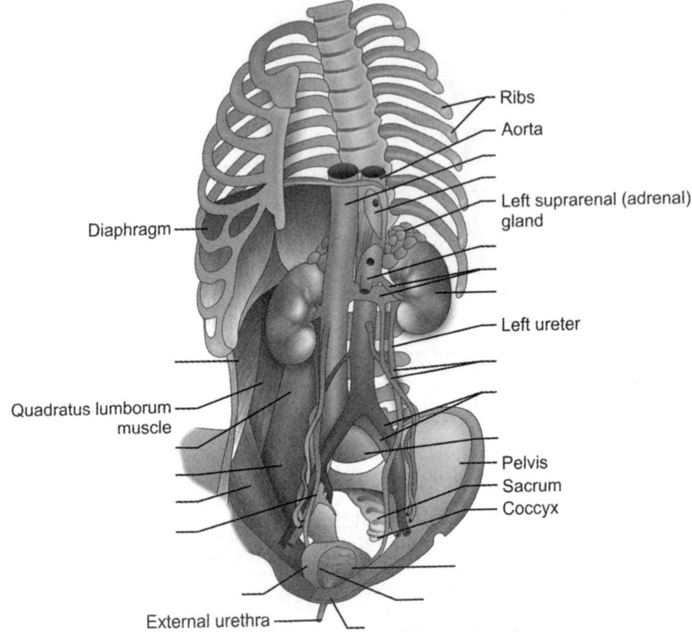

FIG. 10.2 Urinary system comprising names of different parts including kidneys

54. Identify the part name on indicated lines.

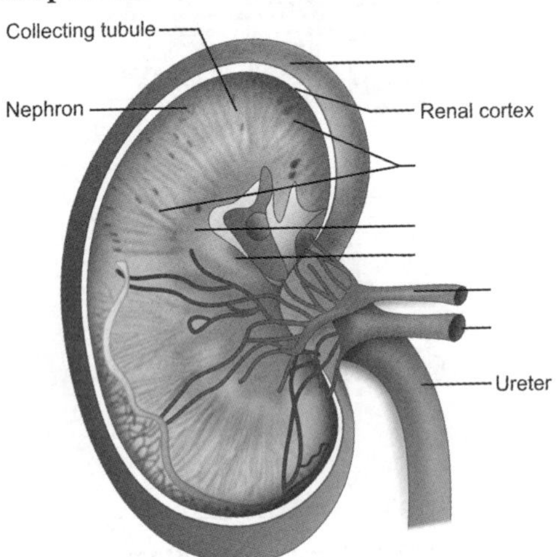

FIG. 10.3 Longitudinal section of right kidney with names of different parts

55. Identify the part name on indicated lines.

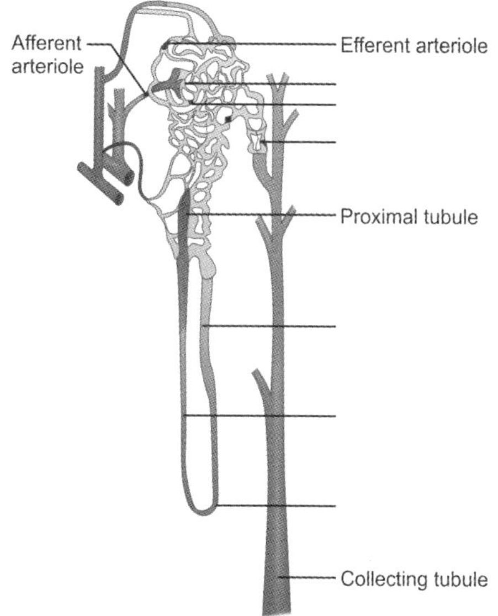

FIG. 10.4 Nephron with the names of different parts

56. Identify the part name on indicated lines.

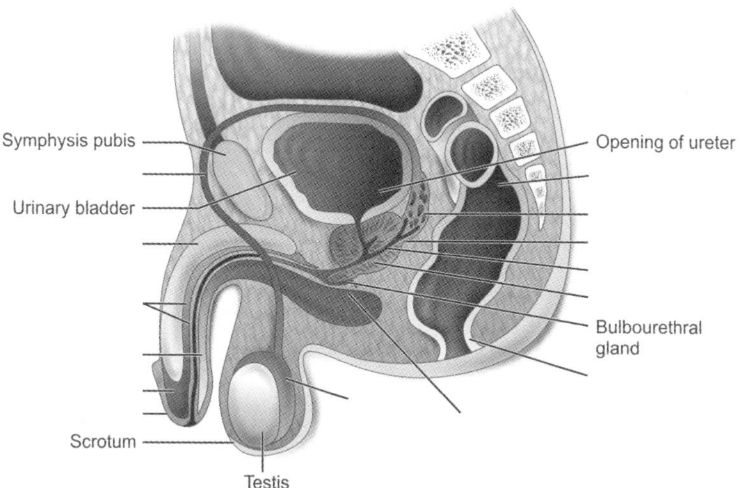

FIG. 11.1 Parts of the male reproductive system

57. Identify the part name on indicated lines.

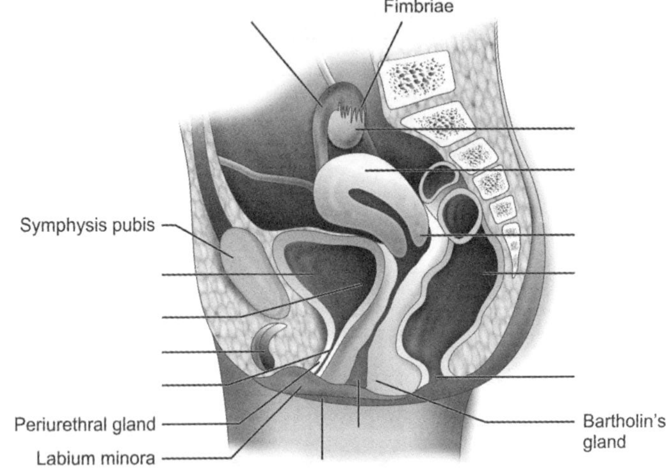

FIG. 11.2 Parts of the female reproductive system (lateral view)

58. Identify the part name on indicated lines.

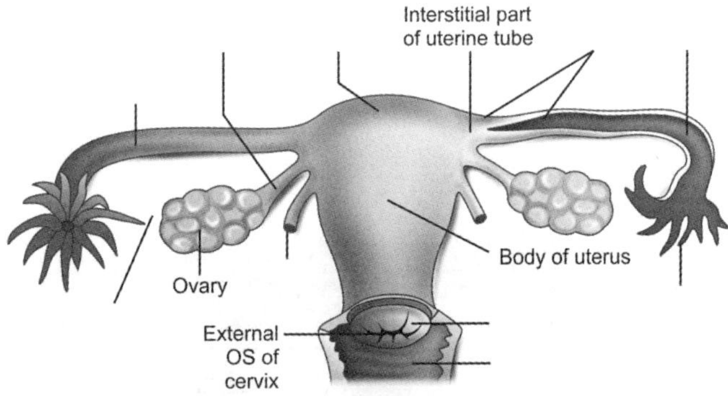

FIG. 11.3 Parts of the female reproductive system (anterior view)

59. Identify the part name on indicated lines.

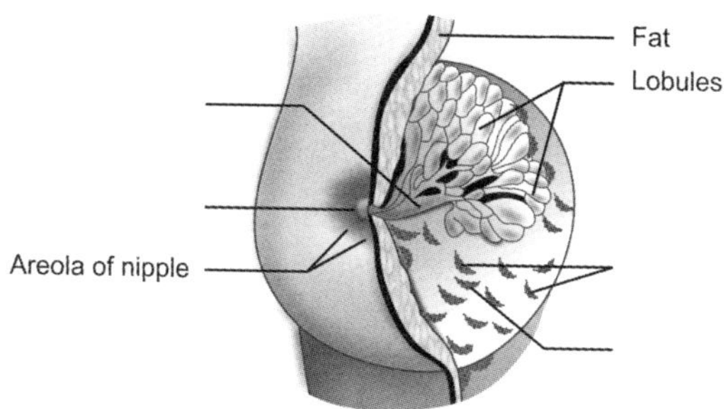

FIG. 11.4 Cross-section of the breast and its parts

Answers

The anatomy and physiology figures located under the figure numbers given below to enable the student to record right name of the part.

Chap. No.	Fig. No.	Exer. No.	Content	Answer Page No.
1	1	1	Evolution of human body	xix
1	1.1	2	Structure of cell	2
1	1.2	3	Parts of cell	2
1	1.3	4	Overview of the body structure and organs	9
1	1.4	5	Body cavities	13
1	1.5	6	Anatomical division of the body	14
1	1.6	7	Clinical divisions of the abdomen	15
1	1.7	8	Anatomical division of the back (spinal column)	16
1	1.8	9	Planes of the body	17
2	2.1	10	Cross-section of skeletal muscle with names of important points of the muscle	22
2	2.2	11	Muscles—(anterior view)	28
2	2.3	12	Muscles—(posterior view)	29
2	2.4	13	Bones—(anterior view)	31
2	2.5	14	Bones—(lateral view)	32
2	2.6	15	Anatomical division of abdominopelvic region with location of hypochondrial lumbar and inguinal region	37
2	2.7	16	Anatomical division of upper and lower, right and left quadrants	38
2	2.8	17	Longitudinal section of long bone with names of different inner parts of long bone	39
3	3.1	18	Important arteries	55
3	3.2	19	Important veins	57
3	3.3	20	Structure of heart	58
3	3.4	21	Exterior section of heart with blood flow and names of parts	59

Contd...

Contd...

Chap. No.	Fig. No.	Exer. No.	Content	Answer Page No.
3	3.5	22	Interior section of heart with blood flow and names of different parts of the heart	60
3	3.7	23	Systemic circulation	61
4	4.1	24	Blood cell	75
4	4.2	25	Blood in the test tube shows the percentage of composition of plasma and cells	75
4	4.3	26	Lymph nodes and their locations	82
5	5.1	27	A motor or efferent neuron	96
5	5.2	28	Parts of brain	98
5	5.3	29	Cross-section of brain	99
5	5.4	30	Peripheral parts of nervous system	102
5	5.5	31	Anatomical nervous system—comprising names of different parts of nerves of the body	105
5	5.6	32	Cross-section of brain with cranial nerves	106
6	6.1	33	Organs of the digestive system	118
6	6.2	34	Parts of the digestive system	119
6	6.3	35	Cross section of oral cavity	120
6	6.4	36	Parts of tooth—crown, neck and root	122
6	6.5	37	Salivary glands comprising names of different ducts and glands	123
6	6.6	38	Organs of the abdominal region with names of different parts	125
6	6.7	39	Liver, gallbladder, pancreas, ducts with associated names of blood vessels and ducts	129
7	7.1	40	Endocrine system with location of glands that produce hormones	143
7	7.2	41	Endocrine glands of human body with their names and location	144
7	7.3	42	Hormones of pituitary gland—direct and indirect effect on target organs	149

Contd...

Contd...

Chap. No.	Fig. No.	Exer. No.	Content	Answer Page No.
8	8.1	43	Cross-section with names of different parts of respiratory system	162
8	8.2	44	Important parts of organs of respiratory system	162
8	8.3	45	Mechanism of internal or tissue respiration	166
9	9.1	46	Parts of the eye	178
9	9.2	47	Parts of the ear	180
9	9.3	48	Cross-section of structure of the skin	183
9	9.4	49	Parts of the tongue	186
9	9.5	50	Cross-section of the structure of olfactory mucosa with different parts names	187
9	9.6	51	Centers of smell and taste	188
10	10.1	52	Excretory system	199
10	10.2	53	Urinary system comprising names of different parts including kidneys	201
10	10.3	54	Longitudinal section of right kidney with names of different parts	202
10	10.4	55	Nephron with the names of different parts	202
11	11.1	56	Parts of the male reproductive system	210
11	11.2	57	Parts of female reproductive system (lateral view)	213
11	11.3	58	Parts of female reproductive system (anterior view)	214
11	11.4	59	Cross-section of breast and its parts	216

16 CHAPTER Recapitulation

CHAPTER 1: CELL

LEVELS OF ORGANIZATION

The *cell is the fundamental unit of life.* As such it must carry on all the functions associated with life. Among these functions are reproduction, respiration, excretion, and adaptation to the environment. In highly complex organisms, cells are modified to carry on a specific activity. In addition to all of the other basic, life functions. Muscle cells are designed for contraction, nerve cells transmit electrical impulses; and red blood cells carry oxygen to body tissues.

Groups of cells that perform the same basic activity are called tissues. Tissue types include epithelial (covering), connective (supporting and protecting), muscular (contracting), and nervous (conducting impulses) tissues. In addition, a variety of cell types compose the specialized tissue of blood.

Groups of tissues that work in close association and perform a special function are called organs. Besides performing specialized functions, organs also have a more or less definite shape. For example, the shape of the stomach somewhat resembles a sack. The stomach composed primarily of much tissue and epithelial tissue. The muscle tissue provides for the mixing of ingested food with gastric juice. These juices are secretion from the epithelial tissue in order to aid in the digestive process.

The next higher level of organization is a system. ***A system is composed of group of organs that work together to perform a common function.*** For example, the mouth, pharynx, esophagus, stomach, small intestine, and colon, along with accessory organs, constituted with digestion. Other body systems are -integumentary, gastrointestinal, respiratory, cardiovascular, hematic and lymphatic, musculoskeletal, urogenital, reproductive, endocrine, nervous, and sense organs.

The ***highest level of organization is the organism***, which is living entity composed of all the body systems. These systems provide for all the processes associated with the life. They are responsible for its autonomous existence.

The levels of organization can be represented as follows:

Cells → Tissue → Organs → Systems → Organism

ANATOMICAL POSITION

The anatomical position places the body in a stance that is accepted by all anatomical throughout the world. In this position, the body is erect, and the eyes are looking straight to the front. The upper limbs hang to the sides, with palm facing forward. The lower limbs are parallel, with the toes opining forward. Whether the body lays face upward or downward, or whether the limbs are placed in any fashion, the positions and relationships of a structure are always described as if the body were in the anatomical position.

PLANES OF THE BODY

A plane of the body is an imaginary flat surface that passes through the body at different places in order to divide it for anatomical purposes.

BODY CAVITIES

The body is divided into four major cavities. ***A coronal plane divides these four cavities into two dorsal cavities and two ventral cavities.***

The **dorsal cavities** include the *cranial cavity*, which contains the brain, and the spinal cavity, which contains the spinal cord.

The **ventral cavities** include the *thoracic cavity*, which contains the heart, lungs, and associated structures, and the *abdominopelvic cavity*, which contains the digestive, excretory, and reproductive organs. The thoracic cavity is separated from the abdominopelvic cavity by a muscular wall, the diaphragm.

Abdominopelvic Region

The abdominopelvic region may be divided into nine major sections by constructing an imaginary "tic-tac-toe" over this region. This provides anatomical with divisions to locate the placement of visceral organs. Detailed operative reports sometimes reference these divisions. The nine regions, from left to right and top to bottom, are as follows:

1. *Right hypochondriac:* Upper right region beneath the ribs
2. *Epigastria:* Region of the stomach
3. *Left hypochondriac:* Upper left region beneath the ribs
4. *Right lumbar:* Right middle lateral region.
5. *Umbilical:* Region of the novel.
6. *Left lumbar:* Left middle lateral region
7. *Right inguinal (iliac):* Right lower lateral region
8. *Hypo gastric:* Lower middle region beneath the navel.
9. *Left inguinal (iliac):* Left lower lateral region.

For purposes of clinical evaluation, the abdominopelvic region may be divided into four quadrants (sections) by an imaginary cross:

1. Right upper quadrant (RUQ)
2. Left upper quadrant (LUQ)
3. Right lower quadrant (RLQ)
4. Left lower quadrant (LLQ)

Back

The back is divided into sections corresponding to the vertebra, which are located in the spinal column. These divisions are as follows:

- Cervical (neck)
- Thoracic (chest)
- Lumbar (loin)
- Sacral (lower back)
- Coccyx (tailbone)

DIRECTIONAL TERMS

In order to explain where a structure is located in relation to one that is already known, anatomists use directional terms. These terms avoid confusion by expressing in only one word a specific position relative to another. In learning the following list, you should consider opposing terms for ease in memorization. The following directional terms are presented in such a fashion.

- Superficial—Toward the surface of the body
- Deep (Internal)—Away from the surface of the body
- Abduction—Movement away from the median plane of the body or one of its parts.
- Adduction—Movement toward the medium plane of the body
- Medial—Pertaining to the middle of the body or structure
- Lateral—Pertaining to a side
- Superior (cephal or cranial)—Toward the head or upper portion of a structure
- Inferior (caudal or caudad)—Away from the head, or toward the tail or lower part of a structure
- Proximal—Near the attachment of an extremely to the trunk or a structure
- Distal—Farther from the attachment of an extremity to the trunk or a structure
- Anterior (ventral)—Near the front of the body
- Posterior (dorsal)—Near the back of the body
- Visceral—pertaining to the covering of an organ
- Prone—Lying horizontal with the face downward, or denoting the hand with palms turned downward
- Spine—Lying on the back with the upward, or denoting the position of the hand or foot with the palm or foot facing upward
- Inversion—Turning inward or inside out
- Eversion—Turning outward.

CHAPTER 2: MUSCULOSKELETAL SYSTEM

ANATOMY AND PHYSIOLOGY OF MUSCULOSKELETAL SYSTEM

The musculoskeletal system consists of bones, joints, and muscles. Bones are the principal organs of support and protection for the body, joints are the places at which two bones meet (articulate). Because bones are incapable of movement without the help of muscles, contraction must be provided by muscular tissue. In the human skeleton, muscles are usually attached to two articulating bones, and during contraction, one bone is drawn toward another. Muscles, therefore, produce movement by exerting a force on the bones to which they are attached. Stated more simply, skeletal muscles produce movement by pulling on bones.

SKELETAL SYSTEM

Functions: Besides support and protection of the vital organs from injury, the skeletal system provides a number of other important functions. Movement is possible because bones act as points of attachment for muscles, joints, tendons, and ligaments. Bone marrow, which is found within larger bones, is responsible for blood cell formation, or hematopoiesis. Bone marrow continuously produce millions of red and white blood cells to replace worn out cells. The bones serve as a storehouse for minerals, particularly phosphorus and calcium. When the body experiences a deficiency in a mineral salt, such as calcium during pregnancy, it is withdrawn from the bones.

STRUCTURE AND TYPES OF BONES

Bones consists of mineral deposits embedded with living cells that must continuously receive food and oxygen. Bone cells also require a system to carry away accumulated waste products. In order to provide these vital functions, there is an extensive vascular system within bones. Fundamentally, all bones can be distinguished from each other by classifying them in four main categories; long bones, short bones, flat bones, and irregular bones. Long bones are found in the extremities of the body, for example, arms and legs.

1. **Diaphysis**, which is the shaft, or long main portion, of the bone, consists mainly of compact bone.
2. **Epiphyses**, which are the two ends, or extremities, of the bones have a somewhat bulbous shape to provide space for muscle and ligament attachments near the joints. Proximal and distal epiphyses are the two terms used for the ends of a long bone.
3. **Articular cartilage** is a thin layer of resilient hyaline cartilage. The elasticity of the hyaline cartilage provides the joints with a cushion against jars and blows.

4. **Periosteum**, which is a dense white fibrous membrane that covers the remaining surface of the bone, contains numerous blood and lymph vessels and nerves. In growing bones, the inner layer contains the bone-forming cells, or osteoblasts. Since the blood vessels and osteoblasts are located here, the periosteum provides a means for bones repair and general bone nutrition. It also serves as a point of attachment for muscles, ligaments and tendons.

Flat bones are exactly what their name suggests. They provide broad surfaces for muscular attachment and extensive protection for internal organs. Examples are bones of the skull, shoulder blades, and sternum.

Short bones are irregular shaped and consist of a core of cancellous, or spongy, bone enclosed in a thin layer of compact tissue. Examples are bones of the ankles, wrists, and toes.

Irregular bones are all of the other's bones that cannot be grouped under the previous headings because of their particular shapes. Examples are the bones of the ear and the vertebrae.

DIVISIONS OF SKELETAL SYSTEM: AXIAL AND APPENDICULAR SKELETON

The skeleton can be divided into two main parts: the axial skeleton and the appendicular skeleton.

1. The **axial skeleton** comprises the bones of the skull, the thorax, and the vertebral column. These bones contribute to the formation of body cavities and provide protection for internal organs.
2. The **appendicular skeleton** consists of the bones of the shoulder, the upper extremes, the hips, and the lower extremities. They attach to the axial skeleton as appendages.

Vertebral Column

The vertebral column of the adult is composed of 26 bones called vertebrae. The vertebral column supports the body and provides a bony canal for the passage of the spinal cord.

Intervertebral disks which are composed of fibrocartilage nous substance with a gelatinous mass in the center (nucleus pulposus).

When the disk material protrudes into the neural canal, pressure on the adjacent nerve root is manifested by pain. This condition is referred to as herniation of intervertebral disk, herniated nucleus pulposus (HNP), ruptured disk, or slipped disk.

Basically, the vertebral column is divided into five groups of bones, and each group derives its name from the location within the spinal column. The seven cervical vertebrae form the skeleton framework of the neck. The first cervical vertebrae is the called the (3) atlas and supports the skull. The second cervical vertebra, the (4) axis, makes possible rotation of the skull on the neck. Under these are the twelve (5) thoracic, or dorsal vertebrae, which support the chest and serve as a point of articulation for the ribs. The next five vertebrae, the (6) lumbar vertebrae, are situated in the lower back area and carry most of the weight of the torso. Below this area, the five sacral vertebrae are fused into a single bone in the adult and are referred to as the (7) sacrum. The tall of the vertebral column consists of four or five fragmented vertebrae fused together to as (8) Coccyx.

Thorax

Two of the most important organs of the chest are the heart and lungs. Together with other soft tissue, they are enclosed and protected by the thorax, or ribs cage.

The ribs, the (1) sternum or chest plate, and the thorax vertebrae from the skeletal framework of the cage. The normal set of ribs in both sexes consists of 12 pairs, or a total of 24 ribs. Twelve ribs are situated on each side of the thoracic cavity. The (2) true ribs are the first seven parts of the ribs. These are attached directly to the sternum by a strip of (3) costal cartilage (hyaline cartilage). The costal cartilage of the next five pairs of the ribs re not fastened directly to the sternum. These are known as (4) false ribs. The last two pairs of false ribs are not joined, even indirectly, to the sternum but attach posteriorly to the thoracic vertebrae and are known as (5) floating ribs.

Pelvic Girdle (Pelvis)

The pelvis is basin-shaped structure that supports the sigmoid colon, the rectum, the urinary bladder, and other soft organs of the abdominopelvic cavity. It also provides a point of attachment for the legs.

Male and female pelvis differs considerably in size and shape. Some of the differences are attributable to the function of the female pelvis during the stages of childbearing. The female pelvis is shallower than the male pelvis but wider in every direction. Not only does the female pelvis support the enlarged abdomen as the fetus matures, but it also must provide a large enough opening to allow the infant to pass through during the process of birth.

Both the female and male pelvis is divided into the (1) ilium, (2) ischium, and (3) pubis. These are fused together in the adult to form a single bone called the innominate bone. Nevertheless, the individual names are retained in order to identify the respective areas of the hipbone. The bladder is located behind the (4) symphysis pubis; the rectum is in the curve of the (5) sacrum and (6) coccyx. In the female, the uterus, fallopian tubes, ovaries, and vagina are located between the bladder and the rectum.

Bone Markings

Surfaces of bones have both protection and depressions to provide attachments for muscles, to join one bone to another, or to furnish cavities and pathways for nerve and blood supplies.

The portion of the bone that projects is called a process. Various types of projections, or processes, are evident in bones. They may be rounded, sharp, and narrow or have a larger ridge, called crest. The anatomical terms for most common types of processes are discussed below.

A condyle is a rounded process at the end of a bone that forms an articulation. An example is the condyles of the humerus. A tubercle is a small, rounded elevation from the surface of a bone, while the larger counterpart is known as a tuberosity. These elevations provide points of attachments for muscles and ligaments. The foramen is an opening, or orifice, for passage of blood vessels and nerves. Fissure (also called sulcus) indicates a narrow slit, often between two bones. A fossa is a depression in a bone surface. The line of bone union in an immovable articulation, as in between the skull bones, is known as a suture. Fontanelle is a soft spot-one of the membrane-covered spaces remaining at the junction of the sutures in the incompletely ossified of the fetus or infant.

Joints or Articulations

In order to allow body movements, all bones must have articulating surfaces. These surfaces form joints, or articulations, with various degrees of mobility. Some are freely movable (diarthroses); others are only slightly movable (amphiarthroses); and the remaining are totally immovable (synarthroses). All three types are necessary for smooth coordinated body movements.

Every joint is covered with connective tissue and cartilage. The ligaments and connective tissue in these areas permit bones to be connected to each other. Muscles attached to freely movable joints permit a great deal of body movement. The synovial membrane that lines the joint cavity secretes synovial fluid, which acts as lubrication of the joints. The bones in a synovial joint are separated by a joint capsule. The joint capsule is strengthened by ligaments (fibrous bands, or sheets, of connective tissues) that often anchor bones to each other. All of the above factors, working together in a complementary manner, make a various body movements possible.

MUSCLES

Muscular tissue refers to all of the contractive tissue of the body. It includes the cardiac muscle of the heart, the smooth muscles that compose the viscera, and the skeletal muscles that attach to bones. The first two categories of muscles are referred to as involuntary, because there is no discretionary control over them. In contrast, the skeletal muscles are voluntary, since their contractions are fully controllable. Some examples of other types of voluntary muscles are those that move the tongue or eyeball and those that contract facial expressions.

All muscles through contraction provide the body with motion or body posture. The less apparent motions provided by muscles are the passage and elimination of food through the digestive system, propulsion of blood through the arteries, and contraction of the bladder to eliminate urine.

Motions such as running and lifting originate with the skeletal muscles, which act upon the system of levers formed by the bones and joints. This engineering relationship needs further explaining. One ends of a muscle, usually the proximal end (also called the original), must attach to a rather immovable bone surface, while the remaining part spans across a joint. The other end of the muscle, the distal end (or insertion) is attached in a movable bone.

As the muscle contracts, the insertion pulls toward the origin and draw the secured bone toward the immovable or first bone. This produces motion. Often, motion is produced when several muscles spanning over the same joint are contracted. Each of these muscles provides for slight variations in a particular movement.

Whether acting singly or in groups, the muscle or muscles that produce the movement are referred to as prime movers or agonists. Once a motion has occurred, such as bending an arm at the elbow, the arm does not return to its original position even after the contraction has stopped. Instead, an opposing muscle, called the antagonist, must contract to bring the arm back to its original position. The need for both agonist and antagonist muscles imply that muscles process only contracting, or pulling, capabilities, not those of pushing. This means that a prime mover is not able to reverse it activity and push a bone away from the origin. Opposite motions are accomplished by muscles that act antagonistically to the prime **movers.**

When other muscles contribute indirectly to as specific movement, they are called synergists. They aid the prime movers in their activity, but indirectly. Finally, a fixator is a muscle that stabilizes, or fixes, one end of a muscle, so that all of the force exerted by it occurs only at one end.

CONNECTIVE TISSUE COVERING

Skeletal muscles are enclosed in a sheath of connective tissue. This connective tissue is part of the deep fascia of the body, which is continuous with adjacent muscles, periosteum and subcutaneous connective tissue. The outer sheath of the muscle is the epimysium. Within a given muscle, a perimysium surrounds small bundles of muscles. The endomysium covers each single muscle fiber.

These layers of connective tissue contain the nerves and supply blood to the muscles.

ATTACHMENTS

Muscles attach to bones either by fleshy or fibrous attachments. In fleshy attachments, muscle fibers arise directly from bone. These fibers distribute force over wide areas, but a fleshy attachment is weaker than a fibrous attachment. In fibrous attachments, the connective tissue of the epimysium, perimysium, and endo mysium converges at the end of the muscle to become continuous and indistinguishable from the periosteum. In some instances, this connective tissue penetrates the very bone itself. When these connective tissue fibers form a cord or strap. It is referred to as a tendon. This provides for a great deal of force to be localized in a small area of bone. Ligaments are composed of connective tissue and attach one bone to another. When the fibrous attachment spans over a large area of a particular bone, the attachment is called an aponeurosis. Such attachments are found in the lumbar region of the back.

CHAPTER 3: CARDIOVASCULAR SYSTEM

ANATOMY AND PHYSIOLOGY OF CARDIOVASCULAR SYSTEM

Discussions in earlier chapter addressed the anatomy and physiology of various body systems. Each of these systems, composed of millions of cells, requires a constant supply of food and vital products in order to function. In addition, each cell within these systems must be cleansed and purified of accumulated waste products. Since body cells are not always located near the source of the products they require and they are not always near the organs necessary for elimination of waste, a transportation system is required. Two distinct body systems, the cardiovascular system and the lymphatic system, are responsible for transportation of products to and from the cells of the body.

The cardiovascular system is composed of the heart, blood vessels, and blood. The lymphatic is composed of lymph glands, lymph vessels, and lymph.

Only the heart and blood vessels are discussed in this chapter. Blood is considered with the lymphatic system because of the similarity between them.

VASCULAR SYSTEM

Three types of vessels carry blood throughout the body. Each differs in structure, depending on its function. These vessels are the arteries, capillaries, and veins.

Arteries

Arteries carry blood from the heart to body tissues and organs. The blood is propelled through the arteries by the pumping action of the heart. Consequently, arterial walls are thick and muscular and capable of expanding of the arterial walls at each heartbeat is referred to as a pulse. Because of the pressure against the arterial walls associated with the pumping action of the heart, a cut or severed artery is a serious condition.

The blood in the arteries (except for the pulmonary artery contains a high concentration of oxygen (O_2). Such blood is referred to as oxygenated blood. It is characterized by bright red color.

Arteries branch to form smaller vessels called arterioles (little arteries). Arterioles further divide to form the smallest vessels of the circulatory system, the capillaries.

Capillaries

Capillaries are microscopic vessels that join the arterial system with the venous system. Although seemingly the most insignificant of the three vessel types because of size (only one blood cell of at a time is able to pass through the lumen). They are functionally the most important. The walls of the capillaries are composed of a single layer of endothelial cells. The thinness of these walls make it possible for substances to pass quite readily into and out of the vessels. Consequently, the primary function of the vascular system-providing cells with vital products is accomplished by the capillaries.

It is important to note that the vast number of capillaries makes their combined diameter so great that blood flows through them very slowly. This allows sufficient time for the exchange of materials to occur between blood and body cells. The pathway for this exchange is as follows:

$$\text{Blood} \; \frac{\text{Vital products}}{\text{Waste products}} \; \text{Body cells}$$

Veins

Veins carry blood to the heart from body organs and tissues. Veins are smaller vessels called ventricles (little veins), which develop from the union of capillaries blood to the heart. Since the extensive network of capillaries throughout the body absorbed the propelling pressure exerted by the heart. Capillaries connect arterioles to venules. This connection provides a gateway for the return of, the blood in veins now must rely on other methods of propulsion in order to return to the heart. These methods include skeletal muscle contraction (especially in the legs), gravity (in the upper areas of the body) and respiratory activity (in the thoracic area). In addition, valves aid in the return of blood to the heart. Valves are small structures within the vein that prevent the backflow of blood. Valves are especially important in the legs because blood must travel a long distance against the force of gravity in order to reach the heart.

Blood carried in the veins (except for the pulmonary vein) contains high concentration of carbon dioxide (CO_2). This gas is waste product of cell metabolism and is produced by all cells of the body. When CO_2 is present in blood, the blood takes on characteristic, purple color. Such blood is said to be deoxygenated. Deoxygenated blood is continuously transported to the lungs, where the CD2 is expelled.

HEART

The heart is a hollow, muscular organ that pumps blood through the arteries, capillaries and veins. It is enclosed in a fibroserous sac called the pericardium. The heart has three distinct layers of tissue:

1. The **endocardium**, which is serous membrane that lines the four chambers of the heart and its valves. It is continuous with the arteries and veins.

2. The **myocardium**, which is the muscular layer of the heart.
3. The **epicardium**, which is the outermost layer of the heart.

The heart is divided into four chambers. These chambers are the right atrium, right ventricle, left atrium, and left ventricle. The two upper chambers, the atria, collect blood; the two lower chambers, the ventricles pump blood from the heart. The right side of the heart provides for the oxygenation of blood (pulmonary circulation) and the left side is responsible for the transportation of blood to body cells, which compose all the systems of the body (systemic circulation). The muscular wall dividing the right side of the heart from the left is called the septum.

Blood Flow through the Heart and Major Blood Vessels

Body cells produce waste product during metabolism. These waste products include carbon dioxide (CO_2) a gas that must be removed or tissue death will occur. The thin-walled capillaries allow CO_2 to enter the blood, where it is transported to the heart by way of two huge veins; the superior vena cava, which collects and carries blood from the top portion of the body; and the inferior vena cava, which collects and carried blood from the lower portion of the body. The superior and inferior vena cava deposits the deoxygenated blood into the right upper chamber of the heart, the right atrium. From the right atrium, blood passes through the tricuspid valve to the right ventricle. The tricuspid valve prevents blood from returning to the right atrium during contraction of the ventricle. When the heart contracts, blood leaves the right ventricle by way of the pulmonary artery. The pulmonary semilunar valve (pulmonary valve) in the pulmonary artery restrains blood from passing back into the right ventricle. In the lungs, this artery branches into millions of capillaries, each lying in close proximity to the alveoli. Here CO_2, in the blood is replaced by O_2 that has been drawn into the lungs during inhalation. The blood is now oxygenated and takes on a bright red appearance.

The pulmonary capillaries unite to form the pulmonary veins, which carry blood back to the heart. The right and left pulmonary veins carry oxygenated blood into the left atrium of the heart. The blood passes from the left atrium through bicuspid valve (also called the mitral valve) to the left ventricle. Upon contraction of the heart, the oxygenated blood leaves the left ventricle through the largest artery of the body, the aorta. Within the aorta is a valve called the aortic semilunar valve or aortic valve? This valve permits blood to flow in only one direction from the left ventricle to the aorta. The aorta branches into many smaller arteries that carry blood to all parts of the body. Some arteries derived their name from the organs or areas of the body that they vascularize. For example, the coronary arteries vascularize the heart muscle; the renal arteries vascularize the kidneys, and so forth.

It is important to recognize the O_2 present in the blood passing through the chamber of the heart cannot be used by the myocardium. Instead an arterial system called the coronary arteries, branches from the aorta and provides the heart muscle with its own blood supply. If the flow of blood the coronary arteries are diminished, myocardial damage may result. When severe damage occurs, necrosis of muscle tissue results.

Blood Pressure

Each heart beat is composed of two phases, the contraction phase, or systolic, the blood is forced out of the heat, and a relaxation phase, or diastole. Blood pressure measures the force exerted by the blood against the arterial walls during these two-phases. Systole indicates the maximum force exerted by the blood against the arterial walls; diastole, the weakest. These are recorded as two figures separated by a diagonal line; the systolic pressure is given first, followed by the diastolic pressure. For example, a blood pressure may be recorded as 120/80; 120 is the systolic pressure, and 80 is the diastolic pressure.

Several factors influence the blood pressure, including the resistance of blood flow in the blood vessels, the pumping action of the heart, the viscosity, or thickness, of the blood, the elasticity of the arteries, and the quantity of blood in the vascular system. Elevated blood pressure is called hypertension; decreased blood pressure is called hypotension.

Conduction System of Heart

Within the heart is a specialized cardiac tissue known as conductive tissue. Its sole function is the initiation and propagation of contraction impulses.

The conductive tissue consists of four masses of highly specialized cells

1. Sinoatrial node, or SA node
2. Atrioventricular node, or AV node
3. Bundle of His
4. Purkinje fibers

The SA node, which is located in the upper portion of the right atrium, possesses its own intrinsic rhythm. Without being stimulated by external nerves. It has the ability to initiate and propagate each heartbeat, thereby setting the basic pace for the cardiac rate. For this reason, it is commonly known as the pacemaker. Cardiac rate may altered by impulses from the autonomic nervous system. Such an arrangement allows outside influences to accelerate or decelerates the rate of the heartbeat. For example, during a period of physical exertion the heart beats faster, and during a restful interval the rate becomes slower.

Each electrical impulse discharged by the SA node is transmitted to the AV node, causing the atria to contract. The AV node is located at the base of the right atrium. From this point, a tract of conduction fibers called the bundle of His, composed of a right and left branch, relays the impulse to the Purkinje fibers. These fibers extend up the walls of the ventricles, causing them to contract. The blood is now forced out of the heart through the pulmonary artery and the aorta.

In summary, the sequence of involvement of the four structures in the heart that are responsible for the conduction of a contraction impulse is as follows:

SA node → AV node → Bundle of His → Purkinje fibers

Impulse transmission through the conduction system generates weak electrical currents that can be detected on the surface of the body. These electrical impulses can be electrocardiograph produces waves or peaks designated by the letters P, Q, R, S, and T, each of which is associated with a specific electrical event. The P wave is the depolarization (contraction) of the atria, and the QRS complex is the depolarization (contraction) of the ventricles. The T wave, which appears a short time late, is the repolarization (recovery) of the ventricles.

CHAPTER 4: BLOOD AND LYMPHATIC SYSTEM

ANATOMY AND PHYSIOLOGY OF HEMATIC AND LYMPHATIC SYSTEMS

Blood and Lymph are specialized tissues of the body. Each is composed of cells that are suspended in a liquid medium. Both of these tissues play a vital role in defending the body against infection. Since blood and lymph have the ability to move throughout the entire body, they provide a transportation system for body cells. They transport nourishment, water, vitamins, electrolytes (sodium, potassium, and calcium), immune substances, heat and oxygen to all parts of the body. Conveyance of waste products to appropriate body organs for removal, and distribution of hormones from the endocrine glands to numerous organs are some of the other vital functions performed by blood and lymph.

BLOOD

Blood is composed of liquid medium called plasma and a solid portion that consists of three major blood cells; red blood cells (erythrocytes), white blood cells (leukocytes), and platelets (thrombocytes). All blood cells develop from an undifferential cell, the hemocytoblast, also called stem cell. The maturation of the different blood cells is called hematopoiesis. The immature forms are found in the bone marrow; the mature forms circulate in the peripheral blood. The composition of blood is represented by the following diagram:

Whole blood = Liquid portion + Solid portion

- *Liquid portion:* Plasma
- *Solid portion:* Erythrocytes, leukocytes, thrombocytes (platelets)

Plasma accounts for about 55% and blood cells account about 45% of the total blood volume.

Erythrocytes

Erythrocytes are the most numerous of the circulating blood cells. They are formed in the red bone marrow (my tissue) of the sponge bones of the skull, ribs, sternum, vertebrae, pelvis, and at the ends of the long bones of the arms and legs. Red blood cell development is called erythropoiesis.

During erythropoiesis, red cells develop a specialized compound called hemoglobin, which is an iron-containing pigment that gives the erythrocyte its red color. Hemoglobin carries oxygen (O_2) to body tissues, where it is exchanged for carbon dioxide (CO_2). The fact that there are millions of hemoglobin molecules in each of the trillions of red blood cells can help you to appreciate the magnitude of the job that is accomplished by erythrocytes. The size of the red cell and its nucleus decreases during erythropoiesis. Just prior to maturity, the nucleus is extruded from the cell, leaving behind a small vestige of nuclear material (DNA). This DNA resembles a fine, lacy net, giving this cells its name, reticulocyte. Eventually, the DNA disappears and the now mature erythrocytes enter the circulatory system.

The mature erythrocyte appears as a smooth, biconcave structure with the cytoplasm filled with hemoglobin. It is thin in the center where the nucleus was extruded, while the periphery of other cell is thicker.

Erythrocytes live about 120 days and then rupture, releasing hemoglobin and cell fragments. The hemoglobin breaks down into hemosiderin, a compound that contains iron, and several bile pigments. Most of the hemosiderin returns to the bone marrow and is re-used to manufacture new blood cells. The bile pigments are eventually excreted by the liver.

Leukocytes

The chief function of the leukocytes is protection of the body against invasion by bacteria and other foreign substances. Their amoebic nature permits them to leave the blood stream in order to search for and destroy harmful substances. Leukocytes also play a role in tissue repair, but this activity is still not fully understood.

Leukocytes are classified into two categories, the granulocytes (those with granules in the cytoplasm) and the agranulocytes (those without granules). Each of these categories can be further subdivided. Granulocytes: Neutrophils, eosinophil's, and basophils. Agranulocytes: Monocytes and lymphocytes.

Granulocytes

Granulocytes are formed in the red bone marrow from stem cells, which give rise to myoblasts. Myoblasts differentiate into neutrophils, eosinophils and basophils. These names are derived from a polychromatic dye used to stain blood smears in the laboratory. The dye imparts specific colors to the granules of each of these cell types; eosinophil's take up the acid dye eosin; basophils stain with a basic, or alkaline, dye; and neutrophils stain with both the acid and basic dyes and hence are "neutral" in their staining preference. In addition to the presence of granules, these cells are further characterized by a nucleus that is composed of several lobes in their mature form, hence these cells are also called polymorphonuclear cells.

The neutrophil is the most numerous of the circulating white cells. It is very motile and highly phagocytic, permitting it to ingest and devour bacteria and other particulate matter. In some infections, it is not uncommon to find that one neutrophil has ingested as many as 20 bacteria.

The eosinophils and basophils, although capable of phagocytosis, rarely display this activity. Eosinophils protect the body by releasing many substances that are capable of detoxifying foreign protein and other material, especially of a chemical nature. They also are capable of destroying antigen/antibody complexes. Heir number usually increases during allergic reactions.

Eosinophil's release histamines and heparin in the area of damaged tissue. Histamines initiate the inflammation reaction, which increases blood flow. Therefore, additional neutrophils for phagocytosis are brought to the damaged area.

Agranulocytes

Granulocytes include both monocytes and lymphocytes. These cells are characterized by the absence of granules in their cytoplasm. In addition, they both have a single large nucleus and are therefore called mononuclear cells. Granulocytes develop from reticuloendothelial cells, the same cells that give rise to both erythrocytes and granulocytes. However, in early development monocytes and lymphocytes migrate from the bone marrow and enter the lymphatic system, where they undergo change and maturation. Some of these changes still are not fully understood.

Monocytes provide protection from the body in much the same manner as neutrophils, that is, they engage in phagocytosis. Monocytes migrate into tissue to become macrophages. In this form, they are able to consume large numbers of bacteria or other invaders. They can phagocytes as many as 40 or 50 bacteria or other invaders.

Lymphocytes, on the other hand, provide protection through immunologic activity. An immune response is the body's ability to distinguish foreign material as harmful and invasive, and then neutralize, eliminate, or metabolize it, thereby rendering it harmless. The harmful invader is called the antigen; the defense provided by the body is called the antibody.

The immunologic response can be divided into two categories; humoral immunity and cellular immunity.

Humoral immunity is provided by a specialized type of lymphocytes called B-cells or B-lymphocytes. Humoral immune involves the production of a substance called an antibody, which seeks out and renders harmless the invading substance called an antigen. As a general rule, the antigen-antibody reaction is specific, that is the antibody reacts only with the antigen that induces its formation. For example, if the body has developed antipolio antibodies in response to the presence of polio antigens (a situation that occurs after the administration of polio vaccine), these antipolio antibodies provide no protection against any other antigen except polio. In order to produce antibodies, certain B-cells are activated in the presence of an antigen to become plasma cells. Plasma cells synthesize and export antibodies. Some activated B-cells do not develop into plasma cells but remain as "memory cells". These cells stay in the lymphoid tissue. In the event of a future encounter by the same antigen, the memory cells immediately produce the plasma cells that are capable of manufacturing a specific antibody. It is believed that each plasma cell can manufacture specific antibodies at a rate of 2,000 per second for about 4 or 5 days.

The other type of protection provided by lymphocytes is cellular immunity. This immunity is function of T-lymphocytes, also called T-cells. T-cells mature in the thymus gland; hence the designation T-cells. When they encounter an antigen, T-cells become sensitized and change into "killer cells". They produce a lymphotoxin or cytotoxin that damages or ruptures the cell membranes of the antigen. T-cells also aid in production of interferon, a protein released from cells that have been invaded by a virus or other antigen. Interferon includes noninfected cells to form an antiviral protein that inhibits viral multiplication within the cell.

Thrombocytes

The smallest formed elements within the blood are thrombocytes, or platelets. They are known as platelets because of their small platelike appearance. Their chief function is to initiate blood clotting when injury occurs.

Blood clotting is not a single reaction, but rather a chain of interlinked reactions. At least 13 separate steps are involved, but this complex reaction can be described as essentially three major reactions.

Thromboplastin is either released by traumatized tissue at the site of injury or formed when platelets rupture. The action of thromboplastin causes prothrombin, a blood protein, to convert to thrombin. Eventually, thrombin converts a soluble blood protein, fibrinogen, to fibrin, an insoluble protein. Fibrin forms a meshwork in which blood cells become entangled. This jellylike mass of protein and blood cells is a blood clot.

The following reaction, simplified below. Shows the formation of a clot.

$$\text{Prothrombin} \xrightarrow{\text{Thromboplastin}} \text{Thrombin}$$

$$\text{Fibrinogen (soluble)} \xrightarrow{\text{Thrombin}} \text{Fibrin (insoluble)}$$

Plasma

Plasma is the liquid portion of the blood in which the corpuscles are suspended. It is composed of about 92% water and contains the plasma proteins (albumins, globulins, and fibrinogen), gases, nutrients, salts, hormones, and excretory products. Plasma makes possible the chemical communication between all body cells by carrying these products to different parts of the body. When free of corpuscles, plasma is thin and colorless or has a faint yellow tinge.

Blood serum is product of blood plasma. It differs from plasma in that serum does not contain fibrinogen. This can be represented as follows:

Plasma – Fibrinogen = Serum

When a blood sample is placed in a test tube and permitted to clot, the resulting clear fluid that remains after the clot from the test tube is serum. The formation of the clot has removed fibrinogen from the plasma.

BLOOD GROUPS

Human blood is divided into four groups based on the presence of absence of blood and antigen on the surface of the red blood cells. These four groups are A, B, AB, and O. Type A blood has A antigen; type B blood, B antigen; type AB blood, both A and B antigens; and Type O has neither A nor B antigens. In each of these four blood groups, the plasma does not contain the antibody against the antigen that is present on the red cells. Rather the plasma contains the opposite antibodies. For example, A blood contains A antigen on the surface of the red cells, therefore, its plasma contains B antibodies. B blood contains B antigen on the surface of the red blood cells; therefore its plasma contain A antibodies.

In clinical situation the mode in which an antibody antigen interacts provides a more specific way of identifying the antibody antigen complex. The mode in which this antigen/antibody complex reacts when the clinician serologically identifies blood types is agglutination (clumping); therefore, the antigen may be called an agglutinogen and the antibody may be called an agglutinin. Hence, type B blood contains B agglutinogens (antigens) on the surface of the red blood cells and A agglutinins (antibodies) in the plasma.

BLOOD GROUPS	
Agglutinogen on RBC (antigen)	**Agglutinin in plasma (antibody)**
A	B
B	A
AB	None
O	A and B

In addition to the blood groups listed above, there are numerous other antigens that may be present on the red blood cells. One such factor includes the Rh-hr system. This particular factor may be involved in hemolytic diseases of the newborn because of an incompatibility existing between the maternal blood and the fetal blood.

Although more than 90 blood factors have been identified by hematologists, most of these are not highly antigenic. Consequently, these factors generally do not cause concern in pregnancy of in a clinical situation in which blood is transfused into a patient.

LYMPHATIC SYSTEM

The lymphatic system consists of lymph, a network of transporting structures called lymph vessels, lymph nodes, and the spleen, thymus and tonsils. The primary function of the lymphatic system is to drain fluid from tissue spaces and return it to the blood. Other functions provided by the lymphatic system include transporting materials (nutrients, hormones, and oxygen) to body cells and carrying waste products from body tissue back to the blood stream. It also conveys lipids, or fats, away from the digestive organs. Finally, it aids in the control of infection by providing lymphocytes and monocytes, which are used to defend against infections caused by microorganisms.

Lymph originates from blood plasma. As whole blood circulates through the capillaries, some of the plasma seeps out of these thin-walled vessels. This fluid, now called interstitial or tissue, fluid, resembles plasma, except it contains less protein.

Interstitial fluid nourishes and cleanses the body tissues through which it circulates. It also collects cellular debris, bacteria, and particular matter. Eventually, interstitial fluid enters into blind-ended vessels called lymph capillaries. Once it enters a capillary it is called lymph. Lymph passes from the capillaries to larger vessels and finally to lymph nodes, which serve as depositories for cellular debris. As lymph passes through the nodes it is filtered and replenished with lymphocytes, globulins, and antibodies. Bacteria and debris are phagocytized by macrophages that line the nodes. At times, the number of bacterial entering a node is so great that the node enlarges and become tender.

Lymph vessels from the right chest and arm join the right lymphatic duct. This duct drains into the right subclavian vein, a major vessel in the cardiovascular system. Lymph from all other parts of the body enters the thoracic duct, which drains into the left subclavian vein. In this fashion, lymph is redeposited into the circulating blood in order to begin the cycle, once again, throughout the body.

Three organs are associated with the lymphatic system; the spleen, thymus, and tonsils. Like the lymph nodes, the spleen acts as a filter for lymph. Phagocytic cells within the lining of the spleen remove cellular debris, bacteria, parasites, and other infectious agents, thereby cleansing the lymph. The spleen also functions in the destruction of old red blood cells and serves as repository for healthy blood cells, to be put into circulation when needed.

The thymus gland is located in the mediastinum, the upper part of the chest. It partially controls the immune system. The thymus changes lymphocytes to T-cells, which provide cellular immunity.

Three sets of tonsils, the palatine, pharyngeal, and lingual tonsils, contain T and B lymphocytes. They guard against infection at the entrance of the digestive and respiratory tracts.

CHAPTER 5: NERVOUS SYSTEM

ANATOMY AND PHYSIOLOGY OF NERVOUS SYSTEM

The nervous system is one of the most complicated systems in the body. Along with the endocrine system, it controls many body activities. The nervous system senses changes in both internal and external environments, interprets these changes, and then coordinates appropriate responses that are designed to maintain homeostasis, which is a state of equilibrium in the internal environment.

DIVISIONS OF NERVOUS SYSTEM

The brain, spinal cord, and nerves all interact in relaying information. The nervous system has two major divisions; the central nervous system (CNS), which is composed of the brain and spinal cord; and the peripheral nervous system (PNS), which includes all other nervous tissue of the body found outside of the CNS.

The PNS includes 12 pairs of cranial nerves, which emerge from the base of the skull, and 31 pairs of the spinal nerves, which emerge from the spinal cord. All of these nerves consist of fibers that may be either sensory or motor, or mixture of both sensory and motor fibers.

Sensory nerves receive impulses from the sense organs, such as the eyes, ears, nose, tongue, and skin, and then transmit the impulses to the CNS. Because they conduct impulses toward a specific site—the central nervous system - they are also known as afferent nerves.

Motor nerves conduct impulses away from the CNS; thus, they are known efferent nerves. These impulses travel to muscles and other body organs causing them to respond in some manner.

Nerves composed of both sensory and motor fibers are called mixed nerves examples of a hen mixed nerve is the facial nerve. When it supplies the facial muscles with impulses for smiling or frowning, the facial nerve is functioning as a motor nerve. But when the tongue transmits a taste impulse to the brain through this nerve. It is responding in a sensory capacity.

Functionally, the PNS is divided into two specialized systems; the somatic nervous system (SNS) and the autonomic nervous system (ANS). The somatic component is under the direct control of the individual. It innervates (supplies with nerves) the extremities and the body wall, including the skeletal muscles and the skin. Since the somatic nervous system produces movement only in the skeletal muscles, it is under conscious control of the organism and is therefore voluntary. Examples of a voluntary activity include walking, talking, and playing tennis. In contrast, the autonomous component conveys impulses to glands, smooth muscles, and cardiac muscles. This division is therefore considered involuntary since it operates without conscious control. Examples of autonomic activity include digestion, heart contraction, and vasoconstriction

The autonomic nervous system is further specialized into two subdivisions: the sympathetic and parasympathetic divisions. To a large extent, these subdivisions function in opposing the action of each other, although in certain instances, they may be exhibit independent action. In general, sympathetic nerve fibers produce vasoconstriction, increased heart rate, elevated blood pressure, and depressed gastrointestinal activity, while the parasympathetic system generally conveys impulses to bring about vasodilation, a slower heart rate, a decrease in blood pressure, and a return to normal gastrointestinal activity. These autonomic functions are evident in "fight or flight" situations. Blood flow increases in skeletal muscles to prepare the individual to either fight or run away from a threatening situation. When the danger passes, more blood is directed to the internal organs.

NERVOUS TISSUE

In spite of its complexity, the nervous system is composed of only two principal types of nerve cells neurons and neuroglia. Neurons, the functional cells of the nervous system, are responsible for impulse conduction. All neural circuits are composed of neuron chains. In contrast to neurons neuroglia do not transmit impulses. Neuroglia is specialized nervous tissue that functions as connective tissue supporting and binding neurons. During infection, neuroglia is capable of performing certain phagocytic activities.

Neurons

Neurons consist of three major structures:

1. Dendrites, which are branching cytoplasmic projections that receive impulses and transmit them to the cell body.
2. Cell body, which contains the cell nucleus.
3. Axon, which is a long single projection that transmits the impulse from the cell body.

Many axons in both the PNS and CNS are covered with a white, lipoid sheath called myelin. This wrapping acts as an electrical insulator that reduces the possibility of impulses stimulating adjacent nerves. In addition, myelin accelerates impulses through the axon. The presence of myelin on axons in the brain and spinal cord gives a white appearance to these structures, and they make up what is called the white matter of the CNS. Unmyelinated fibers, dendrites and nerve cell bodies make up the gray matter.

On peripheral nerves, a thin cellular membrane called **neurolemma**, or **neurolemmal** sheath, wraps around the myelin sheath. The neurolemmal sheath permits a damaged axon to regenerate. Since neurolemma is not found in the CNS served nerves in the CNS cannot regenerate; therefore, nerve function is permanently lost unless alternate pathways are established.

Neurons are not continuous with one another. Instead, a small space, known as a synapse, is found between the axon of one neuron and the dendrite or cell body of another. In order for the impulse to travel along a nerve path, it must be transmitted at the synapse. This transmission is facilitated by certain chemical substances called neurotransmitters.

Neuroglia

The term neuroglia literally means nerve glue. It was once believed that neuroglia served only a supporting role for neurons. But it is now known that different shaped neuroglia cells perform many other functions. Astrocytes, as their name suggests, are star-shaped neuroglia and are believed to be involved in the transfer of substances from the blood to the brain. Oligodendrocytes are calls with only a few processes. They are believed to help in the development of myelin on neurons of the CNS. Microglia, the smallest of the neuroglia, possesses phagocytic properties and may become very active during times of infection.

Brain

In addition to being one of the largest organs of the body, the brain is also the most complex in structure and function. It integrates almost every physical and mental activity of the body. This organ is also the center for memory, emotion, thought, judgement, reasoning, and consciousness.

The brain is composed of four major section; the cerebrum, cerebellum, diencephalon (interbrain), and brain stem. In order to develop a better understanding of the anatomy of the brain, read the following material.

The (1) cerebrum is the largest and uppermost portion of the brain. It consists of two hemispheres divided by a deep longitudinal fissure, or groove. The fissure does not completely separate the hemispheres. A structure called the corpus callosum joins them medially on their inferior surfaces. Each hemisphere is further divided into five lobes.

Four of these lobes are named for the bones that lie directly above them. The fifth lobe of the cerebrum is hidden from view and can only be seen upon dissection.

Numerous folds, or convolutions, called gyri are found on the cerebral surface. These are separated by furrows or fissures called sulci. A thin layer of gray matter, the cerebral cortex, which is composed of millions of cell bodies, covers the entire cerebrum and is responsible for its bray color.

The reminder of the cerebrum is composed primarily of white matter (myelinated axons). Major functions of the cerebrum include sensory perception and interpretation, muscular movement, and the emotional aspects of behavior and memory.

The second largest part of the brain, the (2) cerebellum, occupies the back portion of the brain. It is attached to the brain stem. When the cerebrum initiates muscular movement, the cerebellum coordinates and refines the movement. The cerebellum also aids in maintaining equilibrium and balance of the body.

The (3) diencephalon, or interbrain, is composed of many smaller structures two of which are the (4) thalamus and the (5) hypothalamus. All sensory stimuli, except olfactory, are received by the thalamus. Here they are processed and transmitted to the proper area of the cerebral cortex. In addition impulses from the cerebrum are received by the thalamus and relayed to efferent nerves. Beneath the thalamus is a small structure called the hypothalamus? Its chief function is the integration of autonomic nerve impulses and the regulation of certain endocrine functions

The (6) brain stem completes the last major section of the brain. It is composed of three structures; the (7) medulla oblongata, the (8) pons, and the (9) midbrain (mesencephalon). In general, the brain stem serves as a pathway for impulse conduction between the brain and the spinal cord. The brain stem also serves as the origin of 10 of the 12 pairs of cranial nerves. The brain stem is the center that controls respiration, blood pressure, and heart rate.

Spinal Cord

Bones protect both the brain and the spinal cord against injury. The brain is enclosed within the skull, and the spinal cord is enclosed within the vertebral column. In addition, both the brain and the spinal cord receive limited protection from a set of three coverings called meninges. The outermost coat, the dura mater, is tough and fibrous. Immediately beneath the dura mater is a cavity called the subdural space? It is filled with serous fluid. The next layer of the meninges is the arachnoid. As its name suggests, the arachnoid has a spider-web appearance. A subarachnoid space, with filled cerebrospinal fluid, provides additional protection for the brain and spinal cord by acting as a shock absorber. Finally, the innermost layer, the pia mater, contains numerous blood vessels and lymphatics, which provide nourishment for the underlying tissues.

Cerebrospinal fluid circulates around the spinal cord and brain and through spaces called ventricles. These ventricles are located within the inner position of the brain. This clear, colorless fluid contains proteins, glucose, urea, salts, and some white blood cells. As it circulates, this fluid provides nutritive substance to the central nervous system. Normally, cerebrospinal fluid is absorbed as rapidly as it is formed. Any interference with absorption results in hydrocephalus.

CHAPTER 6: DIGESTIVE SYSTEM

ANATOMY AND PHYSIOLOGY OF DIGESTIVE SYSTEM

The two-fold purpose of the digestive system is to prepare the food that we eat for absorption by millions of body cells and to eliminate 8 waste materials from the body.

When food is ingested, it is in a form that cannot reach the cells because of its inability to pass through the intestinal mucosa into the bloodstream. Therefore, the consume food must be altered not only physically but also chemically. Thus, digestive can be defined as the complete process of changing the chemical and physical composition of food in order to facilitate assimilation of the nourishing ingredients of food by the cells of the body.

The organs of the gastrointestinal (GI) system form a tube that begins at the mouth and terminates at the anus. This tube referred to as the alimentary canal or the digestive tract. It measures approximately 30 feet in adults.

MOUTH (ORAL CAVITY, BUCCAL CAVITY)

The gastrointestinal (GI) tract is continuous tubular passageway that begins at the oral cavity, or mouth. The structures within the oral cavity are the cheeks, or bucca, and the tongue and its muscles, which extend across the floor of the mouth. The main functions of the tongue are manipulation of food during the chewing process, deglutition (swallowing), speech production, and determination of taste. The surface of the tongue has rough elevations, these elevations are taste buds. These sense organs are called papillae and are capable of perceiving a variety of flavors found in our foods, such as bitterness, sweetness, selfishness, and sourness.

The teeth are also found in the oral cavity and play an important role in the initial stages of digestion. The teeth that are located in the front of the oral cavity, the incisors and cuspids, cut and tear the food into small pieces. The teeth located in the rear of the oral cavity are called molars. They further crush and grind the food into finer particles. Teeth are covered by hard enamel, which gives them a white and smooth appearance. Beneath the enamel is the main structure of the tooth, the dentin. Dentin is surrounded by a thin layer of modified bone called cemented. In the innermost part of the tooth is the pulp, which stores the nerves and blood vessels of the tooth. The teeth are embedded in pink fleshy tissue known as gums, or gingiva.

Two of the other structures located within the mouth are the hard and soft palates. The hard palate lied in the anterior portion of the roof of the oral cavity, while the soft palate lies in its posterior portion. The soft palate forms a partition between the mouth and the nasopharynx and is continuous with the hard palate. The entire oral cavity, like the rest of the digestive tract, is lined with mucous membrane.

After the food is chewed, it is formed into a round, sticky mass called a bolus. The bolus is pushed by the tongue from the mouth into pharynx (also called the throat). Its downward movement is guided into the pharynx by the soft, fleshy V-shaped tissue called the uvula. The uvula hangs from the superior rood of the oral cavity. The pharynx is a muscular tube. It is divided into three major sections.

1. The **nasopharynx** (the part of the throat behind the mouth)
2. The **oropharynx** (the part of the throat behind the mouth

3. The **laryngopharynx** (the part of the throat above the larynx). The laryngopharynx is further divided into two tubes; one that leads to the lungs, called the trachea; and one that leads to the stomach, called the esophagus.

A small flap of tissue, the epiglottis, covers the trachea. The main function of the epiglottis is to prevent food from entering the trachea, thus allowing all food to be channeled to the stomach though the esophagus.

STOMACH

The stomach is a saclike structure located in the abdominal cavity directly below the diaphragm. It is continuous with the esophagus. Thus, food continuous its descent downs the stomach. The stomach mixes the undigested food with gastric juices to further break it down for digestion. Within the stomach, there are a considerable number of folds, called rugae. The rugae appear only when the stomach is empty. As the stomach fills the interior walls becomes smooth. The interior lining of the stomach is composed of mucous membranes and contains the glands that secrete hydrochloric acid (HCl) and gastric juices. Once the food or bolus mixed with gastric juices and HCl, it forms a semi-creamy fluid called chyme.

There are two valves in the stomach. The first valve is called the **cardiac valve**, or **cardiac sphincter,** and is located at the top of the stomach. It connects the esophagus to the stomach. The second valve is called the pyloric valve, or pyloric sphincter, and is located at the base of the stomach. It connects the stomach to the small intestine. Both valves are composed of a round band of muscles called sphincters, which contract and expand to allow food to enter and leave the stomach.

SMALL INTESTINE

The small intestine is approximately 1 inch in diameter and is continuation of the gastrointestinal tube. The small intestine consists of three parts.

1. The **duodenum**, the uppermost division, which is about 10 inches long.

2. The **jejunum**, which is approximately 8 feet long.
3. The **ileum**, which is about 12 feet long. Most of the absorption of food takes place in the ileum, by tiny figure like projections called villi. Inside the villi is a network allows the absorption of food into the bloodstream.

There are also many other intestinal digestive glands located in the mucous membrane lining the small intestine. These microscopic glands secrete additional digestive juices.

The **pancreas** and **liver** produce digestive secretions, and these secretions are added to the chyme at the beginning of the small intestine. With the exception of some forms of fat, water, and waste products, all of the food ingested into the body is absorbed through the walls of the small intestine.

Colon

The colon is a continuation of the gastrointestinal tube and is attached to the ileum by the ileocecal valve. This valve is composed of sphincter muscles that serve to close the ileum at the point at which the small intestine is connected to the colon.

The large intestine has an average diameter of 2½ inches and is approximately 5 feet long. It is divided into two major divisions, the cecum and the colon.

The cecum is the first 2–3 inches of the large intestine. Attached to the cecum is a wormlike projection, the vermiform appendix, which performs no function in the digestive system.

The colon consists of the following parts.

- The **ascending colon**, which extends from the cecum to the lower border of the liver (hepatic flexure).
- The **transverse colon**, which passes horizontally across the abdomen to the left toward the spleen (splenic flexure)
- The **descending colon**, which continuous down to form the **sigmoid colon**.
- The **rectum**, which serves as storage area for the waste products of digestion, leads to the orifice called the **anus**. The anus is kept closed by internal and external sphincters, or muscles, except during the process of defecation (elimination of feces).

ACCESSORY ORGANS AND DIGESTION

Liver

The liver is the largest glandular organ in the body and weighs approximately 3–4 pounds. It is located beneath the diaphragm in the right upper quadrant (RUQ) of the abdominal cavity.

The liver performs so many vital functions that people cannot survive without it. Some important functions of the liver include the following:

1. Produce bile, which is used in the small intestines to emulsify and absorb fats.
2. Removes glucose (sugar) from blood, which it synthesis and stores as glycogen (starch).
3. Stores vitamins, such as B, A, D, E, and K
4. Breaks down or transforms some toxic products into less harmful compounds.
5. Maintains normal levels of glucose in the blood
6. Destroys old erythrocytes and releases bilirubin
7. Produced various blood proteins, such as prothrombin and fibrinogen, which aid in the clotting of blood.

Pancreas

The **pancreas** is an elongated somewhat flattened organ that lies posterior and slightly inferior to the stomach. The pancreas acts as both an endocrine gland and an exocrine gland. In the digestive system, it provides digestive juices that pass through the **pancreas duct**, thereby giving it its exocrine function. These enzymatic juices aid in the digestive process. The pancreatic duct extends along the gland and enters the duodenum in the company of the bile duct from the liver. By secreting digestive juices through a duct, the pancreas functions as an exocrine gland in the GI system. But in the endocrine system, the pancreas releases hormones directly into the bloodstream and functions as an endocrine, or ductless gland. The endocrine function of the pancreas is related to the islets of Langerhans, whose beta cells secrete the hormone insulin and alpha cells secrete the hormone glucagon, which regulate blood sugar levels.

Gallbladder

The gallbladder serves as a storage area for bile. During the process of digestion, when there is a need for some bile, the gallbladder releases it into the duodenum through the common bile duct. Bile is also drained from the liver through the hepatic ducts. The hepatic ducts connect with the cystic duct from the gallbladder, forming the common bile duct.

CHAPTER 7: ENDOCRINE SYSTEM

ANATOMY AND PHYSIOLOGY OF ENDOCRINE SYSTEM

Both the endocrine system and the nervous system regulate the basic metabolic activities of the body. Their functions are closely related because they work together to maintain homeostasis (the state of equilibrium in the internal environment of the body). The endocrine system is essentially a chemical communication system and is composed of endocrine glands, which are responsible for secretions of hormones. Included in the endocrine system are a number of ductless glands located in various parts of the body. These glands are called endocrine glands because they release their secretions directly into blood vessels that run through the glands. They are not to be confused with exocrine glands, such as the sweat and oil glands of the skin, which release their secretions externally through ducts. This chapter includes the function of the pituitary, thyroid parathyroid, adrenals, pancreas and pineal glands.

PITUITARY GLAND

The pituitary gland, or hypophysis, is no larger than a pea and is located at the base of the brain. It is known as the "master gland" because it regulates many body activities and stimulates other glands to secret their own specific hormone (Table 16.1).

The gland consists of three distinct portions—an anterior lobe (adenohypophysis or pars distalis), or middle lobe (pars-distalis), and a posterior lobe (neurohypophysis or pars-distalis). All these lobes secrete a number of hormones.

TABLE 16.1 Hormones of the pituitary gland

Gland	Hormone	Major effects
Adeno hypophysis (anterior lobe)	Growth hormone (GH), or somatotropin	Stimulates bone and body growth
	Thyroid-stimulating hormone (TSH), or thyrotropin	Controls secretions of hormones from the thyroid gland
	Prolactin	• Promotes, growth of breast tissue • Stimulates milk production after birth
	Adrenocorticotropic hormone (ACTH)	Stimulates secretions by the adrenal cortex, especially cortisol
	Gonadotropin; Follicle-stimulating hormone (FSH)	• Stimulates development of eggs in the ovaries • Stimulates secretion of estrogen in females • Stimulates production of sperm cells in the testes
	Luteinizing hormone (LH), or interstitial cell-stimulating hormone (ICSH) in male	• Promotes the secretin of sex hormones in both males and females • Plays a role in the release of the egg cell in females
Neurohypophysis (posterior lobe)	Antidiuretic hormone (ADH), or vasopressin	• Decrease volume of urine excreted • Increases volume of water reabsorbed in kidney
	Oxytocin	• Causes contraction of the uterus during labor and childbirth • Stimulates milk secretion

THYROID GLAND

The thyroid gland is the largest gland of the endocrine system. It is an H-shaped organ located in the neck just below the larynx. This gland is composed of two fairly large lobes that are separated by a strip of tissue called an isthmus.

The function of the thyroid gland is to produce, store and release thyroxin (T3) and triiodothyronine (T4) the major thyroid hormones.

Both T3 and T4 regulate metabolism and are responsible for a person's energy level. They increase the rate of oxygen consumption and thus the rate at which fats are utilized. In addition both hormones work with the growth hormone (GH) and stimulate activity in the nervous system.

PARATHYROID GLANDS

The **parathyroid glands** consist of a least four separate glands located on the posterior surface of the thyroid gland. The only hormone known to be secreted by the parathyroid glands is a protein called parathyroid hormone (PTH), or parathormone. PTH helps to regulate the metabolism of calcium by influencing three types' organs-the bones, the intestine, and the kidneys. PTH seems to stimulate the formation of new bone cells (osteoblasts). As a result of this increased activity calcium and phosphates are released from the bones, and the blood concentrations of these substances increase. Thus, the calcium that is necessary for the proper functioning of body tissues is present in the bloodstream. At the same time, PTH enhances the absorption of calcium and phosphates from foods in the intestine, and this action also produces a rise in the blood levels of calcium and phosphates. PTH causes the kidneys to conserve blood calcium and to increase the excretion of phosphates in the urine.

ADRENAL GLANDS

The adrenal glands are paired structures located superior to the kidneys. Because of their location a top the kidneys, the adrenal glands are also known as suprarenal glands. Each adrenal gland is structurally and functionally differentiated into two sections: the outer adrenal cortex, which makes up the bulk of the gland, and the inner adrenal medulla. Although these regions are not sharply divided, they represent distinct glands that secrete different hormones. Steroids are secreted by the cortex. Cells of the adrenal medulla secrete two closely related hormones, epinephrine (adrenaline) and nor-epinephrine (noradrenaline).

The hormones of the adrenal cortex are all steroids (and are essential to life. In fact, in the absence of cortical secretions, a; person usually does within a week unless extensive electrolyte therapy (sodium, potassium, and calcium levels are carefully controlled).

Histologically, the cortex is subdivided into three zones. Each zone has a different cellular arrangement and secretes different groups of hormones. The three groups are as follows:

1. **Mineralocorticoids** which help to regulate water and mineral salts (also called electrolytes) that are retained in the body. One of the mineralocorticoids of major importance in humans is aldosterone. Like all of the hormones of the adrenal cortex, aldosterone is a stored. This hormone acts mainly through the kidneys to maintain the homeostasis of sodium and potassium. More specifically, aldosterone causes the kidneys to conserve sodium and to excrete potassium. At the same time, it promotes water conservation and reduces urine output.
2. **Glucocorticoids** which influence the metabolism of carbohydrates, fats and proteins. The glucocorticoid with the greatest activity is cortisol. It helps to regulate the concentration of glucose in the blood, protecting against low blood sugar between meals. Another effect of cortisol is to stimulate the breakdown of fats in adipose tissue and release fatty acids causes many cells to use relatively less glucose.
3. **Gonadocorticoids** (sex hormones), which affect sexual characteristics. Although the sex hormones are primarily male type (adrenal androgens), small quantities of female hormones (adrenal estrogens and progesterone) are also present. The normal functions of these hormones are not clear, but they may supplement the supply of sex hormones from the gonads and stimulate dearly development of the reproductive organs. Also, there is some evidence that the adrenal androgens play a role in controlling the female sex drive.

Epinephrine (adrenaline) and norepinephrine (noradrenaline) are two closely related hormones secreted by the adrenal medulla. The effects of the medullary hormones resemble those of the sympathetic nervous system. The adrenal medulla, like the rest of the sympathetic nervous system, is not essential to life, but it is important to the ability of the organism to meet emergencies.

PANCREAS (ISLETS OF LANGERHANS)

The pancreas lies inferior to the stomach in a bend of the duodenum. It functions both as an exocrine and endocrine gland. A large pancreatic duct runs through the gland carrying enzymes and other exocrine digestive secretions from the pancreas to the small intestine. The pancreas has groups of cells called islets of Langerhans, which produce endocrine secretions. There are two main kinds of cells in the islets; A-cells (alpha cells) produce glucagon and constitute about 25% of the islet cells; B-cells (beta cells) produce insulin and constitute about 75% of the islet cells. Both of these hormones, glucagon and insulin, play an important role in the proper metabolism of sugars and starches in the body.

PINEAL GLAND

The pineal gland is shaped like a pine cone and is attached to the posterior part of the third ventricle of the brain. Although the exact functions of this gland have not been established, there is evidence that it secretes melatonin hormone. It is believed that melatonin may inhibit the activities of the ovaries. When melatonin production is high, **ovulation is** blocked and there may be a delay in puberty development. The pineal gland starts to degenerate at about 7 years of age; in the adult, it consists mostly of fibrous tissue.

CHAPTER 8: RESPIRATORY SYSTEM

ANATOMY AND PHYSIOLOGY OF RESPIRATORY SYSTEM

Respiratory activity consists of two separate simultaneous operations that involve the exchange of oxygen (O_2) and carbon dioxide (CO_2).

EXTERNAL RESPIRATION

The first operation, external respiration refers to the exchange of O_2 and CO_2 between the organism and the external environment. In this operation, oxygen-rich air from the environment is brought into the lungs during inspiration (inhalation). And CO_2 is removed from the body during expiration (exhalation). For more familiarity, external respiration is called lung breathing.

INTERNAL RESPIRATION

The second operation, internal respiration, refers to the exchange of O_2 and CO_2 at the cellular level. Oxygen contained in the red blood cells is exchanged for the waste carbon dioxide in the tissues. This exchange is also called tissue breathing. Just as the organism as a while requires exchange of gases to maintain life, each individual cell must also exchange gases for the metabolic process. Ultimately, CO_2 will be transferred to the lungs to be expelled.

STRUCTURES ASSOCIATED WITH BREATHING

The following will provide a better understanding of the anatomy and physiology of the respiratory system.

During the breathing process, air from the environment is drawn into the nose and **passes** through the nasal cavity (turbinate's) to the pharynx (throat). The pharynx is a muscular tube that constitutes the first major section of the air passages to the lungs. It is about 5 inches long and consists of three sections:

1. The **nasopharynx,** posterior to the nose
2. The **oropharynx**, posterior to the mouth
3. The **laryngopharynx**, above the larynx.

Within the nasopharynx is a collection of lymphatic tissue known as adenoids, or pharyngeal tonsils. Another collection of lymphatic tissue called palatine tonsils, or more commonly, tonsils, is located in the oropharynx.

Beneath the laryngopharynx is the larynx (voice box). This structure is responsible for sound production, or phonation. A leaf-shaped flap on top of the larynx, the epiglottis, seals off the air passage to the lungs during swallowing to ensure that food or liquids do not obstruct the flow of air to the lungs.

The extension of the new air passage tube beneath the larynx is the trachea. It is composed of smooth muscle embedded with C-shaped cartilage rings. These rings provide the necessary rigidity to keep the air passage open at all times. The trachea divides into two branches called bronchi (singular form bronchus). One bronchus leads to the right lung and the other to the left lung. Like the trachea, the bronchi contain C-shaped cartilage rings. Without them, the trachea or bronchi may possibly collapse and endanger life.

Each bronchus divides into small branches called bronchioles (little bronchi), which terminate in air sacs called alveoli (singular from alveolus). An alveolus resembles a small balloon because it expands and contracts with inflow and outflow of air. Capillary beds of the circulatory system lie adjacent to the thin tissue membranes of the alveoli. Carbon dioxide passes from the blood within the pulmonary capillaries into the alveolar spaces; while oxygen from the alveoli passes into the blood. After the blood becomes oxygenated, it returns to the heart where it is pumped to all body tissues. At the tissue level O_2 from the blood is exchanged for tissue CO_2. This exchange of gases is called internal respiration.

The diaphragm assists in changing the volume of the thoracic cavity. As the diaphragm contacts, the intercostal muscles elevate the rib cage. Both of these activities result in enlarging the thoracic cavity. Consequently air from the environment passes into the lungs. The reverse activity causes the air to pass from the lungs into the environment.

CHAPTER 9: SENSE ORGANS

ANATOMY AND PHYSIOLOGY OF SPECIAL SENSES

The special senses of the body include the senses of taste, smell, equilibrium, sight, and hearing. These senses allow us to detect changes in our environment, and each of them has a structurally complex receptor organs.

Taste

The ability to taste is accomplished by numerous structures located on the tongue, the taste buds. In order for the taste buds to be stimulated, substances must be dissolved in saliva. When this occurs, the solution containing the dissolved substances enters the taste bud and stimulates the particular receptor, producing taste. Despite the fact that we believe that taste many flavors, the taste buds of the tongue respond to only four sensations; sour, salty, bitter, and sweet.

Tall other "tastes" are actually odors that stimulating the olfactory bulb in the nose.

Smell

Olfactory sensation or the sensation of the smell, is accomplished by a highly, specialized collection of nervous tissue, the olfactory bulb. Odors emitted from substances enter the nasal passageways and stimulate the olfactory bulb, producing the sensation of smell, not taste.

Equilibrium

The ability to maintain equilibrium is accomplished, to a large extent, by a complex structure located in the inner portion of the ear. The semi-circular canals. The posture and orientation of the body is sensed by this structure which transmits impulses to the brain. As the brain integrates these impulses, it makes the necessary physiologic adjustments that are required to maintain equilibrium.

EYE

The eye functions in a manner similar to that of a camera. Light rays pass through a small opening and are focused by a lens upon a photoreceptive surface. In a camera, the surface is a photographic film; in the eye, it is the retina.

The eye is a globe shaped organ that is composed of three distinct layers. Its outermost layer is the sclera. As the name suggests, it is a tough fibrous tissue that serves as a protective shield for the more sensitive structures beneath. The sclera is also known as the white of the eye. A highly vascular middle layer, the choroid, provides the blood supply for the entire eye. The innermost layer of the eye, the retina, is composed of nerve endings that are responsible for the reception and transmission of light impulses.

A specialized portion of the sclera, the cornea, passes in front of the lens. Rather than being opaque, it is transparent and thus permits the entrance of light into the interior of the eye.

One of the two major humors, or fluids, of the eye is the **aqueous humor.** The iris divides the aqueous humor into two small chambers, the **anterior chamber** and the **posterior chamber**. A colored, contractile membrane, the iris, functions as a sphincter. Its perforated center is the **pupil**. The amount of light entering the eye is regulated by the size of the pupil. As the environmental light increases the pupil constrict; as the light decreases, the pupil dilates.

Located behind the posterior chamber is the **lens**. This crystalline structure is suspended between the ciliary muscles. As these muscles relax or contract, they alter the shape of the lens, making it thicker or thinner, respectively, thus enabling the light rays to focus upon the retina. This process is called accommodation.

The second major humor of the eye is the vitreous humor. This clear, jelly-like fluid occupies the entire orbit of the eye behind the lens. The vitreous humor, the lens, and the aqueous humor are the refractive structures of the eye. They are responsible for the bending of light rays so that they focus sharply on the retina, if any one of those structures does not function properly, vision is impaired.

The retina is extremely delicate eye membrane. It is continuous with the optic nerve and has two types of light receptors upon, its surface, rods and cones. Rods function in dim light and provide black-and-white vision. Cones function in bright light and provide color vision.

Both the optic nerve and the blood vessels of the eye enter the eyeball at the optic disc. Its center is referred to as the blind spot because the area has neither rods nor cones.

Six muscles control the movement of the eye; the superior, inferior, lateral, and medial rectus muscles, and the superior and inferior oblique muscles. These muscles are coordinated to move both eyes in a synchronized manner.

The front of the eye is protected by two movable folds of skin, the eyeballs. Hair edges are lined with two or three rows of eyelashes, which protect the surface of the eye.

A thin mucous membrane called the conjunctiva lines the inner surface of the eyelids and passes over the cornea. Lying superior and to the outer edges of each eye are the lacrimal glands. They produce tears to bathe and lubricate the eyes. The tears collect at the inner edges of eyes, the canthi (singular, canthus), and pass through pinpoint openings, the lacrimal canaliculi, to the nose.

EAR

The ear is the sense organ of hearing. It consists of three major sections; the external or outer ear; the middle ear, or tympanic cavity; and the inner ear, or labyrinth. Although each of these sections transmits sound waves, each accomplishes the task in a different way. The external ear conducts sound waves through air, the middle ear through bone, and the inner ear, through fluid. As will be subsequently explained, this series of transmissions plays an integral part in hearing.

The external ear is designed to channel sound waves from the environment to the middle and inner ears. An auricle, or pinna, is the external structure designed to collect waves traveling through air. The auricle channels the waves through the ear canal, which is a slender tube that leads to the middle ear. The canal is lined with glands that produce a waxy secretion called cerumen. Cerumen prevents foreign particles from entering the ear. A flat membranous structure, the tympanum (tympanum membrane, or ear drum) is drawn over the end of the canal. Sound waves that enter the ear canal strike against the tympanum.

In the middle ear, vibrations of the tympanum are picked up by three tiny articulating bones called **ossicles**. These bones are responsible for the transmission of sound waves through the middle ear. The three bones are the malleus (hammer), the incus (anvil), and the stapes (stirrups). These bones form a chain that stretches from the inner surface of the tympanum to an inner ear structure called the **cochlea.**

A tube called the e**ustachian tube**, connects the nose and the throat with the cavity of the middle ear. Its purpose is to equalize pressure on the outer and inner surfaces of the eardrum. In situations in which sudden pressure on the outer and inner surfaces of the eardrum. In situations in which sudden pressure changes occur, equalization of pressure is achieved by deliberate swallowing.

The inner ear, sometimes referred to as the labyrinth because of its complicated maze like design, is composing of three structures; a snail shaped **cochlea**, the **semicircular canals**, and the **vestibule,** which is a chamber that joins the cochlea and the semicircular canals.

The cochlea is filled with fluid. Lining its inner surface are tiny nerve endings called the hairs of Corti. There is a membrane-covered opening on the external surface of the cochlea, called the **oval window**.

It is on this membrane that the stapes is attached to the cochlea. Transmission of sound along the ossicles in the middle ear causes the stapes to exert a gentle pumping action against the oval window. The pumping action forces the cochlear fluid to move. Disturbance of the fluid stimulates the hairs of Corti, causing them to generate a series of nerve impulses. The impulses are transmitted to the brain by way of the auditory nerve, where they are interpreted a sound.

CHAPTER 10: EXCRETORY SYSTEM

ANATOMY AND PHYSIOLOGY OF UROGENITAL SYSTEM

The male and female urinary systems consist of four major structures; a pair of kidneys; two ureters, a bladder, and a urethra. This chapter presents information on these structures. In addition, it includes a discussion of the male reproductive system, since some of the male reproductive organs use urinary structures.

URINARY SYSTEM

The urinary system acts as the regulator of extracellular products of the body by determination the harmful products in the blood plasma and selectively filtering them from the blood. Included in the products that must be removed from the body are nitrogenous wastes and excess fluid electrolytes (sodium, potassium, and calcium). One of the nitrogenous products is urea. This substance is produced when body tissues metabolize protein. High concentrations of urea in the blood cause a toxic condition known as uremia. The blood collects urea and other waste materials from body tissues and conveys these materials to the kidneys. In the kidneys, microscopic structures called nephrons filter these substances from the blood as they form complex fluid called urine. Urine is eventually expelled from the body.

Macroscopic Structures of the Urinary System

Two kidneys, each about the size of a fist, are located in the retroperitoneal area of the abdominal cavity. A concave medial border gives the kidney its beanlike shape. Near the medial border is a slit like aperture, the hilus or hilum. It serves as an opening for a renal vein and a renal artery to enter the kidney. The renal artery carries blood that is laden with waste products to the microscopic filtering tubules located within the kidney for purification. After the blood is cleansed, it leaves the kidney by way of the renal vein. The waste material, now in the form of urine, is carried in a hollow chamber, the renal pelvis, located at the hilus. This chamber is an enlarged funnel shaped extension of the ureter at the entrance to the kidney. Each ureter is a slender tube about 10–12 inches long that conveys urine, in peristaltic waves, to the bladder. The bladder, which is an expandable hollow organ, acts as a temporary reservoir for urine. During micturition (voiding), urine is expelled from the bladder through the urethra, a membranous tube that terminates at the urinary meatus. The urethra is approximately 1 1/2 inches in women and about 7 inches in men.

Microscopic Structures of the Urinary System

Microscopic examination of kidney tissue reveals the presence of approximately 1 million tiny functional structures called nephrons. These little filtering units are responsible for maintaining homeostasis (a stable optimal internal environment) by continually adjusting the conditions necessary for survival. When the level of various products in the blood becomes elevated beyond a normal range, or reaches the renal threshold, nephrons selectively remove those products from the blood to re-establish a level that can sustain life. The substances that are removed by nephrons are the end products of metabolism-urea, uric acid, and creatinine. Nephrons also extract any excess electrolytes. Some pathological states may cause certain undesirable substances to appear in the blood. This maul so be removed by the nephrons. For example, when the blood sugar level becomes elevated, as in diabetes mellitus, the excess sugar is filtered from the blood and is removed from the body in the urine.

Each nephron includes a **renal corpuscle** and a **renal tubule**. The renal corpuscle to compose of a tuft of capillaries, the glomerulus, and a modified funnel-shaped end of the renal tubule, **Bowman's capsule**. This capsule encases the glomerulus. An **afferent arteriole** conveys blood to the glomerulus, and a smaller efferent arteriole carries blood away from the glomerulus. As the efferent arteriole passes behind the renal corpuscle, it forms the **peritubular capillaries.**

Each renal tubule consists of four sections; the **proximal tubule**, followed by the narrow **loop of Henle**, then a larger portion, the **distal tubule**, and finally the **collecting tubule**.

The nephron removes waste products from the blood by three physiological activities filtration, reabsorption, and secretion. All of these activities are performed by different sections of the nephron.

The phase of urine production, filtration, takes place in the renal corpuscle. Here, water, electrolytes, sugar, amino acids, and other compounds pass from the blood in the glomerulus into Bowman's capsule. The fluid that is formed is called filtrate. The next phase of urine production starts with the passing of filtrate through the four sections of the tubule. As the filtrate travels the long and twisted pathway, most of the water and some of the electrolytes and amino acids are absorbed by the peritubular capillaries, thus re-entering the circulating blood. The final stage of urine production occurs when specialized cells of the collecting tubules secrete ammonia, uric acid, and other substances directly into the lumen of the tubule. The formation of urine is now completed. It is passed from the collecting tubules to the renal pelvis, or the basin of the kidney.

CHAPTER 11: REPRODUCTIVE SYSTEM

ANATOMY AND PHYSIOLOGY OF UROGENITAL SYSTEM

This chapter presents information on the male and female reproductive system.

MALE REPRODUCTIVE SYSTEM

The male reproductive system serves two important functions. First, it produces sperm, the male sex cell, which contains one half of the genetic material necessary to produce a living being. Second, it provides the structures necessary to transport and maintain viable sperm.

The primary male reproductive organ consists of pair of testes (singular testis), which are located in an external sac, the scrotum. Within the testes are numerous small tubes that twist and coil to form the seminiferous tubule. These structures produce a sperm, which is the male sex cell. The testes also secrete testosterone, an androgenic hormone that develops and maintains secondary sex characteristics and influences adult male sexual behavior. Lying over the superior surface of each testis is a single, tightly coiled tube, the epididymis. This structure stores sperm after it leaves the seminiferous tubule. The epididymis is the first duct through which sperm passes after its production in the testes. Tracing the duct upward, the epididymis forms the vas deferens (seminal duct or ducts deferens), which is a narrow tube that passes through the inguinal canal into the abdominal cavity. The vas extends over the top and down the posterior surface of the bladder, where it joins a duct leading from an accessory sex gland, the seminal vesicle. The union of the vas and the duct from the seminal vesicle forms the ejaculatory duct.

The seminal vesicle secretes approximately 60% of the fluid that ultimately ejaculated during sexual climax. This fluid contains nutrients that support sperm viability.

The ejaculatory duct passes at an angle through the prostate gland, which is triple lobed organ fused to the base of the bladder where it joins the urethra. The prostate secretes a thin, alkaline substance that account for about 30% of the seminal fluid. Its alkalinity helps protect the sperm from the acidic environments of both the male urethra and the female vagina. Two pea-shaped glands, Cowper's glands, or bulbourethral glands, are located below the prostate. They are connected by a small duct to the urethra. Cowper's glands also provide an alkaline fluid that is necessary for the viability of the sperm. The penis is the male organ of copulation. It is cylindrical organ composed of erectile tissue, and it encloses the urethra. The urethra expels both semen and urine from the body. During ejaculation, the sphincter at the base of the bladder is closed. This not only stops the urine from being expelled with the semen, but also prevents the sperm from entering the bladder.

The enlarged tip of the penis is the glans penis. It contains the urethral orifice (meatus). A movable hood of skin, called prepuce of foreskin, covers the glans penis.

FEMALE REPRODUCTIVE SYSTEM

The female reproduction system consists of internal and external organs of reproduction. The internal, or essential, organs of the reproduction are the ovaries, fallopian tubes, uterus, and vagina.

The external genitalia include the labia majora, labia minora, clitoris, vestibule of the vagina, and the greater vestibular glands, or Bartholdi's glands. The combined structures of the external genitalia are known as the vulva.

Both the cervix and vagina are lubricated by the mucus secretions of the Bartholdi's glands. These glands provide lubrication during sexual intercourse by secreting a mucoid acid substance.

Ovaries

The ovaries are almond-shaped glands located in the pelvic cavity. One on each side of the uterus. They produce both the ovum, and eggs, which is the female reproductive cell, and various hormones.

Two of the hormones secreted by the ovaries are estrogen and progesterone. These hormones are responsible for the menstrual cycle and menopause. In addition, both hormones prepare the uterus for implantation of the fertilized egg, help maintain pregnancy, and promote growth of the placenta. Estrogen and progesterone also play an important role in the development of secondary se characteristics.

Fallopian Tubes or Oviducts

Two fallopian tubes or oviducts extend laterally from superior angles of the uterus. They transport the ovum by a wavelike current (peristalsis) from the ovary to the uterus. In addition to conveying the ovum an oviduct provides a passageway through which sperm travel from the uterus toward the ovary. Union of the ovum and sperm results in fertilization. Thus a 9-month period of development (gestation, pregnancy within the uterus) begins with the fertilization of the egg.

Uterus and Vagina

The uterus is an organ that contains and nourishes the embryo from the time the fertilized egg is implanted until the fetus is born. It is a muscular, hollow, pear-shaped structure and is located in the pelvic area between the bladder and rectum. The uterus is normally in a position of anteflexion (bent forward), and it consists of three parts: the fundus, which is the upper-rounded part; the corpus, or body, which is the central part; and the cervix. The cervix is sometimes referred to as the neck of the uterus and it extends into the top portion of the vagina.

The vagina is a muscular tube about 7 1/2 cm long, and its lining consists of a mucous membrane fold that gives the organ an elastic quality. The vagina extends from the cervix to the exterior of the body. Besides serving as the organ of sexual intercourse and the receptor of semen, the vagina discharges the menstrual flow. The vagina also as passageway for the delivery of the fetus.

Menstrual Cycle

The menstrual cycle consists of approximately 28 days and can be groups into four phases, which are used in describing the events of the cycle (Table 16.2). The initial menstrual period (menarche) occurs between the ages of 9 and 18, the average being 12 to 13 years of age.

Following ovulation, the Graafian follicle collapses and forms a clot which is absorbed by the remaining follicular cells. These follicular cells enlarge, change character, and from the corpus luteum, or yellow body. The corpus luteum then secretes increasing quantities of estrogens and progesterone.

It fertilization and implantation do not occur, the decreased secretions of progesterone and estrogens (by the corpus luteum) then initiates menstrual cycle.

TABLE 16.2 Phases of menstrual cycle

Phase 1: Menstrual phase (first 5 days)	A discharge that is a mixture of endometrium, blood, mucous, and vaginal cells passes from the uterine cavity to the cervix, through the vagina, and ultimately to the exterior
Phase 2: Preovulatory phase (days 6–13)	Ovarian follicles produce more estrogen, which stimulates the repair of the endometrium. During his phase, one of the secondary follicles matures into a graafian follicle, which is ready for ovulation
Phase 3: Ovulation (day 14)	About the 14th day, the graafian follicle ruptures (ovulation), and the egg cell leaves the ovary and enters the peritoneal cavity. The egg cell is then drawn into the uterine tubes
Phase 4: Postovulatory phase (days 15–28)	This represents the time between ovulation and the onset of the next menses

TABLE 16.3 Climacteric period	
Premenopausal	Nervousness; irregular menses; vasomotor symptoms (due to an effect o the diameter of the blood vessels) Instability (hot flashes)
Menopausal	Frequent vasomotor symptoms; atrophy of genitourinary fissure Wasting's decrease in size of an organ or tissue)
Postmenopausal	Occasional vasomotor symptoms atrophic vaginitis Atrophy of genitourinary tissue with decreased support osteoporosis

MENOPAUSE

Menopause is the cessation of menses for the reminder of a woman's lifetime. It is usually diagnosed if amenorrhea (absence of menses) has persisted for 1 year and there are no other problems. The period of time in which symptoms of approaching menopause occur is knows the climacteric period. Some common manifestation during the climacteric is as follows (Table 16.3).

PREGNANCY

Pregnancy is the condition in which a zygote (fertilized ovum) develops in the uterus. The normal gestation period is approximately 9 calendar months. The product of conception up to the month of pregnancy is referred to as the fetus.

During pregnancy, the uterus changes its shape, size and consistency. The peritoneal covering becomes enlarged, and there is an enormous increase in the muscle mass. The vaginal canal becomes elongated by the rise of the uterus in the pelvis. The mucosa thickens and secretions increase, and there is rise in the vascularity and elasticity of both the cervix and vagina.

Pregnancy also causes enlargement of the breasts, sometime to the point of painfulness. On the whole, many changes are evident in all of the body systems in order to accommodate the development and birth of the fetus.

Labor and Birth

Labor is the physiological process by which the fetus is expelled from the uterus. Labor occurs in three stages as follows: The first is the stage of dilation, which begins with uterine contractions and terminates when there is complete dilation (10 cm) of the cervix. The second is the stage of expulsion. This is the time from complete cervical dilution to the birth of the baby. The last is the placental stage, or afterbirth. It begins shortly after childbirth, when the uterine contractions discharge the placenta from the uterus. Barring complications, the actual birth usually occurs in a relatively short period.

CHAPTER 12: ONCOLOGY

Oncology is the study of tumors. It includes both malignant and nonmalignant growths. The purpose of his chapter is to provide a comprehensive understanding of oncology.

CHARACTERISTICS OF NEOPLASMS

In healthy individuals, cell division is an orderly process in which body cells are produced for growth of the individual or for replacement of cells that are destroyed or worn out. In some instances, however, cell division is without purpose. The newly formed cells increase at an uncontrolled rate, producing a lump or swelling known as tumor on neoplasm. These neoplasms may be benign or malignant.

Benign Neoplasms

Benign neoplasms are new growths that develop in body tissues. They are composed of the same type of cells as the tissue in which they are growing. For example, a benign tumor of a gland is composed of the glandular tissue form which it is developing. Benin neoplasms are continued within a capsule and do not invade the surrounding tissue. They harm the individual only insofar as they place pressure on surrounding structures. If the benign neoplasm remains small and places no pressure on other organs or structures, excision is necessary. Benign brain tumors are always very serious since the cranial cavity is enclosed and pressure on other parts of the brain inevitably results. As a general rule, however, benign tumors are not life-threatening. Once they are removed, they usually do not regrow.

Malignant Neoplasms

The cells that compose a malignant neoplasm often do not resemble the tissue in which they are growing. The tumor cells lack specialization in both structure and function. In such cases, the tumor is said to be dedifferentiated. In dedifferentiation, cells lose their ability for specialized function and revert to an immature or embryonic form. More significantly, however, the cells of the malignant neoplasm are not encapsulated and are thus able to spread to normal tissues. This invasive growth develops by either direct extensions or metastasis. In direct extension, the tumor grows directly into normal tissue. This phenomenon is called proliferation. With metastasis, the malignant cells from the primary tumor site find their way into lymph channels or blood vessels and are carried to remote body structures in which secondary malignant neoplasms then develop (Table 16.4).

TABLE 16.4 Characteristics of neoplasms

Benign	Malignant
Encapsulated	Nonencapsulated, having protections infiltrating surrounding tissues
Composed of tissue that closely resembles the tissue in which the neoplasm arises	Composed of tissue that does not resemble the tissue in which the neoplasm arises
Does not spread to remote areas of the body	If left untreated, the cells of the neoplasm metastasis to remote regions of the body
Generally poses little risk, if any, to the patient	If left untreated poses a risk to the patient

BRAINSTORMING QUESTIONS

1. A cell is a mass of protoplasm containing a ___________.
2. The human body is made of ___________ numbers of cells.
3. There are 2 types of cell division-they are Mitosis and ___________ .
4. The fluid inside the cell is called ___________ fluid.
5. The fluid outside the cell is called ___________ fluid.
6. Tissue is made up of a group of ___________.
7. Tissues can be classified into ___________ major groups:
8. Organs are structures of several types of ___________.
9. The medical term of internal organ is ___________.
10. Eye is called cell or tissue or organ.
11. A system is a group of ___________.
12. Muscular, Nervous, Endocrine, called system or organ or tissue ___________.
13. Three types of muscular tissues; Skeletal, Visceral and ___________.
14. Skeletal system contains ___________.
15. How many bones are there in the adult skeletal system? ___________.
16. The nervous system consists of the Brain, ___________ Nerves.
17. Sense organs consist of Eye, Ear, Nose, ___________ Skin.
18. Sex glands (Ovaries and ___________.
19. Blood composition ___________ blood cells.
20. Blood contains: Thrombocytes; what is other name ___________.
21. Blood groups: A, B, ___________ O, Rhesus factor (Rh) (+) and (-).
22. Lymphatic System contains: Lymph vessels, nodes and ___________.
23. ___________ are the primary organs of the respiratory system.
24. What system does Esophagus belong to?
25. Jejunum belongs to ___________ Intestine.
26. The sigmoid colon is part of ___________.
27. Accessory organs: Liver, Gallbladder, ___________.
28. Ureters belong to which system ___________.
29. Ovaries belong to which system ___________.
30. Hymen belongs to which system ___________.
31. The brain is located in the ___________ cavity.
32. The lung is located in the ___________ cavity.
33. Stomach located in the ___________ cavity.
34. Ureters, urinary bladder, urethra located in the ___________ cavity.
35. Nerves runs through vertebra is called ___________ cavity.
36. In front of the body is called ___________.
37. At the back of the body is called ___________.
38. Away from the surface is called ___________.
39. Near the surface is called ___________.
40. Below another structure is called ___________.

41. Above another structure is called ___________.
42. Pertaining to the sides ___________.
43. Lying on the back is called ___________.
44. Lying on the belly is called ___________.
45. Towards the structure.
46. Away from the structure.
47. What type of bones are found in the limbs/extremities: short or long.
48. Short bones are found in the hands/limbs ___________ (carpals).
49. Shoulder blades (scapula and ___________).
50. Irregular bones are found in the Face and the ___________.
51. How many bones are there in Skull?
52. How many bones are there in Face?
53. How many bones are there in the Ear?
54. How many bones are there in Neck?
55. How many bones are in the Thoracic cavity?
56. How many bones are there in Vertebral columns?
57. How many bones are there in Cranial?
58. How many bones are there in Thoracic?
59. How many bones are there in Lumbar?
60. How many bones are there in Sacrum?
61. How many bones are there in Coccyx?
62. Scapula and Clavicle belong to which limb?
63. Humerus belongs to which arm lower or upper.
64. Radius and Ulna part of which arm.
65. Carpal and metacarpal belong to ___________.
66. Fingers bones are called ___________.
67. The femur belongs to the upper or lower limb.
68. Tibia and Fibula are part of the hand or leg.
69. Tarsal belongs to the lower or upper limb.
70. The pelvis belongs to the lower or upper limb.
71. Name which carries various functions such as reproduction, respiration, excretion, and adaptation to the environment.
72. The ___________ is structured, which gives the power of movements.
73. They ___________ conduct impulses all over the body.
74. ___________ give the body the power of movement.
75. ___________ are structures composed of several types of tissues.
76. Groups of organs working together in a human is called ___________.
77. The ___________ system includes the bones, muscles, and joints.
78. Muscles and ___________ make up for most of the body's weight.
79. The adult human skeleton contains ___________ bones.
80. The ___________ consists of the cranium, face, and lower jaw.
81. The ___________ consists of the spinal column, ribs, and stern.
82. The ___________ bones of the skull protect the brain.

83. The vertebral column is composed of ____________ bone.
84. The ____________ is the set of five bones and it is the tailbone.
85. Name vessels that carry oxygenated blood ____________.
86. The ____________ is a conical-shaped hollow muscular organ.
87. The organ is made of cardiac muscle is called ____________.
88. Blood circulation from the heart to the lungs and back known as ____________.
89. ____________ is the liquid portion of the blood.
90. ____________ are formed in the red bone marrow of the spongy bones.
91. ____________ or WBC that work with the immune system.
92. Blood is divided into ____________ groups.
93. Lymph originates from the blood ____________.
94. Injecting antibodies against foreign organisms is called ____________.
95. More than ____________ nerve cells are operating all over the body.
96. The nervous system is made up of innumerable nerve cells ____________.
97. The main function of the ____________ is memory.
98. The medulla oblongata is located at the base of the ____________.
99. The ____________ glands are exocrine glands producing saliva.
100. ____________ is to move the food from the pharynx to the stomach.
101. The stomach, SI and LI together form the ____________ tract.
102. The ____________ has three parts: Duodenum, jejunum, and Ileum.
103. The ____________ is the only organ, which has no anatomy.
104. The ____________ is the largest gland in the body.
105. The ____________ acts as both endocrine and exocrine gland.
106. Thyroxin hormone released by ____________ gland.
107. ____________ occurs when the diaphragm and the intercostal muscles relax.
108. ____________ located below the lungs is the major muscle of respiration.
109. Muscular tube common for respiratory and digestive system ____________.
110. ____________ are two cone-shaped organs help in breathing.
111. The right lung has ____________ lobes and the left has two lobes.
112. Dome shaped muscle sits below the lungs and the heart is known as ____________.
113. Organ that is essential for taste and speech is ____________.
114. The ____________ is the organ for the smell.
115. The ____________ system is also known as the excretory system.
116. Two ____________ convey urine from the kidney to the urinary bladder.
117. The prostatic part is part of the Male or Female: ____________.
118. The female gonads are the ____________.
119. The male gonads are the ____________.
120. The ____________ is filled with a fluid called amniotic fluid.
121. ____________ is the study of tumors.

Answers

1. Nucleus
2. Trillion
3. Meiosis
4. Intracellular
5. Extracellular
6. Cells
7. 4
8. Tissues
9. Viscera
10. Organ
11. Organs
12. System
13. Cardiac
14. Bones
15. 206
16. Spinal cord
17. Tongue
18. Testes
19. Plasma
20. Platelets
21. AB
22. Spleen
23. Lungs
24. Digestive
25. Small
26. Large intestine
27. Pancreas
28. Urinary
29. Reproductive
30. Reproductive
31. Cranial
32. Thoracic
33. Abdominal
34. Pelvic
35. Spinal
36. Anterior
37. Posterior
38. Deep
39. Superficial
40. Inferior
41. Superior
42. Lateral
43. Supine
44. Prone
45. Afferent
46. Efferent
47. Long
48. Wrist
49. Sternum
50. Vertebra
51. 8
52. 14
53. 6
54. 1
55. 51
56. 26
57. 7
58. 12
59. 5
60. 1
61. 1
62. Upper limb
63. Upper
64. Lower
65. Hands
66. Phalanges
67. Lower
68. Leg
69. Lower
70. Lower
71. Cell
72. Muscles
73. Nerves
74. Muscles
75. Organs
76. System
77. Musculoskeletal
78. Bones
79. 206
80. Skull
81. Trunk
82. Cranial

83. 26
84. Coccyx
85. Arteries
86. Heart
87. Heart
88. Pulmonary
89. Plasma
90. Erythrocytes
91. Leukocytes
92. Four
93. Plasma
94. Vaccination
95. 10 billion
96. Neurons
97. Cerebrum
98. Brain
99. Salivary
100. Esophagus
101. GI
102. Small intestine
103. Appendix
104. Liver
105. Pancreas
106. Thyroid
107. Expiration
108. Diaphragm
109. Pharynx
110. Lungs
111. Three
112. Diaphragm
113. Tongue
114. Nose
115. Urinary
116. Uterus
117. Male
118. Ovaries
119. Testes
120. Placenta
121. Oncology

Annexure 1

DEFINITIONS OF MEDICAL SPECIALTIES

Specialty	Specialty focus
Allergy and immunology	Allergic and immunologic diseases and their respirator complications (such as pollen, chemical and food allergies, asthma and AIDS).
Anesthesia	Anesthesia or relief of pain during surgery and childbirth, and control of pain due to various causes.
Bariatric surgery	Weight loss surgery—includes a variety of procedures performed on people who are obese, weight loss is achieved by reducing the size of the adjustable gastric band. Gastric bypass surgery-sleeve gastrectomy.
Cardiovascular disease	Diseases of the heart and blood vessels.
Dermatology	Diseases of the skin.
Emergency medicine	Diseases that are acute medical or surgical conditions or injuries that require urgent or immediate care (usually in a hospital emergency room).
Endocrinology and metabolism	Diseases of the internal glands of the body, including diabetes mellitus.
Family practice	All diseases and related total health care of an individual and the family.
Gastroenterology	Diseases of the digestive tract, including the stomach, bowel, liver and pancreas.
General practice	All diseases and related total health care of an individual and the family.
Geriatric medicine	Disease of the elderly.
Gynecology	See 'Obstetrics and Gynecology'.
Gynecology oncology	Cancer diseases of the female reproductive system.
Hematology	Disorders of the blood and blood-forming organs (including cancerous disorders of the blood) such as anemia, leukemia and lymphoma (see oncology, medical).

Contd...

Contd…

Specialty	Specialty focus
Infectious diseases	Infections of all types.
Internal medicine	All diseases and total health care of adults, usually 18 years of age and older.
Neonatology	Diseases of the newborn child.
Nephrology	Diseases of the kidney, including dialysis.
Neurology	Diseases of the brain, spinal cord, nervous system and related structures.
Neurological surgery	Diseases of the brain, spinal cord, nervous system and related structures requiring surgery.
Obstetrics and gynecology	Normal and abnormal pregnancy, diseases of the female reproductive system and fertility disorders.
Oncology, medical	Cancer and disorders of the blood and blood-forming organs (see hematology).
Ophthalmology	Diseases of the eye.
Orthopedic surgery	Diseases of the bones, joints, muscles and tendons.
Otorhinolaryngology (ear, nose and throat)	Diseases of the ears, nose, sinuses, throat and upper airway passages.
Pathology	Tissues and specimens removed by biopsy and surgery to diagnose normal from diseased tissues and specimens; supervises and interprets laboratory tests on blood, urine and other body fluids.
Pediatrics	All diseases and total health care of newborns, infants, children and adolescents.
Physical medicine and rehabilitation	Diseases with major and minor disabilities requiring restoration of functional ability, such as assistance, retaining and recondition of muscles, tendons and extremities for ambulation and other activities of daily living.
Plastic surgery	Diseases and conditions requiring surgical reconstruction for deformity or loss of a body part, or for cosmetic purposes to improve appearance or function.

Contd…

Contd...

Specialty	Specialty focus
Podiatric medicine (Podiatry)	Diseases of the foot and ankle as they affect the conditions of the feet.
Preventive medicine	Health care and other measures to avoid delay or prevent disease or illness from occurring.
Psychiatry	Diseases affecting mental health including diseases of the brain, nervous system and substance abuse of drugs or chemicals.
Pulmonary disease	Diseases of the lung.
Radiology	Diagnostic X-ray, ultrasound and other imaging techniques, such as computerized tomography (CT) and magnetic resonance imaging (MRI).
Radiology nuclear	Diseases requiring use of radioactive isotopes or as an aid in diagnosis and/or therapy.
Radiation oncology	Cancer and other diseases with X-ray therapy, radioactive isotopes and linear accelerator particle radiation.
Rheumatology	Diseases of the joints including arthritis and autoimmune diseases.
Sports medicine	Diseases and injuries acquired in sports.
Surgery, general	Diseases that require surgical operation for diagnosis or treatment.
Surgery, hand	Diseases and injuries of the nerves, tendons, muscles, bones or skin of the hand requiring surgery.
Surgery, thoracic	Diseases of the chest, including lungs, heart, blood vessels and chest wall that require surgical operation for diagnosis and or treatment.
Surgery, vascular	Diseases of the blood vessels that require surgical operation for diagnosis or treatment.
Surgery, colon and rectal	Diseases of the large intestine (bowel), rectum and anus that require surgical operation for diagnosis or treatment.
Surgery, urology	Diseases of the kidneys, bladder and male reproductive tract that require surgical operation.

Annexure 2

TERMS AND DEFINITIONS USED IN HEALTH CARE MANAGEMENT

The following are some of the important terms and definitions which are required for documenting medical records in general and nursing records in particular.

- **Accident and Emergency Record:** It is used for emergency (casualty) patients in the A/E department. This term is commonly used as A/E record, or casualty record or emergency room record or emergency file. These records are kept in the casualty department for one year and later transferred to medical record department.
- **Admission Waiting List:** A list of names of patients maintained by the admission office waiting for a vacant bed and room for admission to the hospital.
- **Adult Patient:** A patient 12–14 years of age or older.
- **Allergy:** A condition of unusual or exaggerated specific susceptibility to a substance which is harmless in similar amounts for other members of same species. This term embraces all types of human hypersensitiveness.
- **Allied Health Personnel:** Those not involved in the direct care of the patient but are vital in providing health care (such as dietary, social services and medical records personnel).
- **Amalgamation of Records:** Bringing together of two or more files and numbers of one single patient created at different times under one hospital number and one file.
- **Analysis of Hospital Service:** A gross appraisal of the efficiency of the hospital and medical staff primarily for benefit of, and use by, the patient and hospital. It is intended to give a picture of the type of illnesses cared for by the hospital and their end results.
- **Anatomy:** It is the study of different organs which make up the body, their arrangements, and relationships to each other, and the different types of cells recognizable on microscopic examination.
- **Anesthesia:** Loss of feeling or sensation.
- **Angiocardiography:** A diagnostic procedure involving an X-ray dye into the blood stream, followed by chest X-rays to show the dimensions of the heart and the large blood vessels.

- **Anomaly:** It is a structure or organ which is irregular information (malformation). Examples of congenital anomalies are missing fingers or toes and heart defects.
- **Arthroscopy:** Visual examination of the inside of a joint with an endoscope.
- **Assembling of Records:** Arrangement of different forms in a standard prescribed order, e.g. outpatient file and inpatient file as recommended in the work procedures.
- **Assistant Medical Record Technician (AMRT):** It is a trained employee of the Medical Record Department who works under the supervision of a Medical Record Technician (MRT)?
- **Audiometric:** An instrument (audiometer) which delivers acoustic stimuli of specific frequencies to determine the patient's hearing for each frequency. The results are plotted on a graph called an audiogram.
- **Authorized Personnel** are employees of the hospital and are directly involved with the medical care of the patient e.g. medical, nursing, and paramedical staff.
- **Autopsy:** Examination of organs of a dead body (autopsy) to determine the cause of death, is also known as postmortem examination.
- **Autopsy Rate:** The ratio during any given period of time of all autopsies to all deaths.
- **Average Daily Census:** The total number of inpatients days (exclusive of newborn) care rendered for a period is computed and divided by the total number of days in that period.
- **Average Length of Stay:** The total number of inpatient day's care rendered to discharge patients (exclusive of newborn) in a given fiscal period divided by the total number of patients (exclusive of newborn) who were discharged or who died during the same period. In computing the length of stay, the day of admission should be counted but not the day of discharge.
- **Bacteriology:** The study of bacteria and diseases caused by them.
- **Bassinet:** For the use of infant other than newborns. Bassinets used for newborn infants are not considered to be hospital beds and should not be included in the bed complement of a hospital.
- **Bed Complement:** It is the total number of hospital beds, exclusive of newborn bassinets, normally available for 24 hours service to inpatients in the hospital.

- **Bed Occupancy Board:** This board is maintained by the admission office, is also termed as the 'bed control board' or the 'bed utilization board' for keeping the account of occupied and vacant beds in different wards of the hospital.
- **Benign Tumor:** A benign tumor is a slow growing neoplasm and does not metastasize. Benign tumors are limited in extent and often are surrounded by a capsule.
- **Biochemistry:** The science which deals with the chemistry of life.
- **Biopsy:** Excision of tissue from a living body for microscopic examination to establish a diagnosis.
- **Birth:** It is the acceptance of an infant patient newly born in the hospital for inpatient service. This involves occupancy of a newborn infant bassinet and maintenance of a hospital chart during the period of care.
- **Birth Weight:** The first weight of the fetus or newborn obtained after birth. This weight should be measured preferably within the first hour of life before significant postnatal weight has occurred.
- **Burn:** A lesion of the tissues due to chemicals, dry heat, electricity, flame, friction, or radiation. They are usually classified into three types:
  - *First degree burns:* No blisters; superficial lesions mainly in the epidermis; hyperesthesia; and erythema.
  - *Second degree burns:* Damage to the epidermis and corium; blister; erythema; and hyperesthesia.
  - *Third degree burns:* Both the epidermis and corium are destroyed and subcutaneous layer is damaged, leaving charred, white tissue.
- **Carcinomas:** The largest group of solid tumors which are derived from epithelial tissue.
- **Cardiac Catheterization:** A thin flexible tube (catheter) is introduced into a vein or artery and is guided into the heart for detecting pressure and pattern of blood flow. Dye can also be injected and X-rays taken.
- **Cardiology:** The study of the structure, function, and disease of the heart.
- **Casualty:** This term is synonymous to 'Accident and Emergency' or 'Emergency'.

- **Causes of Death:** The causes of death to be entered on the medical certificate of cause of death are all those diseases, morbid conditions, or injuries which either resulted in or contributed to the death and the circumstances of the accident or violence which produced any such injuries.
- **Cauterization:** Burning a part of tissue.
- **Census:** The number of inpatients presents in a hospital or health care facility at any one time. Ward clerk (AMRT) will prepare a daily ward census report and send it to the Medical Record Department.
- **Centralized Filing System:** A system in which all information is filed in one central location. Outpatient and inpatient files are kept in medical record folder and filed in the Medical Record Department.
- **Centralized Serial:** The method of issuing one series of numbers to both the outpatient department and the inpatient department, and storing all records in one place. In addition, a patient is given a new number on each admission either in the outpatient department or in the inpatient department.
- **Centralized Serial Unit:** Same as centralized serial, but the earlier records of the patient are brought to the folder of the latest admission.
- **Central Processing Unit (CPU):** The part of a computer system that contains the circuits which control the interpretation and execution of instructions, including arithmetic, logic, and control functions.
- **Central Registration:** This section works around the clock to register new patients for outpatient and inpatient services. This section also maintains patient master index filing to enable verification of previous registration numbers.
- **Cesarean Section:** Delivery of the fetus by an incision through the abdominal and uterine wall.
- **Cesarean Section Rate:** The ratio of cesarean sections performed to viable births.
- **Chart (Record) Analysis:** Careful review of the entire record (patient file); identification of specific areas that are incomplete or deficient.

- **Chemotherapy:** It is the administration of a drug which destroys microorganisms, parasites, or malignant cells within the body and is utilized in the treatment of infectious diseases.
- **Child Patient:** Any patient less than 12–14 years is called a child patient, excluding newborn infants (born in the hospital).
- **Coding:** A numerical assignment that provides an organized approach to data retrieval. The term coding for disease and operation classification as per International Classification of Diseases and Operations. The medical record staffs are responsible for coding of diseases and operations.
- **Color Coding:** It is used in terminal digit filing system, in which ten different color strips or labels are used for numerals 0–9 to facilitate and to identify the numbers of records filed by color.
- **Communicable Disease:** Causative agents which transfer disease from one person to another directly or indirectly.
- **Completion of Records:** Completing the records (patient files) which are deficient in number of forms or content as per the established standards. The medical record staff reviews each case and notes the deficiencies of physician and other documentation.
- **Complication:** A disturbance occurring in the course of a disease and arising wholly or in part separate from the disease itself.
- **Comprehensive Record:** It is the one which has all the required forms with detailed and complete clinical and other information in a patient file as per established criteria.
- **Computer:** An electronic device which stores, transmits, and manipulates information according to predetermined instructions known as a program.
- **Confidential Information:** A statement made to a physician, an attorney, or a clergyman in confidence with the implicit understanding that it should remain confidential. Patient health records are confidential documents.
- **Confidentiality:** Status accorded to data or information which is sensitive for some reason and therefore must be protected against theft or improper use, and disseminated only to authorized individuals or organizations.
- **Consent:** Concurrence of wills; voluntary yielding of one's will to the proposition of another; acquiescence or compliance.

This is obtained in the hospital generally for rendering treatment and performing surgical procedures to patients.

- **Consultation:** A meeting of two or more physicians at the request of the attending physician or other authorized persons or body for study of a problem case, with necessary examinations to arrive at an accurate diagnosis and a written opinion as to prognosis, therapeutic measures, and recommendations proposed.
- **Contagious Disease:** One communicable by contact with an individual suffering from it or by contact with an object touched by that person.
- **Convalescent Patient:** A patient who is recovering from disease and who is preparing for normal activity.
- **Cribs:** Equipped with sides or guards, for the use of young children (i.e. below 12–14 years of age).
- **Critcria:** Predetermined elements against which aspects of the quality of medical service may be measured; for instance, two criteria for care of urinary tract infection might be the obtaining of a urinalysis and a urine culture.
- **Cross Index:** Cross indexing of diseases and operations may be defined as listing on a card for a specific disease or operation entity, according to recognized classification, all essential data of each patient having that particular condition, with a cross reference on other cards to every other entity involved in the particular case.
- **Cryosurgery:** Using cold temperature to destroy tissue. The cold is usually produced by a probe containing liquid nitrogen.
- **Data Bank:** Computer term for storage of information.
- **Death Rate:** The ratio of total number of deaths in the hospital during any given period of time to the total number of discharges and deaths during that same time.
- **Deficiency:** A nonjustifiable variation from expected standards.
- **Deficiency Check:** Reviewing of outpatient and inpatient files for deficiencies by the Medical Record Department staff.
- **Dermatology:** The science which deals with the skin, its structure, function, disease, and treatment.
- **Detrimental:** Harmful, damaging and undesirable.
- **Diagnosis:** It is made on the basis of extensive knowledge about the patient, such as family history, physical examination, and

investigation including X-rays and laboratory tests. The following are some of different kinds:

- *Clinical diagnosis:* Based upon symptoms shown during life, irrespective of the morbid changes producing them.
- *Final diagnosis:* A statement of opinion arrived at after extensive study, which is complete and accurate and is in conformity with the accepted medical terminology.
- *Pathological diagnosis:* Based on gross and microscopic examinations of the structural lesions present.
- *Differential diagnosis:* Based on symptoms and physical signs of two contrasting diseases.
- *Provisional diagnosis:* Based upon the availability of sources of information but subject to change.
- *Tentative diagnosis:* As above (provisional).
- *Preoperative diagnosis:* Made before operation and based on clinical findings.
- *Postoperative diagnosis:* Based upon findings observed during the operation.

- **Dialysis:** Literally means 'complete separation'. A dialysis machine (artificial kidney) can completely separate out from the blood the harmful waste products of the body which are normally removed in the urine.
- **Dilatation and Curettage:** Dilatation (widening) of the cervical opening is accomplished by inserting a series of probes of increasing size. Curettage (scraping) is accomplished by using a curette (metal loop at the end of along, thin handle) to remove the lining of the uterus.
- **Direct Admission:** A patient admitted onto a ward and occupying a bed without processing through the admission office. This is permitted in emergency and obstetrics cases.
- **Discharge Analysis:** The tabulation of data on discharged hospital patients to reflect the professional services provided in a hospital.
- **Disease:** Any deviation from or interruption of the normal structure and function of any part of the body. It is manifested by a characteristic set of signs and symptoms and in most instances the etiology, pathology, and prognosis are known.
- **Disease and Operation Index:** A numerical index of patient problems, diagnoses, and surgical procedures by individual

categories. This work is performed by the Medical Record Department.

- **Dividers:** Heavy-weight fabric forms of pressboard, used to designate different sections, e.g. 'outpatient', 'correspondence', 'investigations', and 'inpatient' records of the patient folder. Also used to designate alphabetical breaks in the Patient Master Index or numerical divisions of the Disease or Operation Index.
- **Doctor's Conference Room:** Area in the Medical Record Department allocated exclusively for doctors to periodically complete deficient records.
- **Doubtful Cases** are those in which either hospital number or the name of the patient is recorded wrongly.
- **Early Fetal Death or Abortion:** Completed less than 20 weeks gestation (500 g or less).
- **Echocardiography:** A diagnostic procedure in which pulses of high frequency sound waves (ultrasound) are transmitted into the chest and echoes returning from the surfaces of the heart are electronically plotted and recorded. This can show the structure and movement of the heart over time and may be useful in determining structural defects in the heart.
- **Elective Surgery:** A surgical procedure is planned or performed which is subject to the choice or decision of the patient or physician; applied to procedures that are advantageous to the patient but not urgent.
- **Electrocardiography (ECG or EKG):** The record of the electrical activity flows through the heart.
- **Electrocochleography:** A direct recording of the action potential generated following stimulation of the cochlear nerve.
- **Electroconvulsive Therapy (ECT):** A form of physical treatment occasionally used by psychiatrists mainly in the management of depression.
- **Electroencephalography (EEG):** Ultrasonic waves are beamed through the head and echoes coming from brain structures are recorded as a image. This procedure is useful in detecting brain tumors, and hydrocephalus.
- **Electromyography (EMG):** The use of an instrument which records electrical current generated by inactive muscle.

- **Electrooculography (EOG):** The use of an instrument which records eye position and movement.
- **Emergency:** Any condition which could result in serious permanent harm to a patient or aggravation of injury or disease, or in which the life of a patient is in immediate danger, and any delay in administering treatment could add to the danger. Casualty or Accident and Emergency (A/E) or Emergency is synonymous terms.
- **Emergency Record:** Patient file of an emergency or casualty or A/E patient. If the patient is transferred to outpatient or inpatient care, then the emergency record also becomes part of main patient file.
- **Emergency Treatment:** Treatment immediately necessary to save life. For example: treatment of a fracture case is not, whereas the treatment of a shock and hemorrhage case is.
- **Endemiology:** The special study of endemic disease (recurring in an area, e.g. Tuberculosis).
- **Endocrinology:** The study of the ductless glands and their internal secretions (hormones).
- **Endoscopy:** An instrument used for visualization of body cavities or organs.
- **Epidemiology:** A branch of medical science that deals with the incidence, distribution, and control of disease in a group of people (population).
- **Eponym:** A name or phrase formed from or including the name of a person, such as Brigit's disease or Paget's disease.
- **Etiology:** A science dealing with the causation of disease.
- **Evaluation of Medical Record Service:** This evaluation should provide information on how effectively medical record services are being performed, e.g. how accurate is the filing of records or index cards, or how accurate is the disease index, etc.
- **Fetal Death:** A death prior to the complete expulsion or extraction of the product of conception from the mother irrespective of the duration of pregnancy. Death is indicated by the fact that, after such separation, the fetus does not breathe or show any other evidence of life, such as beating of heart, pulsation of the umbilical cord, or definite movement of voluntary muscle.
- **File Folders:** Solid, two sided binders of Kraft, manila, press-board or patent composition used to store paper records. This term relates to a patient file (folder).

- **Filing:** Placing a collection of records or cards in a methodical manner so that they may be instantly available:
  - *Alphabetical Filing:* The method of filing charts or cards in strict alphabetical (dictionary style) sequence.
  - *Serial Number Filing:* The method of filing charts or cards in strict numerical sequence.
- **Follow-Up:** The periodic examination of a patient following disease or injury to determine the progress was being made toward complete recovery and normal health, and to study the end results of treatment.
- **Follow-Up Appointment:** Giving an appointment for an existing patient to attend the relevant clinic on a particular date and time. All referral hospitals have to observe a follow-up appointment system in collaboration with the related health centers and hospitals.
- **Forensic Medicine:** Also called 'legal medicine'. The application of medical knowledge to legal proceedings.
- **Format:** The arrangement of a form, or an organization of forms in a permanent folder, which directs the type of entries, the way entries are made, and the future use of those entries.
- **Fracture:** The breaking of a bone due to injury or disease; some terms describing fractures and related injuries are:
  - *Closed Fracture:* A bone is broken but there is no open wound in the skin (simple fracture).
  - *Open Fracture:* A broken bone with an open wound in the skin (compound fracture).
  - *Comminuted Fracture:* The bone is splintered or crushed.
  - *Impacted Fracture:* The bone is broken, and one end is wedged into the anterior portion of the other.
  - *Greenstick Fracture:* The bone is partially bent and partially broken as when a greenstick breaks.
- **Gastroenterology:** The study of the digestive tract, including the liver, biliary tract, pancreas and the accompanying diseases.
- **Gerontology:** The scientific study of the problems of aging in all their aspects, e.g. clinical, biological, historical, and sociological.
- **Gestational Age:** The duration of gestation is measured from the first day of the last normal menstrual period. Gestational age is expressed in completed days or weeks (e.g. events occurring 280 to 286 days after the onset of the last normal

menstrual period are considered to have occurred at 40 weeks of gestation).

- **Gynecology:** Study of the female reproductive system (organs, hormones, and diseases).
- **Health Center:** Generally, provides primary care and, if requiring further special care, refers the patient with a referral letter to an appropriate hospital.
- **Health Information:** Any data pertains to the physical, mental, or social well-being of an individual or group of individuals.
- **Health Record:** Documentation of direct or indirect health care services to patients or clients by providers and users of the data in any type of health-related institution.
- **Hematology:** The science dealing with formation, composition, function, and disease of the blood.
- **Homonyms:** Word of same forms as another word but with different meaning (different spelling but pronounced alike).
- **Hospital Bed:** A bed installed for regular 24 hour use by an inpatient (other than newborn infant) during his or her period of hospitalization.
- **Hospital Inpatient:** A hospital patient who is provided with a bed, a room, board, medical care, and continuous general nursing service in an area of the hospital where patients generally stay at least overnight.
- **Hospital Number:** It is a unit number allocated to a new patient who visits the hospital for outpatient or inpatient service for the first time. This is a permanent number used for all episodes and subsequent admissions. Patient files including relevant forms are represented by this number.
- **Hospital Record:** A written account of all the services provided to the patient as an outpatient, emergency, or inpatient from the time of the visit or admission until discharge. This identifies the dates, the ward, the bed, and the room where the patient was physically located, the names of the physicians, the nurses, and the other health professionals who provided care, and the results of that care.
- **Immature Infant:** It is a live born infant with a recorded birth weight of 2500 g or less.
- **Immunology:** The study of the immune system of lymphocytes, inflammatory cells, associated cells, and protein which affect the individuals response to antigens.

- **Implied Consent:** That which is given by mutual understanding.
- **Incident Report:** The event of occurrence of an incident in which the patient has suffered during hospitalization that was recorded and intimated to the concerned officials.
- **Incomplete Record:** Any hospital record of an outpatient or a discharged patient was lacking essential data.
- **Index:** An organized and condensed list of data selected and recorded on a designed index for easy and quick retrieval of information.
- **Infectious Disease:** A disease due to organisms ranging in size from viruses to parasitic worms; it may be contagious in origin, result from nosocomial organisms, or be due to endogenous microflora from the nose, throat, skin, or bowel.
- **Information:** Knowledge or intelligence; facts and data.
- **Informed Consent:** That which is documented to show the following: all procedures and treatment explained (including advantages and disadvantages) signed by a person giving consent as a result of their own decision.
- **Inpatient:** It is defined as a person who occupies a hospital bed, crib, or bassinet while housed in a hospital, for observation, care, diagnosis, or treatment.
- **Inpatient Census:** The number of inpatients present at any one time in all of the hospital wards.
- **Inpatient Discharge:** The release of a hospitalized inpatient from the hospital by the admitting physician after providing necessary medical care for a period deemed necessary.
- **Institutional Deaths** are those which occur 48 hours or more after admission.
- **Intermediate Death:** Completed 20 or more week's gestation but less than 28 weeks gestation (501 to 1000 g).
- **International Classification of Diseases (ICD):** A basic system of three-digit categories with four-and five-digit subcategories in some areas as recommended by the World Health Organization.
- **Job Description:** A document contains information about a position, such as required education, training, and experience, as well as lines of authority and designation of supervisor, with a description of general duties and responsibilities and major job functions.
- **Laparoscopy:** Endoscopic examination of the interior of the abdomen by means of a laparoscope.

- **Late Fetal Death or Stillbirth:** Completed 28 weeks gestation and over 1001 g.
- **Legal Liability:** Accepting responsibility before the court of law for reasonable care of the patients with reasonable maintenance of facilities for that purpose.
- **Length of Stay:** The number of days a patient remains in a facility (the day of admission should be counted but not the day of discharge unless the patient was admitted the same day).
- **Live Birth:** It is the complete expulsion or extraction from the mother of a product of conception, which, after such separation, breaths or shows any other evidence of life, such as beating of heart, pulsation of the umbilical cord, or definite movements of voluntary muscles, whether or not the umbilical cord has been cut or the placenta is attached; each product of such birth is considered a live birth.
- **Low Birth Weight:** Less than 2500 g (up to, and including 2499 g).
- **Malignant Tumor:** One that has the properties of invasion and metastasis and that shows a greater degree of anaplasia than do benign tumors.
- **Malpractice:** Improper, careless, or ignorant treatment.
- **Maternal Mortality:** The death of a woman while pregnant or within 42 days of termination of pregnancy irrespective of the duration and the site of the pregnancy, from any cause related to or aggravated by the pregnancy or its management but not from accidental or incidental causes.
- **Medical Audit:** An evaluation system in which established standards are used to measure performance. Once corrective action has been taken on problems identified through this review process, performance is remeasured after an appropriate time period.
- **Medical Board:** A meeting or conference of the medical staff of the hospital held for the purpose of reviewing and analyzing the clinical work of the hospital. This board deals with death cases, unimproved cases, infection, complications, or performance not conforming with the standard. The board also deals with problems concerning organization and management of the various medical services of the hospital.

- **Medical Care Evaluation:** A structured program to measure the quality of care given to patients. It is a global term that encompasses methods used to carry-out such measurement functions as audit, appraisal, peer review, quality assurance, and assessment in various specific forms.
- **Medical Certificate:** It is a document containing disease and injury specifications and duration of treatment of a patient in the emergency, outpatient, or inpatient areas of a hospital and attested to by the treating physician.
- **Medical Consultation:** The response by one member of the medical staff to a request for consultation by another member of the medical staff, characterized by review of the patient's history, examination of the patient, and completion of a consultation report presenting recommendations and opinions.
- **Medical File:** Medical record or patient record or patient file all are synonymous terms. This file contains both outpatient and inpatient records.
- **Medical Record:** It is an orderly written report of the patient's history, physical, laboratory findings, treatment, and hospital course. When complete, it should contain sufficient data to justify the diagnosis and also describe the result of the care rendered.
- **Medical Record Committee:** A committee which ensures that accurate and complete medical records are developed and retained for every patient treated. Also evaluates the work of the Medical Record Department to ensure that the department is functioning efficiently.
- **Medical Record Department (MRD):** It is one of the important departments in the hospital responsible for proper custody of the medical records of the patients, for conducting medical audits, for preparing reports necessary to demonstrate the quantity and quality of medical practice, and for assisting in the advancement of medical science through assuring accurately recorded data.
- **Medical Record Form:** It is a piece of paper or card, which is a formal arrangement of information (usually with spaces for the entry of additional information). A set of 90 basic medical record forms are recommended for adequate patient care in the hospital.
- **Medical Record Officer (MRO):** It is an individual responsible for establishing, organizing, and controlling a Medical Record

Department which initiates medical records for patient care. The MRO is also responsible for developing a good information system to compile and distribute patient or client data. He or she is the chief administrator of the Medical Record Department (MRD).

- **Medical Record Technician (MRT):** It is a trained person who works under the supervision of a medical record officer. He or she is an intermediate supervisory staff person and performs most of the technical jobs in the department and supervises the work of the assistant medical record technicians.
- **Medical Report:** It is a document containing medical information, such as history, physical examination, investigations, diagnosis, and treatment including surgical procedures, end results, duration of treatment, and recommendations about a patient treated in the hospital.
- **Medical Social Service:** The sociological investigation of a patient and his environment to ascertain any factors which might have a bearing on the diagnosis, treatment, and aftercare of the patient, followed in close collaboration with the physician with respect to the findings.
- **Medicine:** (1) The science or art of healing, especially as distinguished from surgery and obstetrics. (2) A therapeutic substance, such as a drug.
- **Medicolegal Case (MLC):** Case which is accidental, suicidal, or homicidal. The casualty medical officer (CMO) determines a case as medicolegal or not. Except in minor injury cases, all cases of traffic accidents, burns, poisonings, and quarrels have to be treated as medico legal cases.
- **Metastasis:** Tumor spreading from its primary location to secondary sites throughout the body.
- **Microbiology:** The science which deals microorganisms.
- **Microfilming:** A process of photographing and reducing a given report to a miniature of the original on film. The Medical Record Department may microfilm certain old records as per the 'record retention schedule' as recommended by regulations.
- **MOH:** Ministry of Health.
- **Morbidity:** The incidence of disease or proportion of diseases in a given population; statistical data that represents rates or ratios of disease.

- **Morphology:** The science which deals with the structure and form of living things.
- **Mortality:** The incidence of deaths or the proportion of deaths in a given population; statistical data that represents rates or ratios of deaths.
- **Mounting of Investigation (Diagnostic) Reports:** Reports of laboratory, X-ray and other investigations mounted on laboratory mount sheets, and X-ray mount sheets or EKG strips. All inpatient reports are received on the ward and mounted by the ward nurse or clerk (AMRT). Reports of outpatient are received and mounted by the Medical Record Department. The reports of A/E department are received by casualty staff and inserted with the relevant casualty record. If patient is transferred to outpatient or inpatient services, the casualty record along with all associated reports become part of the main patient file.
- **Necropsy (Autopsy):** Postmortem examination; see 'Autopsy'.
- **Neonatal Death:** An infant's death occurring less than 28 completed days after delivery.
- **Neoplasm:** New growth; tumor.
- **Nephrology:** The special study of the kidneys and the diseases which affect them.
- **Neurology:** (1) The science and study of the nerves, their structure, function, and pathology. (2) The branch of medicine dealing with diseases of the nervous system.
- **Newborn:** Any infant newly born in the hospital.
- **New Patient:** A new patient is one who visits the hospital for the first time, for whom a new hospital number has to be allocated, or an outpatient record has to be created after obtaining accurate and complete identification data.
- **Noninstitutional Deaths** are those which occur under 48 hours after admission.
- **Numbering System:** An identifying method that utilizes assigned numbers to label each record for filing in a systematic manner to facilitate easy retention and retrieval.
- **Obstetrics:** It is a specialty concerned with pregnancy and delivery of the fetus.
- **Odontology (Dentistry):** The science which deals with the structure, function, and diseases of the teeth.

- **Old (Follow-up) Patient:** It is one who has been treated in the hospital either as an outpatient or inpatient for whom a patient file with hospital number exists.
- **Old Medical Records** are those records which are inactive and kept for a certain duration or period as per the retention schedule for administrative, educational, research, and legal purposes. These include patient files, X-rays, medical registers, reports, index cards, etc.
- **Online:** A device that currently is an operating part of the computer system. A terminal is online if it is logged into the system. An idle service is online if it may be activated by the computer.
- **Oncology:** The scientific study of tumors.
- **Operation Index:** Does a card possess patient information about particular surgical operation undergone by different patients. Operation indexing is performed by the medical record staff.
- **Ophthalmology:** The science which deals with the structure, function, and diseases of the eye.
- **Oral Surgery:** Pertaining to structures found in the mouth.
- **Orthopedics:** Branch of study dealing with all conditions affecting the locomotor system.
- **Otorhinolaryngology (ENT):** The science which deals with the structure, function, and diseases of the ear, nose, and throat.
- **Out Guide Card:** This is also known as the 'tracer card' or 'locator'. This card contains patient identification information which indicates the movement of the patient file.
- **Outpatient:** It is a person who makes use of the diagnostic or therapeutic services of a hospital but does not occupy a regular bed.
- **Outpatient Clinic Schedule:** It is the list of patients new and established to be seen in the clinic. Each unit in consultation with the administration and medical record officer decides upon the number of patients (new and established) to be seen in the clinic and the appointments are booked accordingly.
- **Outpatient Record:** It is a patient file created with a hospital number for treatment as an outpatient and generally comprises: the medical record folder, the outpatient form, the history and physical examination report, the outpatient follow-up form,

laboratory and X-ray mount sheets, and other special forms added wherever required.

- **Paramedical** are those personnel who are qualified to render treatment or assist in patient care under the supervision of the medical staff, e.g. occupational therapists, radiographers, laboratory technicians, and so on.
- **Pathology:** The science which deals with the cause and nature of disease.
- **Patient Day:** A unit of measure for the service rendered an inpatient between the census-taking hours on two successive days, the day of discharge being counted only if the patient was admitted the same day. Only patients admitted, assigned abed, and having a medical record initiated should be counted in the census. When a patient is admitted and discharged the same day, the length of stay should be considered as one patient day.
- **Patient File:** Medical record.
- **Patient Master Index (PMI):** A '5 × 3' card containing patient identification information with hospital number; this card is filed in the central registration section in strict alphabetical order. This process assists in tracing out whether a patient has registered previously or not. This is also known as 'master patient index'.
- **Pediatrics:** Any patient less than 12–14 years of age, treated by a pediatrician on a pediatric unit is considered as a pediatric patient or child patient.
- **Pharmacology:** The science that deals with the origin, nature, chemistry, and uses of drugs, as well as their effects on the body.
- **Physiology:** The science which deals with the normal functions of the body.
- **Policy:** A basic guide of action which prescribes the boundaries within which activities are to take place.
- **Prenumbered Folder:** Patient files with required forms numbered well in advance and kept ready for registration of new cases.
- **Pregnancy:** The condition of having a developing embryo or fetus in the body after union of an ovum and a spermatozoon. In normal pregnancy, the embryos develop within the uterus. In an

ectopic pregnancy, the embryo is implanted outside the uterus, it is most commonly found in the fallopian tubes, and sometimes in the ovary or in the abdominal cavity.

- **Premature Infant:** It is a live born infant with a period of gestation of less than 37 completed weeks, or specified by the obstetrician as 'premature.'
- **Presentation (Obstetrical):** The relationship of the long axis of the fetus to that of the mother. There are two divisions, the longitudinal, in which the head or breech may be present, and the transverse in which the shoulder is the presenting part and may include shoulder, arm, or any other part of the trunk.
  - *Breech:* Presentation of buttocks or feet of the fetus in labor; breech presentation complete mean presentation of the buttocks in labor, with the feet alongside of the buttocks, the feet being in the same position as in vertex presentation, but with polarity reversed.
  - *Cephalic (Head):* Presentation of any part of the fetal head in labor, including occiput, brow, or face.
  - *Transverse:* Shoulder; scapula is the point of direction.
- **Preservation of Records:** Patient files and related documents are preserved in a safe location and well protected area for the period recommended in a 'record retention schedule' furnished by regulations.
- **Privacy:** A right to declare information confidential and to recognize formally the patient's inherent right to privacy.
- **Privileged Communication:** Any information acquired by a physician or surgeon in attending a patient which was necessary to enable him or her to prescribe or act for the patient and which cannot be revealed in a civil action without the consent of the patient.
- **Procedure:** An act or manner of proceeding or method of conducting a business proceeding. A procedure is a series of tasks designed to accomplish work in a given time.
- **Processing of Records:** Reviewing of records (files) to determine whether the records are quantitatively and qualitatively complete. This also refers to effective documentation of the details of the patient's history and physical examination, other diagnostic measures, specific treatment procedures, etc.

- **Prodrome:** Symptoms of disease (such as rash or fever) which appear before and signal the onset of an approaching more severe illness.
- **Prognosis:** A prognosis made by a doctor after diagnosis about the nature of the patient's illness. It is a prediction about the disease.
- **Psychiatry:** The branch of medical study devoted to the diagnosis and treatment of mental illness.
- **Qualitative Analysis:** Retrospective review program by the organized medical staff. It assesses the quality of care as compared to locally or internally developed standards and verifies that the standards or exceptions are met, that deficiencies are corrected, and that the original problem is reassessed on a planned program basis.
- **Quality Assurance:** Activities performed to determine the extent to which a phenomenon fulfills certain values and standards, and to assure changes in practice that fulfill the highest of a predetermined level of values.
- **Quality Assurance Program (QAP):** It is a comprehensive and coordinated network of formal mechanisms that provide ongoing objective assessment of patient care services and the correction of identified problems.
- **Quality Control:** It is defined as those evaluation procedures that are performed systematically to ensure that established policies and standards are being met.
- **Quantitative Analysis:** The responsibility the Medical Record Department to check and analyze the component parts of the medical record to ensure that it is complete, adequate, and accurate, and is available at all times for legitimate needs of the patients, the hospital, and the physician.
- **Radiology:** The study of the diagnosis of disease by using X-rays and other allied imaging techniques.
- **Record Control:** It is the supply of records (patient files) for patient care, administrative, and other reasons and the collection and accounting for that effective control, as well as the safeguarding of the confidentiality of information.
- **Referrals are of two types:** From outside, e.g. from health centers and other hospitals or from inside, e.g. within the hospital from

one department to another. Any referral of a patient must be on a written prescribed document. Referral forms are in triplicate. When a health center refers a patient, two copies are given to the patient to be forwarded to the hospital, and the third copy is retained by the patient. After treatment, the hospital returns one copy with details as feedback information to the health center and retains one copy in the hospital.

- **Relapse:** A relapse is the reappearance of symptoms of disease.
- **Remission:** A remission is the lessening or disappearance of disease symptoms.
- **Reports:** Relating to statistics: Daily, monthly, and yearly. Daily report is the analysis of hospital services which includes the work performed by the different departments, such as outpatient, accident/emergency, inpatient, and allied departments. Monthly report is a cumulative daily report for calendar months with ratios (or percentage rates) of service facilities used, and other statistical data and rates. Annual report is a compilation of the twelve-monthly reports. The figures are cumulated monthly, just as the monthly report figures are cumulated from daily analysis.
- **Responsibility for Medical Certificates of Cause of Death:** Medical certification of cause of death should normally be the responsibility of the attending physician. In the case of deaths certified by coroners or other legal authorities, the medical evidence supplied to the certifier should be stated on the certificate in addition to any legal findings.
- **Retention of Records:** Keeping information for a specific period so that it may be used in the future. Planning, implementation, and control of a system that safeguards physical and information characteristics of medical or health data for future use. The patient files and other documents are retained in accordance with the 'record retention schedule' as suggested per regulations.
- **Review:** Examination of a medical record by a physician to determine if continued hospitalization is medically necessary.
- **Sarcomas:** Rare types of cancer which are derived from supportive and connective tissue, such as bone, fat, muscle, cartilage, bone marrow, lymphatic tissue, or blood cells.

- **Serial Numbering:** A system of numbering in which the patient is assigned a new number each time treatment is received.
- **Sphygmomanometer:** Instrument to measure blood pressure.
- **Stages of Labor:** The act of giving birth to a child. The following three stages are recognized:
  1. *First stage:* From beginning of labor to complete dilatation.
  2. *Second stage:* From complete dilatation to birth of infant.
  3. *Third stage:* From birth of infant to expulsion of placenta.
- **Standard:** Generally, a measure set by a competent authority as the rule for measuring quantity or quality. Conformity with standards is usually a condition of licensing, accreditation, or payment of service.
- **Sterilization:** The act or process of rendering sterile; the process of freeing from germ life. A procedure by which an individual is made incapable of reproduction by undergoing surgery, such as a vasectomy or a tubectomy.
- **Stethoscope:** An instrument used for listening to the various body sounds, especially those of the heart and chest.
- **Stillbirth:** Fetal death
- **Suit:** An action or process in a court of law for the recovery of right or claim.
- **Summons:** A process (document) served on a defendant in civil court action to secure his or her appearance in the action.
- **Surgery:** It is the branch of medicine which treats diseases, deformities, and injuries wholly or partly, by manual or operative procedures.
- **Symbiosis:** Refers to the living together in close association of two organisms, either for mutual benefit or not. The bacteria which normally lie in the digestive tract of humans are an example of symbiosis.
- **Syndrome:** It is a group of signs or symptoms which commonly occur together and indicate a particular disease or abnormal condition. An example of a syndrome is Homer's syndrome, characterized by ptosis of the eyelid, enophthalmos, and cool, dry face on the affected side due to nerve damage.
- **System:** Related elements that are coordinated to form a unified result, specifically people, activities, equipment, materials, plans,

and controls, working together to achieve a unified objective or whole; an array of components that interact to achieve some objective through a network of procedures that are integrated and designed to carry-out a major activity.

- **Terminal Digit Filing:** A method of filing by the last digits of a number instead of by the first digits. The entire number is broken into groups of twos or threes, with the last group being filed first. This system is suggested to all the referral hospitals.
- **Topography:** A description of the regions of the body.
- **Toxicology:** It is the study of harmful chemicals and their dangerous effects on the body.
- **Transfer of Patient:** If a patient is transferred within the hospital (except from casualty) from one unit to another, the same patient file will be continued for the duration of treatment except for change of ward census. In the case of a patient transferred from other hospitals, the case has to be registered and a record has to be created (if he or she is not an established patient).
- **Traumatology:** The branch of surgery dealing with injury caused by accident.
- **Treating Physician:** It is one under whose care, the treatment to the patient is rendered. Physician can be a surgeon, a pediatrician or an obstetrician or gynecologist. This term is synonymous to a medical doctor.
- **Treatment:** The application of any measure to assist in bringing about the cure of disease or relief of symptoms or to correct the disturbances of the function was arising from an infection. Therapeutics or therapy is the general term for all forms of treatment of disease. The kinds of treatment are:
  - *Symptomatic:* Directed towards the removal of the cause based on the treatment of symptoms as they are manifested.
  - *Prophylactic:* Aimed to prevent the occurrence of disease.
  - *Palliative:* Designed to check or to reduce symptoms.
  - *Specific:* Assigned treatment devised for specific action.
- **Underlying Cause of Death:** The underlying cause of death is the disease or injury which initiated the chain of events leading directly to death or the circumstances of the accident or violence which produced the fatal injury.

- **Unit Numbering:** A system in which only one number is assigned to the patient's record and is retained permanently.
- **Unit Numbering System:** Whereby only one serial number is given to the patient irrespective of the number of admissions either in the outpatient department or in the inpatient department and all records of the patient are available in one folder.
- **Unit Record System:** A method that compiles all information on a single patient or subject and records it in one document and file folder.
- **Urology:** The branch of medicine which deals with disorders of the female urinary tract and with disorders the male genital urinary tract.
- **Utilization Review:** The evaluation of the necessity, appropriateness, and efficiency of the use of medical services, procedures, and facilities. In a hospital, this includes review of the appropriateness of admissions, services ordered and provided, length of stay, and discharge practices on a concurrent and retrospective basis. This can be done by a utilization review committee, by peer review, or by any other assigned committee.
- **Venereology (Sexually Transmitted Disease):** The study and treatment of diseases transmitted during sexual intercourse.
- **Viable Infant:** A fetus that has reached a stage of development that has enabled itself to live outside the uterus, usually consider and as 28 completed weeks of gestation or more.
- **Virology:** The study of viruses and the diseases caused by them.

Annexure 3

STANDARDIZED ABBREVIATIONS WITH SINGLE MEANING

Abbreviations	Expansion
A-P	Anteroposterior
A/B	Acid-base Ratio
A/G	Albumin-Globulin Ratio
A2	Aortic Second Sound
AAA	Abdominal Aortic Aneurysm
AAR	Antigen Antiglobulin Reaction
AAS	Aortic Arch Syndrome
AB	Asthmatic Bronchitis
ABD HYST	Abdominal Hysterectomy
ABE	Acute Bacterial Endocarditis
ABO	Blood Groups (Name For Agglutinogens)
ABP	Arterial Blood Pressure
AC	Before Meals (Ante-cibum)
ACC	Adenoid Cystic Carcinoma
ACE	Adrenocortical Extraction
ACH	Adrenal Cortical Hormone

Abbreviations	Expansion
ACM	Albumin-calcium-Magnesium
ACS	Antereticular Cytotoxic Serum
ACT	Activated Coagulation Time
ACTH	Adrenocorticotropic Hormone
ACVD	Acute Cardiovascular Disease
ADA	Anterior Descending Artery
ADH	Antidiuretic Hormore
AD LIB	As Desired (Ad Libitum)
AD	Right Ear (Auris Dextra)
ADS	Antibody Deficiency Syndrome
AEG	Air Encephalogram
AFG	Acid Fast Bacilli
AFT	Acute Follicular Tonsillitis
AGA	Appropriate for Gestational Age
AGL	Acute Granulocytic Leukemia

Contd…

Contd...

Abbreviations	Expansion
AGN	Acute Glomerulonephritis
AHA	Acquired Hemolytic Anemia
AH	Arterial Hypertension
AHD	Arteriosclerotic Heart Disease
AHF	Acute Hemophilic Factor
AHT	Augumented Histamin Test
AI	Aortic Incompetence
AIDS	Acquired Immune Deficiency Syndrome
AIHA	Autoimmune Hemolytic Anemia
AJ	Ankle Jerk
AKA	Above Knee Amputation
AK	Above Knee
ALL	Acute Lymphocytic Leukemia
Alt. Dieb	Every Other Day (Alternis Diebus)
Alt. Hor	Every Other Hour (Alternis Horos)
Alt. Noc	Every Other Night
AMA	Against Medical Advice
AM	Auditory Meatus
AMI	Acute Myocardial Infarction

Abbreviations	Expansion
AML	Acute Myeloblastic Leukemia
AMOL	Acute Monocytic Leukemia
ANA	Antinuclear Antibodies
AN	Antenatal
ANT	Anterior
AOM	Acute Otitis Media
AP	Anterior Pituitary
APC	Aspirin, Phenacetin, Caffeine
APH	Antepartum Hemorrhage
APTT	Activated Partial Thromboplastin Time
AR	Aortic Regurgitation
ARD	Acute Respiratory Disease
ARF	Acute Respiratory Failure
ARM	Artificial Rupture of the Membranes
AS	Aortic Stenosis
ASD	Arterial Septal Defect
ASHD	Arteriosclerotic Heart Disease
ASO	Arteriosclerosis Obliteral
ATD	Asphyxiating Thoracic Dystrophy

Contd...

Contd...

Abbreviations	Expansion
ATS	Antitetanic Serum
AVF	Arteriovenous Fistula
AVH	Acute Viral Hepatitis
B/K	Bladder Kidney (Scan Ratio)
B_{12}	Vitamin B_{12}
BA	Barium
BBA	Born before Arrival
BBB	Bundle Branch Block
BB	Blood Bank
BCG	Bacille Calmette Guerin (Vaccine)
BGTT	Borderline Glucose Tolerance Test
BID	Brought in Dead
BID	Twice a Day (Bis in Die)
BIH	Benign Intracranial Hypertension
BJM	Bones, Joints, Muscles
BKA	Below Knee Amputation
BM	Bowel Movement
BMR	Basal Metabolic Rate
BOM	Bilateral Otitis Media
BP	Blood Pressure
BPH	Benign Prostate Hypertrophy
BR	Bronchitis
BR PN	Bronchopneumonia
BSOM	Bilateral Suppurative Otitis Media
BSR	Blood Sedimentation Rate
BT	Bleeding Time
BUN	Blood Urea Nitrogen
BW	Birth Weight
BX	Biopsy
C1, C2	First, Second Cervical Vertebra
CA	Carcinoma
CAD	Coronary Artery Disease
CAHD	Coronary Atherosclerotic Heart Disease
C and D	Cystoscopy and Dilatation
CAT	Computerized Axial Tomography
CAV	Congenital Absence of Vagina
CBA	Chronic Bronchitis with Asthma
CBC and Diff	Complete Blood Count and Differential
CBC	Complete Blood Count
CB	Chronic Bronchitis
CBD	Common Bile Duct
CC	Chief Complaint

Contd...

Contd...

Abbreviations	Expansion
C	Centigrade (Centum Gradus)
CCF	Congestive Cardiac Failure
CCU	Coronary Care Unit
CDH	Congenital Dislocation of the Hip
CEA	Carcinoembryonic Antigen
CGL	Correction with Glasses
CHA	Congenital Hypoplastic Anemia
CHB	Complete Heart Block
CHD	Congestive Heart Disease
CHF	Congestive Heart Failure
CHS	Chediak-Higashi Syndrome
CLBBB	Complete Left Bundle Branch Block
CLL	Chronic Lymphocytic Leukemia
CM	Costal Margin
CML	Chronic Myelocytic Leukemia
CMR	Cerebral Metabolic Rate
CNS	Central Nervous System

Abbreviations	Expansion
CO_2	Carbon Dioxide
COAD	Chronic Obstructive Airways Disease
COLD	Chronic Obstructive Lung Disease
COPD	Chronic Obstructive Pulmonary Disease
CPD	Cephalopelvic Disproportion
CPK	Creatinine Phosphokinase
CPR	Cardiopulmonary Resuscitation
CRBBB	Complete Right Bundle Branch Block
CRF	Chronic Renal Failure
CRH	Corticotrophin Releasing Hormone
CSF	Cerebrospinal Fluid
CSOM	Chronic Suppurative Otitis Media
CSSD	Central Sterile Supply Department
CST	Convulsive Shock Therapy
CT	Cerebral Thrombosis
CVA	Cardiovascular Accident
CV	Cardiovascular
CVD	Cardiovascular Disease

Contd...

Contd...

Abbreviations	Expansion
D and C	Dilation and Curettage
D and V	Diarrhea and Vomiting
DIC	Diffuse/ Disseminated Intravascular Coagulation
DI	Diabetes Insipidus
DLE	Discoid Lupus Erythematous
DM	Diabetic Mellitus
DNS	Deflected/Deviated Nasal Septum
DOA	Date of Admission
DOB	Date of Birth
DOC	Date of Confinement
DOD	Date of Discharge or Death
DTP	Diphtheria, Tetanus and Pertussis
DUB	Dysfunctional Uterine Bladder
DU	Duodenal Ulcer
DVT	Deep Vain Thrombosis
DX	Diagnosis
EAM	External Auditory Meatus
ECG	Electrocardiogram
ECS	Electroconvulsive Shock

Abbreviations	Expansion
ECT	Electroconvulsive Therapy
EDC	Expected Date of Confinement
EDD	Expected Date of Delivery
EEG	Electroencephalo-gram
EH	Essential Hypertension
EMG	Electromyogram
EMI	Electromagnetic Interference
EN	Emmetropia
ENT	Ear, Nose and Throat
ER	Emergency Room
ERG	Electroretinogram
ESR	Erythrocyte Sedimentation Rate
EUA	Examination Under Anesthesia
F/U	Follow-up
FB	Foreign Body
FBS	Fasting Blood Sugar
FD	Forceps Delivery
FDIU	Fetal Death in Utero
FH	Family History
FHR	Feral Heart Rate
FSH	Follicle-stimulating Hormone
FTM	Fractional Test Meal

Contd...

Contd...

Abbreviations	Expansion
FTND	Full Term Normal Delivery
FUO	Fever of Unknown Origin
G/S	Glucose and Saline
GA	General Anesthesia
GB	Gallbladder
GFR	Glomerular Filtration Rate
GH	Growth Hormone
GIT	Gastrointestinal Tract
GP	General Practitioner
GS	General Surgery
GSH	Glomerular-Stimulating Hormone
GT	Glucose Tolerance
GTT	Glucose Tolerance Test
GU	Gastric Ulcer
H/T	Hypertension
HB	Hemoglobin
HBP	High Blood Pressure
HBW	High Birth Weight
HCG	Human Chorionic Gonadotropin
HCT	Hematocrit
HCVD	Hypertensive Cardiovascular Disease
HD	Heart Disease

Abbreviations	Expansion
HDN	Hemolytic Disease of the Newborn
HF	Heart Failure
HHA	Hereditary Hemolytic Anemia
HHD	Hypertensive Heart Disease
HIV	Human Immuno-deficiency Virus
HPI	History of Present Illness
HVD	Hypertensive Vascular Disease
I and D	Incision and Drainage
I and O	Intake and Output
ICC	Intensive Coronary Care
ICCU	Intensive Coronary Care Unit
ICD	International Classification of Disease
ICM	Intercostal Margin
ICU	Intensive Care Unit
IDK	Internal Derange-ment of Knee
IDKJ	Internal Derangement of Knee Joint
IHD	Ischemic Heart Disease

Contd...

Contd…

Abbreviations	Expansion
IMF	Idiopathic Myelofibrosis
IMP	Improved
IP	Inpatient
IQ	Intelligence Quotient
ITP	Idiopathic Thrombocytopenic Purpura
IUD	Intrauterine Death
IUFB	Intrauterine Foreign Body
IU	Intrauterine
IV	Intravenously
IVP	Intravenous Pyelogram
IVSD	Interventricular Septal Defect
IVU	Intravenous Urography
JBE	Japanese B Encephalitis
KJ	Knee Jerk
KUB	Kidney, Ureter and Bladder
L-1, L-2	First, Second Lumbar Vertebrae
LAG	Lymphangiography
LA	Local Anesthesia
LBBB	Left Bundle Branch Block
LBB	Left Bundle Branch
LB	Live Birth

Abbreviations	Expansion
LBW	Low Birth Weight
LCM	Left Costal Margin
LE	Left Eye
LFT	Liver Function Test
LHF	Left Heart Failure
LIH	Left Inguinal Hernia
LK	Left Kidney
LLE	Left Lower Extremity
LL	Left Lung
LLL	Left Lower Lobe (Lungs)
LMP	Last Menstrual Period
LP	Lumbar Puncture
LSCS	Lower Segment Cesarean Section
LSD	Lysergic Acid Diethylamide
LTH	Luteotropic Hormone
LUE	Left Upper Extremity
LUL	Left Upper Lobe
LVF	Left Ventricular Failure
LVH	Left Ventricular Hypertrophy
LV	Left Ventricle
MA	Mental Age
MCH	Mean Corpuscular Hemoglobin

Contd…

Contd...

Abbreviations	Expansion
MCT	Mean Circulation Time
MCV	Mean Corpuscular Volume
MD	Muscular Dystrophy
MFD	Mid Forceps Delivery
MH	Marital History
MI	Myocardial Infarction
MR	Mental Retardation
MS	Mitral Stenosis
MSW	Medial Social Worker
N/C	No Complaints
NAD	Nothing Abnormal Detected
NBI	No Bone Injury
NBM	Nothing by Mouth
NB	Newborn
NBW	Normal Birth Weight
ND	Normal Delivery
NEC	Not Elsewhere Classified
NED	No Evidence of Disease
NFTD	Normal Full Term Delivery
NOS	Not Otherwise Specified
NS	Neurosurgery
NYD	Not Yet Diagnosed
O/A	On Admission

Abbreviations	Expansion
O and E	Observation and Examination
OA	Osteoarthritis
OBG	Obstetrics and Gynecology
OD	Once a Day
OD	Right Eye (Ocular Dexter)
OE	On Examination
OH	Obstetric History
OMD	Ocular Media
OMI	Old Myocardial Infarction
OM	Otitis Media
OPC	Outpatient Clinic
OP	Outpatient
OR	Operating Room
OS	Left Eye (Oculus Sinister)
OT	Operation Theater
OU	Each Eye (Oculi Uterque)
P and A	Percussion and Auscultation
P and V	Pyloroplasty and Vagotomy
PANT	Postero Anterior
PA	Pernicious Anemia
PAP	Primary Atypical Pneumonia
PAT	Paroxysmal Atrial Tachycardia

Contd...

Contd...

Abbreviations	Expansion
PCV	Packed Cell Volume
PDA	Patent Ductus Arteriosus
PEG	Pneumoencephalog-raphy
PET	Pre-eclamptic Toxemia
PGH	Pituitary Growth Hormone
PH	Past History
PHT	Pulmonary Hypertension
PID	Pelvic Inflammatory Disease
PI	Present Illness
PIVD	Prolapse Intervertebral Disk
PMA	Progressive Muscular Atrophy
PMB	Post Menopausal Bleeding
PMI	Point of Maximum Impulse
PMN	Polymorphonuclear Neutrophil
PM	Post Mortem
PMP	Past Menstrual Period
PMR	Physical Medicine and Rehabilitation
PNC	Postnatal Clinic

Abbreviations	Expansion
PND	Paroxysmal Nocturnal Dyspnea
PN	Postnatal
PO	Postoperative
POP	Plaster of Paris
PP	After Meals (Post Prandial)
PPBS	Post Prandial Blood Sugar
PPH	Postpartum Hemorrhage
PP	Postpartum
PPU	Perforated Peptic Ulcer
PRN	As Required (Pro Renata)
PS	Pulmonary Stenosis
PTH	Para Thyroid Hormone
PT	Pulmonary Tuberculosis
PTT	Partial Thromboplastin Time
PUE	Pyrexia of Unknown Etiology
PUO	Pyrexia of Unknown Origin
PU	Peptic Ulcer
PVC	Premature Ventricular Contraction

Contd...

Contd...

Abbreviations	Expansion
PV	Per Vaginum (Through the Vaginum)
PVP	Portal Venous Pressure
PVR	Pulmonary Vascular Resistance
PVT	Paroxysmal Ventricular Tachycardia
QDH	Quaque Duo Hora (Every Two Hours)
QD	Quaque Die (Every Day)
QH	Quaque Horo (Every Hour)
QID	Quarter in Die (Four Times Daily)
QN	Quaque Nocte (Every Night)
QNS	Quantum Nonsatis (Insufficient Quantity)
QQH	Quaque Quator Hora (Ever)
QS	Quantum Statis (Sufficient Quantity)
QTH	Quaque Tres Hora (Every Three Hours)
QV	Quantum Vis (As Much As Desired)
RAD	Radiation Absorbed Dose

Abbreviations	Expansion
RA	Rheumatoid Arthritis
RBBB	Right Bundle Branch Block
RBC	Red Blood Count
RCA	Right Coronary Artery
RCM	Right Costal Margin
RCU	Respiratory Cardiac Unit
RDH	Right Inguinal Hernia
RD	Respiratory Disease
RDS	Respiratory Distress Syndrome
REM	Rapid Eye Movement
RFB	Retained Foreign Body
RF	Rheumatic Fever
RFT	Renal Function Test
Rh. Neg	Rhesus Factor (Negative)
Rh. Pos	Rhesus Factor (Positive)
RHD	Rheumatic Heart Disease
RHF	Rheumatic Heart Failure
RIA	Radioimmunoassay
RIF	Right Iliac Fossa
RIH	Right Inguinal Hernia

Contd...

Contd…

Abbreviations	Expansion
RIIH	Right Indirect Inguinal Hernia
RK	Right Kidney
RLE	Right Lower Extremity
RLL	Right Lower Lobe
RL	Right Lobe
RM	Radical Mastectomy
RNA	Ribonucleic Acid
ROIH	Right Oblique Inguinal Hernia
ROM	Rupture of Membrane
ROP	Right Occipit Posterior
ROT	Right Occipit Transverse
RPA	Right Pulmonary Artery
RP	Retrograde Pyelogram
RR	Recovery Room
RS	Respiratory System
RT	Radiation Therapy
RUE	Right Upper Extremity
RUL	Right Upper Lobe
RU	Retrograde Urogram
RURTI	Recurrent Upper Respiratory Tract Infection

Abbreviations	Expansion
RVF	Right Ventricular Failure
RVH	Right Ventricular Hypertrophy
RX	Recuoe (Take)
S-1, S-2	First, Second Sacral Vertebrae
SAP	Serum Alkaline Phosphate
SA	Sarcoma
SBE	Subacute Bacterial Endocarditis
SBP	Systolic Blood Pressure
SB	Stillbirth
SCA	Sickle-Cell Anemia
SCC	Squamous Cell Carcinoma
SCI	Spinal Cord Injury
SD	Spontaneous Delivery
SEP	Senile Enlarge Prostate
SGOT	Serum Glutamic Oxalic Transaminase
SGPT	Serum Glutamic Pyruvic Transaminase
SH	Serum Hepatitis
SLE	Systemic Lupus Erythematosus

Contd…

Contd...

Abbreviations	Expansion
SMR	Submucous Resection
SOB	Shortness of Breath
SPE	Serum Protein Electrophoresis
SPP	Suprapubic Prostatectomy
SSE	Soapsuds Enema
SSG	Split Skin Graft
STD	Sexually Transmitted Disease
STOP	Suction Termination of Pregnancy
SVD	Spontaneous Vaginal Delivery
SVG	Saphenous Vein Graft
SVT	Supraventricular Tachycardia
SX	Symptoms
T-1, T-2	First, Second Thoracic Vertebrae
T-3, T-4	Tri-Iodothyronine, Thyroxine
TAH	Total Abdominal Hysterectomy
TAL	Tendo Achilles Lengthening
T and A	Tonsillectomy and Adenoidectomy
TAO	Thrombo Angitis Obliterans
TBM	Tuberculosis Meningitis
TB	Tuberculosis
TEV	Talipes Equinovarus
TIA	Transient Ischemic Attack
TID	Three Times Daily (Ter in Die)
TKR	Total Knee Replacement
TMJ	Temporomandibular Joint
TPR	Temperature, Pulse and Respiration
TPUR	Transperineal Urethral Resection
TSH	Thyroid Stimulating Hormone
TS	Thoracic Surgery
TTH	Thyrotropic Hormone
TTP	Thrombotic Thrombocytopenic Purpura
TT	Tetanus Toxoid
TURP	Transurethral Resection of Prostate
TUR	Transurethral Resection
TVH	Total Vaginal Hysterectomy

Contd...

Contd...

Abbreviations	Expansion
TVP	Transvesical Prostatectomy
TX	Therapy
U/A	Urinalysis
UC	Ulcerative Colitis
UDT	Undescended Testicle
UD	Urethral Discharge
UGI	Upper Gastrointestinal
UL	Upper Lobe
UNG	Ointment
URI	Upper Respiratory Infection
URTI	Upper Respiratory Tract Infection
US	Ultrasound
UTI	Urinary Tract Infection
V and D	Vomiting and Diarrhea
VA	Visual Acuity
VDRL	Veneral Disease Research Laboratory
VD	Veneral Disease
VE	Visual Efficiency
VF	Ventricular Fibrillation
VHD	Valvular Heart Disease
VMR	Vasomotor Rhinitis
VRI	Viral Respiratory Infection
VSD	Ventricular Septal Defect
VS	Vital Signs
VT	Ventricular Tachycardia
V V	Varicose Veins
WBC	White Blood Count
WCC	White Cell Count
WC	Whooping Cough
WNL	Within Normal Limits
WPWS	Wolff-Parkinson-White Syndrome
WR	Wassermann Reaction
X-MATCH	Cross Match
XDP	Xeroderma Pigmentosum
XR	X-ray
YF	Yellow Fever
Y	Year

Symbols	Expansion
A	Above
B	After
~	Approximate
@	At
*	Birth
( )	Combined with
+	Death
↓	Decrease
^	Diastolic Pressure
X	End of Operation
=	Equal
♀	Female
ft	Foot
>	Greater than
″	Inch
↑	Increase
∞	Infinity
L	Left

Symbols	Expansion
<	Lesser than
♂	Male
UG	Microgram
UL	Microliter
U	Micron
M	Murmur
–	Negative
+	Not Definite
OZ	Ounce
/	Per
+	Positive
:	Ratio
R	Right
.	Start of Operation
V	Systolic Pressure
RX	Take
C	With
S	Without

Index

Page numbers followed by *f* refer to figure, *fc* refer to flowchart, and *t* refer to table.

A

Abdomen, clinical divisions of 14, 15*f*, 258*f*
Abdominal cavity 13, 340
Abdominal pain 233
Abdominal region, organs of 125*f*, 281*f*
Abdominopelvic cavity 298
Abdominopelvic region 37*f*, 265*f*, 298
Abduction 42
Abortion 365
Absorption 3, 118
Accident 358
Acidosis stimulates respiration 166
Acquired immunodeficiency syndrome 84
Acromegaly 150
Adam's apple 162
Addison's disease 147
Adduction 42
Adenohypophysis 148, 330, 331
Adipose tissue 6, 7
Admission waiting list 358
Adrenal androgens 333
Adrenal estrogens 333
Adrenal medulla 147
Adrenaline 147, 332, 333
Adrenocorticotropic hormone 148
Affective disorders 232
Afferent arteriole 341
Agglutinin 318
Agranulocytes 78, 79, 87, 315
Albumin 76, 317
Alcohol consumption 236
Alcoholism, chronic 236
Alkalosis inhibits 166
Allergy 358
Allied health personnel 358
Alopecia 183
Amino acids 204
Amphiarthroses 40, 305
Amylase 131
Anabolism 131
Anaphase 4
Angiocardiography 358
Angular movements 42
Anomaly 359
Anoxia 166
Anteflexion, position of 344
Antianemic factor 126
Antibody 79, 316, 319
Antidiuretic hormone 150
Antigen 316, 318
Anus 128, 328
Anxiety disorders 232
Aortic blood 62
Aponeurosis 24
Appendicular skeleton 44, 302
Aqueous humor 176, 337
Arachnoid mater 98
Areolar tissue 7
Arm and hand, bones of 38
Arterial pulse 63
Arterioles 202
Artery 54, 65, 308
  carry blood 308
  important 54, 55*f*, 56*t*, 267*f*
  microscopic structure of 54
  small 202
Arthroscopy 359
Articular cartilage 7, 301
Articulations 305
Artificial intelligence 240
Assistant medical record technician 359
Auditory meatus, external 179
Authorized personnel 359
Automatic rhythmic contraction 8
Autonomic nervous system 8, 105*f*, 276*f*, 321
Autopsy 359, 373
  rate 359
Average daily census 359
Axial skeleton 34, 44, 302

B

B agglutinogens 318
B lymphocytes 83
Back 26, 299
  anatomical divisions of 14, 15*t*, 16*f*, 158*f*
  lower 299
Bacteria 79
Bacteriology 359
Baldness 183
Barbiturates 236
Basophils 78, 79
Bassinet 359
B-cell lymphocytes 84

Bed
- complement 359
- occupancy board 360

Behavior
- accounting for 248
- analysis of 251
- states 239
- therapy 233

Bile 130
Bilirubin 77
Binocular vision 178
Biochemistry 360
Biological psychology 239
Biopsy 360
Birth 360
Blood 11, 74, 85, 313
- and lymph 74
- and lymphatic system 74, 313
- cell 75*f*, 271*f*, 313, 314
  - manufacturers of 29
- clotting 317
  - mechanism 80
- flow through heart 310
- functions of 75
- group 11, 80, 80*t*, 89, 318
- oxygenation of 310
- plasma 81
- pressure 63, 68, 311
- serum 76
- vessels 129*f*, 226, 281*f*
  - major 310

Body 150
- anatomical divisions of 12, 14*f*, 257*f*
- cavities 12, 13*f*, 13*t*, 257*f*, 298
- cells 226
  - transportation system for 313
- directional terms of 17, 17*t*
- hair 212
- parts of 21, 233
  - nerves of 105*f*
- planes of 16, 16*t*, 17*f*, 259*f*, 298
- portion of 310
- structure and organs 9*f*, 256*f*
- tissues 226
- weight 21

Bone 28, 31*f*, 32*f*, 263*f*, 264*f*
- cancellous 30
- condyle 33
- crest 33
- depressions 33
- describe 32
- different locations of 33
- epicondyle 33
- facet 33
- flat 30, 44, 302
- formation of 29
- functions of 30
- group of 21
- head 32
- innominate 304
- irregular 31, 44, 302
- long 30, 266*f*
- mandibular 36
- markings 304
- marrow 83, 227
  - red 29, 313
  - yellow 29
- maxillary 36
- meet 300
- names of 34
- occipital 36
- parietal 35
- process 32, 33
- sesamoid 32
- short 30, 44, 302
- sphenoid 36
- structure of 43, 301
- surfaces of 304
- trochanter 33
- tubercle 33
- tuberosity 33
- types of 30, 34*t*, 43, 301
- union, line of 304
- vomer 36

Bowman's capsule 199, 204, 341
Brain 97, 109, 323
- activity 240
- cross-section of 99*f*, 274*f*
- parts of 98, 98*f*, 100, 274*f*, 324
- small 100
- stem 324
- with cranial nerves, cross-section of 106*f*, 277*f*

Brainstem 98
Brainstorming questions 349
Branch of medicine 232
Breast 189, 215
- cross-section of 215*f*, 293*f*
- development 212

Breathing, structures with 168, 335
Bronchi 163
- left 163
- little 336
- right 163

Buccal cavity 118, 326
Burn 360
Bursae 41

C

Calcitonin 144
Calcium 301, 313, 340
  blood levels of 332
Calices 200
Camera lens 175
Cancer treatment 229
Capillaries 54, 65, 203, 308
  connect arterioles 309
  structure 163
Carbohydrates 117
Carbon dioxide 160, 166, 336
  concentration of 309
  exchange of 163
Carcinomas 226, 360
Cardiac catheterization 360
Cardiac circulation 60*f*
Cardiac cycle 59
Cardiac rate 312
Cardiac sphincter 327
Cardiac valve 327
Cardiology 360
Cardiovascular system 10, 53, 307
  anatomy and physiology of 307
Cartilage 7
  tissues 29
Casualty 360
Catabolism 131
Catecholamine 146
Cauda equina 101
Cauterization 361
Cell 1, 297
  alpha 329
  basal layer 182
  blood 75*f*, 271*f*, 313, 314
  body 226
  bone 28, 332
  component parts of 2*f*
  deep-lying 183
  division 4, 5
  fat 183
  fragments 314
  functions of 3
  groups of 297
  killer 316
  malignant 226
  mediated immunity 84
  membrane 1, 95, 317
  mononuclear 315
  nerve 95, 96
  parent 4
  parts of 255*f*
  plasma 316
  polymorphonuclear 315
  receptor 186
  red 165
  sex 208
  sperm 210
  stem 313
  structure of 1, 2*f*, 255*f*
  suppressor 84
  T8 84
  thyroid 145
  tumor 228
  type of 226, 347
  white blood 74, 78, 313, 315
Census 361
Central nervous system 97, 320
Central processing unit 361
Central registration 361
Centralized filing system 361
Centralized serial unit 361
Cerebellum 100, 324
Cerebral cortex 178, 186
Cerebral hemispheres 98
Cerebrospinal fluid 99, 325
  secrete 97
Cerebrum 98
  functions of 99
Cerumen 339
Cervical vertebra 15, 36
  first 303
  second 303
Cervix 347
  occurs 216
Cesarean section 361
  rate 361
Chart analysis 361
Cheeks 120
Chemotherapy 229, 362
Chest 299
  pain 233
Child patient 362
Child psychology 243
Cholecystokinin 127
Choroid 175
Chromosomes 3
Chromtin 3
Ciliated epithelium 6
Circulatory system 10
Cisternae 3
Clavicle 37
Climacteric period 346*t*
  menopausal manifestations during 220
Clinical neuropsychology 239

Clinical psychology 239
Cocaine 236
Coccygeal 15
Coccyx 37, 304
Cochlea 180, 339
  canal of 181
Coding 362
  color 362
Cognitive psychology 240
Collecting tubule 342
Colon 128, 134, 328
  ascending 128, 328
  descending 128, 328
  sigmoid 328
  transverse 128, 328
Columnar epithelium 6
Communicable disease 362
Communication, privileged 376
Community psychology 240
Comparative psychology 241
Computational neuroscience 240
Computer 362
Conception, product of 216
Confidential information 362
Connective tissue 6, 41, 121, 227, 305
  binding 41
  covering 47, 306
Consent 362
Consultation 363
Contagious disease 363
Contraction, power of 21
Convalescent patient 363
Corium 183
Cornea 175, 176
Corpus
  callosum joins 323
  spongiosum 202
Costal cartilage 303
Counseling psychology 241
Cranial bones 33
Cranial cavity 13, 298
Cranial nerve 103, 103*t*, 105, 121
  consists of 102
  pairs of 105
  position of 103
Creatinine 203
Cribs 363
Crista 3
Critical psychology 242
Cryosurgery 363
Curettage 364
Cushing's disease 147
Cytoplasm 1, 314

D

Data bank 363
Death
  causes of 361
  intermediate 369
  rate 363
  underlying cause of 380
Deficiency 363
Delirium 235
Dementia 235
Deoxygenated blood 61
Deoxyribonucleic acid 229
Depressed gastrointestinal activity 321
Dermatology 363
Dermis 183
Desmosome 3
Detoxifying foreign protein 315
Diabetes insipidus 150
Dialysis 364
Diaphragm 135, 163, 164, 298, 336
Diaphysis 29, 301
Diarthroses 305
Diarthrosis 41
Diastole 59
Diazepam 236
Digestion 118
  accessory organs of 128, 135, 329
Digestive enzymes 123
  secrete 127
Digestive system 11, 117, 325
  accessory organs of 128
  anatomy and physiology of 325, 330
  organs of 118, 118*f*, 278*f*
  parts of 119*f*, 279*f*
Digestive tract 325
Dilatation 364
Dilation stage 216
Diphtheria 84
Direct admission 364
Disassociate disorders 233
Discharge analysis 364
Disease 364
  and operation index 364
Distal tubule 342
Distress 239
Doctor's conference room 365
Dorsal cavities 298
Dorsal vertebrae 303
Doubtful cases 365
Drug
  dependence 236
  hallucinogen-type 236
  therapy 233

Ducts 123*f*, 129*f*, 280*f*, 281*f*
  deferens 343
  ejaculatory 209, 210, 343
Duodenum 126, 129*f*, 281*f*, 327
Dura mater 98
Dwarfism 150
Dysfunction 239

E

Ear 8, 95, 178, 192, 321, 339
  drum 339
  external 180
  functioning of 181
  middle 180
  parts of 179*f*, 287*f*
    external 178
    inner 180
    middle 180
  pinna of 7
Early fetal death 365
Echocardiography 365
Edema 76
Educational psychology 243, 247
Efferent neuron 96*f*, 273*f*
Egg cell, single 212
Ejaculated semen, volume of 210
Elasticity 22
Elective surgery 365
Electrocardiography 365
Electrocochleography 365
Electroconvulsive therapy 365
Electroencephalography 365
Electrolytes 199, 333
Electromyography 365
Electro-oculography 366
Electroshock therapy 233
Emergency 366
  record 358, 366
  treatment 366
Endocardium 57, 309
Endocrine 329
  secretions, produce 334
  system 10, 142, 143*f*, 282*f*, 330
Endocrinology 366
Endolymph 181
Endometrium 214
Endomysium converges 307
Endoplasmic reticulum 2
Endoscopy 366
Eosinophils 78, 315
  release histamines 315
Epicardium 310
Epidermis 182
Epididymis 208, 210
Epiglottis 7, 123, 162, 333
Epinephrine 332
Epiphyses 29, 301
Epithelial tissues, types of 5
Epithelium 5
Eponym 366
Equilibrium 190, 337
Erectile tissue 343
Erythrocyte 74, 77, 85, 313-315
  mature 314
Esophagus 10, 119, 123, 124, 327
Estrogen 213
Ethmoid bone 36
Eustachian tube 180, 339
Evolutionary psychology 243
Excretory system 198, 198*f*, 289*f*, 340
Exhibitionism 234
Expiration 26, 165
Expiratory center 166
Expulsion stage 216
External respiration, mechanism of 164
Eye 8, 25, 95, 174, 191, 321, 337
  accessory organs of 176
  anatomy of 175
  fluids of 176
  functions 174, 337
  humors of 176
  parts of 177*f*, 286*f*
  physiology of 178
Eyeball 305
Eyelashes 176
Eyelids 176

F

Facial bones 36
Facial expressions 305
Fallopian tube 214, 216, 218, 344
Family therapy 233
Fat 117
  digestion of 127
Fatigue 22
Fatty acids 117
Feces, elimination of 328
Feet 27
Female reproductive system 212, 213, 218, 343
Femur 39
Fetal death 366
Fetishism 234
Fetus, delivery of 216
Fibrinogen 76, 317

Fibrocartilage 7
Fibrous
- attachment 307
- bands 305
- tissue 6, 334

Fibula 40
Fingers 27
Flagellum, consisting of 211
Flat cells, layer of 5
Flexion 42
Floating ribs 303
Fluid
- electrolytes 340
- part 74
- types of 181

Follicle-stimulating hormone 148
Forearm 27
Forebrain 98
Foreign antigens 79
Forensic
- medicine 367
- psychology 244

Fracture 367
Frontal bone 35

G

Gallbladder 128, 129*f*, 130, 136, 281*f*, 330
Gastric juice 125, 297, 327
Gastroenterology 367
Gastrointestinal activity, normal 322
Gastrointestinal system 117, 325
Gastrointestinal tract 118, 119, 124, 326
Gelatinous mass 302
Genitalia
- external 213, 213*t*, 214
- internal 213, 213*t*

Gerontology 367
Gestational age 367
Gigantism 149
Glands 123*f*, 181, 184, 189, 280*f*
- adrenal 143, 146, 153, 202, 332
- Bartholin's 214, 215
- bulbourethral 211
- ceruminous 189
- Cowper's 211, 343
- ductless 10, 329
- endocrine 142
- exocrine 142
- lacrimal 142, 177
- location of 143*f*, 282*f*
- lymph 307
- mammary 142
- parathyroid 142, 145, 152, 332
- pea-shaped 211
- pineal 143, 150, 155, 330, 334
- pituitary 143, 145, 148, 152, 330
- prostate 202, 209, 210
- salivary 123, 123*f*, 280*f*
- sebaceous 184, 189
- submaxillary 123
- sudoriferous 184, 189
- suprarenal 202
- sweat 142, 184, 189
- thymus 143, 320
- thyroid 142-145, 152, 331
- types of 184

Glans penis 211
Gliding movements 41
Global psychology 244
Globulin 76, 317, 319
Glomeruli 203
Glucocorticoids 146, 154, 333
Glucose 54
Glycerol 117
Golgiosome 3
Gonad, union of male 216
Gonadocorticoids 146, 154, 333
Gonadotropic hormones 148
Graafian follicle
- collapses 216
- ruptures 216

Granulocytes 78, 86, 315
Graves' disease 145
Group therapy 233
Growth 3
- hormone 142, 148

Gums 122
Gynecology 368
Gyrus 324

H

Hair 181, 183, 188
- follicle 183
- root 183

Hand 8, 25, 25*t*, 58
Health
- care management 358
- center 368
- information 368
- psychology 245
- record 368

Healthcare organizations 242
Heart 8, 55, 66, 309
- and blood circulation, functioning of 63*fc*
- beat 311
  - rate of 312

conduction system of 68, 311
cycle 59, 60*f*
parts of 59*f*, 60*f*
pulses, electrical conduction of 64
structure of 58*f*, 269*f*
valves of 58
with blood flow
exterior section of 59*f*, 269*f*
interior section of 60*f*, 270*f*
Hematic and lymphatic systems, anatomy and physiology of 313
Hematology 368
Hemoglobin 77, 165, 314
carries oxygen 314
Hepatic artery 63
Hepatitis B 84
Herniated nucleus pulposus 303
Heroin 236
Hindbrain 98
Hip 26
Histone, primarily 3
Homeostasis 330
Homonyms 368
Hormone 142, 144, 319, 332
epinephrine, types of 147
insulin 329
secretions of 330
Horse tail 101
Hospital
bed 368
inpatient 368
number 368
record 368
service, analysis of 358
Human body 142
endocrine glands of 144*f*, 283*f*
evolution of 254*f*
part 254
Human brain 238*f*
Human immunodeficiency virus 84
Human mind, growth of 242
Human skeleton 33, 300
Human welfare 242
Human-computer interaction 240
Humoral immunity 84, 87, 316
Hyaline cartilage 7, 301, 303
C-shaped rings of 163
Hydrochloric acid 125, 327
Hypercalcemia 146
Hyperthyroidism 145
Hypnosis 233
Hypochondriac regions 265*f*
location of 37*f*
Hypochondriasis 233
Hypothalamus 100
functions of 101
Hypothesis generation 249
Hypoxia 166
Hysterical neurosis 233

I

Ileum 126, 328, 304
Immature infant 368
Immune substances 313
Immunity 84
acquired active 84
Immunoglobin
D 84
E 84
M 84
Immunoglobulin
A 76
G 76
Immunology 368
Implied consent 369
Inappropriate antidiuretic hormone 150
Incident report 369
Industrial psychology 245
Infantile autism, facilitated communication for 251
Infectious disease 369
Informed consent 369
Inguinal regions 265*f*
location of 37*f*
Inpatient 369
census 369
discharge 369
Inspiration 26, 164
Institutional deaths 369
Insulin
hypersecretion of 148
hyposecretion of 147
Interatrial septum 64
Interferon's 84
Interleukins 84
Internal respiration, mechanism of 165*f*, 286*f*
Interstitial fluid 319
Intervertebral disk 302
herniation of 303
Intestine 9
Intracellular fluid 5
Iris 175
Ischium 304
Islets of Langerhans 154, 334
Isthmus 331

J

Jejunum 126, 328
Joint 40, 46, 305
- ball and socket 41
- capsule 41
- cartilaginous 40
- cavity 305
- condyloid 41
- elbow 41
- fibrous 40
- hinge 41
- hip 41
- movements of 41
- pivot 41
- saddle 41
- shoulder 26
- socket 41
- synovial 41, 305

K

Kidney 199, 204, 227
- left 199
- part of 199
  - including 200*f*, 290*f*
- right 199, 201*f*, 290*f*

Knee 27

L

Labia majora, vulva consists of 214
Labor
- and birth 216, 221, 346
- stages of 379

Lacrimal bones 36
Lacrimal duct 177
Lacrimal sac 177
Laparoscopy 369
Large intestine 10, 127
- first part of 128
- functions of 128

Laryngopharynx 124, 162, 327, 335
Larynx 162, 335
Late fetal death 370
Leg 8
- and foot, bones of 39

Legal liability 370
Legal psychology 245
Lens 175, 176, 338
Leukocytes 74, 78, 86, 313, 314
Life, fundamental unit of 297
Ligaments 41
Limbs originate, nerves of 101
Linguists 240
Lipase 131
Lipocytes 183
Lips 25, 120
Live birth 370
Liver 9, 128, 129, 129*f*, 135, 281*f*, 328, 329
Lobe
- anterior 331
- posterior 331

Loin 299
Long bone, inner parts of 39*f*
Loop of Henle 342
Low birth weight 370
Lower limb 25, 35, 58
- muscles of 25*t*

Lower right quadrants, anatomical division of 265*f*
Lumbar puncture 99
Lumbar regions 265*f*
- location of 37*f*

Lumbar vertebrae 15, 37, 303
Lung 8, 163
Luteinizing hormone 148
Lymph 307
- capillaries 319
- channels 226
- nodes 81, 82*f*, 82*t*, 272*f*, 319, 320
- originates 81
- vessels 121, 307, 319, 320

Lymphatic nodules 81
Lymphatic organs, related 83
Lymphatic system 11, 81, 89, 319
Lymphatic tissue 122, 227
Lymphocytes 79, 87, 319
Lysosomes 3

M

Malpractice 370
Mammary papilla 215
Manic depressive illness 232
Mastication 25
Maternal mortality 370
Mathematical and statistical modeling, application of 247
Mathematical psychology 247
Measles 84
Meatus 343
Medical audit 370
Medical board 370
Medical care evaluation 371
Medical certificate 371
- of cause of death, responsibility for 378

Medical consultation 371

Medical file 371
Medical psychology 237
Medical record 371
  committee 371
  department 371
  form 371
  officer 371
  service, evaluation of 366
  technician 372
Medical report 372
Medical social service 372
Medical specialties 355
Medicine 372
Medicolegal case 372
Medulla 199, 200
  oblongata 100
  secretes hormones 146
Meiosis 5
Melanin 183
Melatonin hormone, secretes 334
Memory recovery techniques 251
Meninges 111
Menopause 212, 346
  manifestations 220
Menses, absence of 346
Menstrual cycle 213, 215, 219, 345
  phases of 345*t*
Menstrual discharge 215
Menstrual phase 215, 216
Mental health 245
Mental illness, prevention of 232
Mental processes 247
Mental states 239
Metabolism 131, 166
  products of 198
Metaphase 4
Metastasis 226, 228, 372
Metatarsals 40
Microbiology 372
Microfilming 372
Micturition 204
Midbrain 98, 100
Mineral salts 117
Mineralocorticoids 146, 153, 333
Mitochondria 2
Mitosis 4
Mitral valve 59, 62, 310
Mixed tissue tumors 227
Monocytes 79, 87
Mood, disorder of 232
Morbidity 372
Morphine 236
Morphology 373
Mortality 373
Motor neuron 96*f*, 273*f*
Mountain sickness 166
Mouth 10, 118, 132, 326
Muscles 28*f*, 29*f*, 46, 261*f*, 262*f*, 300, 305
  agonist 306
  antagonist 306
  attachment of 24
  cardiac 8, 23, 56
  ciliary 175
  contracts 306
  fiber, single 306
  functions of 24, 25*t*
    different 24
  important parts of 22, 260*f*
  involuntary 8, 23
  nonstriated 23
  properties of 21
  skeletal 21, 23, 24, 306
  smooth 23
  striated 23, 24
  tissue, types of 7
  tone 23
  type of 56
  visceral 23
  voluntary 7, 23
Muscular system 10
Muscular tissue 7, 23, 305
  characteristics of 23
  types of 23
Muscular tone 22
Musculoskeletal system 21, 300
  anatomy and physiology of 300
Myelinated axons 324
Myocardium 57, 214, 310

N

Nails 181, 185, 188
Nasal bones 36
Nasal cavity 160, 335
Nasolacrimal duct 178
Nasopharynx 124, 162, 180, 326, 335
Nausea 233
Neck 25, 25*t*, 58, 299
Necropsy 373
Neonatal death 373
Neoplasm 226, 373
  benign 226, 227*t*, 347
  characteristics of 347, 348*t*
  malignant 226, 227, 227*t*, 348
Nephrology 373
Nephron 199, 201*f*, 291*f*

Nerve
auditory 181
autonomic 104
cells 95, 96
microscopic 95
cranial 103
endings 121
facial 121
fibers, bundle of 96
glossopharyngeal 121, 186
impulses 95
motor 107
optic 174, 176, 178
parasympathetic 97
sensory 107, 321
somatic 97, 104
spinal 104
sympathetic 97
tissue 97
tracts 100
Nervous system 10, 95, 96, 320
anatomy and physiology of 320
divisions of 107, 320
peripheral parts of 102*f*, 275*f*
structure of 96, 97*fc*
Nervous tissue 8, 108, 322
Neuroglia 109, 323
Neurohypophysis 148, 149, 330, 331
Neuroimaging tools 239
Neurolemma 322, 323
Neurolemmal sheath 322
Neurological illness 245
Neurology 373
Neuron 96, 108, 322
chains, composed of 322
Neuropsychology 239
Neuroticism 246
Neutrophil 78, 315
Newborn 373
Nipple, opening of 215
Nitrogen 165
Nitrogenous waste 203
Nodes 228
Noninstitutional deaths 373
Noradrenaline 147, 332, 333
Norepinephrine 333
Nose 8, 95, 160, 186, 321
Nucleus 3
pulposus 302
Numbering system 373
Nutrients 319
Nutrition 3

O

Obstetrics 373
Occupational health psychology 246
Odontology 373
Old medical records 374
Olfactory mucosa, structures of 288*f*
Olfactory sensation 337
Oligodendrocytes 323
Oncology 226, 347, 374
Operation index 374
Ophthalmology 374
Opioids 236
Oral cavity 120, 326
cross-section of 120*f*, 279*f*
posterior part of 123
Oral surgery 374
Organ 8, 297
group of 297
structures 8
Organizational psychology 245
Oropharynx 124, 162, 326, 335
Orthopedics 374
Ossicles 339
Osteoblasts 332
Osteocytes 28
Otorhinolaryngology 374
Outpatient 374
clinic schedule 374
record 374
Ovaries 143, 150, 213, 218, 227, 344
Oviducts 218, 344
Ovulatory phase 216
Ovum 150, 208
fertilization of 211, 346
union of female 216
Oxygen 160, 319
exchange of 163
Oxyhemoglobin 77

P

Pacemaker 312
Palate 120
Pancreas 128, 129*f*, 131, 135, 143, 147, 154, 281*f*, 328, 329, 334
duct 329
functions of 131
Pancreatic disorder 147
Panhypopituitarism 150
Papillae 185, 326
types of 186
Paranasal sinuses 162
Paranoic disorders 236

Parathormone 145
Parathyroid hormone
  hypersecretion of 146
  hyposecretion of 146
Pars
  distalis 330
  intermedia 149
  nervosa 148
Passive aggression 235
Patella 39
Patient
  day 375
  file 375
  master index 375
  transfer of 380
Pediatrics 375
Pelvic bones
  female 39*t*
  male 39*t*
Pelvic cavity 13
Pelvic girdle 33, 38, 45, 303
Pelvis 37, 45, 303, 313
  bones of 38
  female 304
  floor of 26
  male 304
Penis 209, 211
  enlarged tip of 343
Pericardium 57
Perilymph 181
Perimetrium 214
Periosteum 302, 306
Peripheral nervous system 97, 102, 320
Peristalsis 214, 344
Peritubular capillaries 341
Personal distress 238
Personality
  disorders 235
  psychology 246
Personnel psychology 245
Pharynx 119, 124, 162, 335
Phosphates, blood levels of 332
Phosphorus 301
Pia mater 98
Pinna 179
Pituitary
  anterior lobe of 148, 148*t*
  middle lobe of 149
  posterior lobe of 149, 150*t*
Pituitary gland 143, 145, 148, 152, 330
  anterior 149
  hormones of 149*f*, 284*f*, 331*t*
  hypersecretions of 149
  hyposecretions of 149
  posterior 150
Placenta 344
Placental stage 216
Plasma 74, 76, 88, 313, 317
  and cells, composition of 75*f*, 271*f*
  proteins 77, 317
Platelets 74, 79, 313
  function of 79
Play therapy 233
Pleural sacs 163
Plexus 96
Policy 375
Polio vaccine 316
Poliomyelitis 84
Pons 100
Portal circulation 62
Potassium 313, 340
Pregnancy 212, 216, 220, 346, 375
Premature infant 376
Prenumbered folder 375
Preovulatory phase 215
Prodrome 377
Progesterone 213, 333
Prolactin 148
Prophase 4
Protein 2, 117
  compound 126
Prothrombin 76
  activator 80
Protoplasm 1
Proximal tubule 342
Psychiatry 232, 377
  disorders 232
Psychoanalysis 233
Psychology 237
  abnormal 238
  developmental 242
  disciplines, list of 238
  encompasses 237
  topics 238
Psychosexual disorders 234
Psychotherapy, types of 233*t*
Psychoticism 246
Pubis 304
Pulmonary artery 60
Pulmonary capillaries 310
Pulmonary circulation 61, 62, 310
Pulmonary valve 62, 310
Pulp 326
Pulse 63
Pupil 175, 338

Q

QRS complex 312
Qualitative analysis 377
Qualitative research 250
Quality assurance 377
    program 377
Quality control 377
Quantitative analysis 377
Quantitative psychology 247
Quantitative research 250

R

Radiation therapy 229
Radiology 377
Recapitulation 297
Record
    amalgamation of 358
    completion of 362
    control 377
    preservation of 376
    processing of 376
    retention of 378
Rectum 128, 328
Red blood cells 74, 77, 167, 313, 318, 320
    development of 77
Relapse 378
Remission 378
Renal corpuscle 341
Renal tubule 199, 341
Renin 204
Reproduction 3
Reproductive system 12, 208, 342
    male 208, 217, 342
    parts of
        female 212*f*, 213*f*, 292*f*
        male 209*f*, 291*f*
Research methods 249
Respiration
    external 160, 334
    internal 160, 168, 335
    mechanism of 164*fc*
Respiratory system 11, 160, 334
    anatomy and physiology of 334
    factors influencing 166
    organs of 161*f*, 285*f*
    parts of 160, 161*f*, 285*f*
Retina 175, 176, 178
Rhesus factor 80
Rhythmic respiration, normal 166
Ribosomes 3
Ribs 38, 313
    pairs of 303
    parts of 303
Right atrium 312
Root ganglion, posterior 104
Rugae 125
Ruptured disk 303

S

Sacral vertebrae 15
Sacrum 37, 304
Sarcomas 227, 378
Scalp 25
Scapula 25, 31, 37
Schizophrenic disorders 235
School psychology 248
Sclera 175
Scrotum 208, 209
Secrete wax 184
Sedatives 236
Seeks, critical psychology 242
Semen 211
Semicircular canals 180, 339
Semilunar valve 59, 62
Seminal duct 343
Seminal vesicle 209, 210
Seminiferous tubules 208, 210
Sense organs 10, 95, 174, 336
Sex cell 208
    female 208
    male 208, 211
Sex chromosomes, pair of 5
Sex hormones 154, 333
Sex therapy 233
Sexual masochism 234
Sexual sadism 234
Sexually transmitted disease 381
Shoulder 25, 25*t*
    blades 31
    girdle 33
Simple squamous epithelium 5
Single nucleus 23
Singular testis 342
Sinoatrial node 64
Skeletal muscle 21, 23, 24, 306
    cells 21
    contraction 309
    cross-section of 22*f*, 260*f*
Skeletal system 10, 28, 43, 301
    divisions of 302
Skin 95, 181, 321
    functions of 181
    structure of 182, 182*f*, 287*f*
    subcutaneous layer of 183
Skull, bones of 313
Slipped disk 303

Small infants, mental processes of 243
Small intestine 10, 125, 126, 134, 327
 functions of 127
 layers of 126
Smallpox 84
Smell 190, 337
 and taste, centers of 187*f*, 289*f*
 sensation of 337
Social and cognitive psychology, elements of 248
Social behavior 247
 causes of 248*f*
Social psychology 243, 247
Sodium 313, 340
Soft spots 33
Soft tissue, V-shaped 121
Somatic nervous system 321
Somatoform disorders 233
Sound production 162
Special senses 174, 190
 anatomy and physiology of 336
Speech 162
Sperm 208, 211
 development of 210
 motile 211
Spermatozoa 210
Spermatozoon 211
Sphygmomanometer 379
Spinal cavity 13
Spinal column 14, 15*t*, 16*f*, 258*f*
Spinal cord 101, 110, 302, 324
 functions of 102
Spinal nerves 104
 consists of 102
 pairs of 104
Spinal puncture 99
Spleen 9, 83, 319, 320
Sterilization 379
Sternum 31, 37, 313
Steroids 146
Stethoscope 379
Stillbirth 370, 379
Stomach 8, 10, 124, 133, 327
 functions of 126
 parts of 125
Stratified squamous epithelium 6
Subarachnoid space 98, 101
Subclavian vein, left 320
Subcutaneous connective tissue 306
Subdural space 325
Substance induced disorders 236
Sulcus 304
Summons 379
Surgery 229, 379
Swelling 76
Symbiosis 379
Sympathomimetic agents 147
Synarthroses 40, 305
Syndrome 379
Synovial joint 41, 305
 varieties of 41
Synovial membrane 41
Systemic circulation 61, 61*f*, 270*f*, 310
Systole 60

T

T cell 83, 84, 316, 320
 lymphocytes 84
T lymphocytes 83
T wave 312
Tactile touch 100
Tailbone 299
Tarsals 40
Taste 190, 336, 337
 buds 121
Teeth 121, 132
 parts of 122*f*, 280*f*, 326
Telophase 4
Temporal bone 36
Tendons 24
Terminal digit filing 380
Test tube, blood in 75*f*, 271*f*
Testes 143, 151, 208, 209, 227
 pair of 209
Testosterone 209
Tetanus 84
Thalamus 100
Thick-walled ventricles 56
Thigh 58
Thoracic cavity 13, 34, 55, 58, 298
 side of 303
Thoracic duct 81
Thoracic vertebrae 15, 37, 303
Thorax 45, 303
 bones of 37
Throat 335
 part of 327
Thrombocytes 74, 79, 88, 313, 317
Thromboplastin 80, 317
Thumb 27
Thymus 83, 319
Thyroid
 cartilage 162
 gland 142-145, 152, 331
  function of 332

hormone 332
hypersecretion of 145
hyposecretion of 145
stimulating hormone 145, 148
Thyroxine 143, 144, 332
Tibia 40
Tic-tac-toe 298
Tissue 5, 297
fluid 5
groups of 297
respiration 165
mechanism of 165*f*, 286*f*
T-lymphocytes, function of 316
Toes, phalanges of 40
Tongue 9, 25, 95, 121, 185, 305, 321
functions of 326
parts of 185*f*, 288*f*
Tonsils 83, 122, 319
Topography 380
Toxic
condition 340
goiter 145
Toxicology 380
Trachea 123, 163, 327
Transitional epithelium 6
Transsexualism 234
Transvestism 234
Traumatology 380
Tricuspid valve 59, 62
Triiodothyronine 143, 144, 332
Trochoid 41
Trunk 25, 25*t*
Trypsin 131
Tuberculosis 84
Tubules, small-coiled 210
Tumor 226, 228
benign 347, 360
malignant 370
solid 226
types of 226
Tympanic cavity 180
Tympanic membrane 179, 180, 339
Typhoid fever 84

U

Ultraviolet radiation, harmful effects of 183
Unit numbering system 381
Unit record system 381
Upper left quadrants, anatomical division of 265*f*
Upper limb 25, 35, 58
muscles of 25*t*
Upper right quadrants, anatomical division of 38*f*, 265*f*
Urea 203
Uremia 340
Ureters 202
Urethra 202, 209-211, 341
Urethral meatus 214
Urethral orifice 343
Urinary bladder 202, 210
Urinary meatus 202
Urinary system 12, 198, 199, 205, 340
comprising 200*f*, 290*f*
macroscopic structures of 340
microscopic structures of 341
parts of 199
Urine 340
excretion process of 202, 203*fc*
Urogenital system, anatomy and physiology of 340, 342
Urology 381
Uterine
contractions 347
wall 216
Uterus 214, 216, 218, 344
Uvula 121

V

Vagina 214, 218, 344, 345
Vas deferens 209, 210
Vascular system 65, 308
Veins 54, 66, 309
carry blood 309
important 54, 57*f*, 58*t*, 268*f*
pulmonary 59, 309
Vena cava, inferior 310
Venereology 381
Ventilation 165
Ventral cavities 298
Ventricles 309
Vertebrae 313
Vertebral column 45, 302
bones of 36
Vessels carry blood, types of 308
Vestibule 180, 181, 339
Viable infant 381
Villi 127
Virology 381
Viruses 79
Visceral receptors 100
Vital capacity 166
Vitamin 117
B_{12} 126

Vitreous humor 176
Voice box 335
Voluntary muscles 7, 23
    types of 305
Vomiting 233
Voyeurism 234
Vulva 214
    parts of 215

W

Waste products, conveyance of 313
Water 117
White fibrous tissue 6
Windpipe 123, 163

Y

Yellow elastic
    cartilage 7
    tissue 6

Z

Zygomatic bones 36
Zygote 346